Nurse's Fast Facts:

Your Quick Source for Core Clinical Content

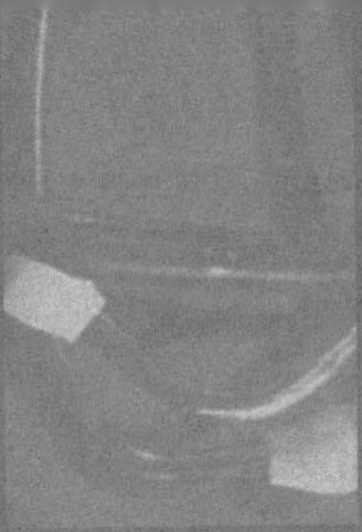

Nurse's Fast Facts:

Your Quick Source for Core Clinical Content

Third Edition

BRENDA WALTERS HOLLOWAY, CRNP, FNP, MSN
Clinical Assistant Professor
University of South Alabama
College of Nursing
Mobile, Alabama

F. A. DAVIS COMPANY
Philadelphia

F. A. Davis Company
1915 Arch Street
Philadelphia, PA 19103

Printed in Canada

Last digit indicates print number: 10 9 8 7 6 5 4 3

Acquisitions Editor: Robert G. Martone
Developmental Editor: Alan Sorkowitz
Art & Design Manager: Joan Wendt

As new scientific information becomes available through basic and clinical research, recommended treatments and drug therapies undergo changes. The author and publisher have done everything possible to make this book accurate, up to date, and in accord with accepted standards at the time of publication. The author, editors, and publisher are not responsible for errors or omissions or for consequences from application of the book, and make no warranty, expressed or implied, in regard to the contents of the book. Any practice described in this book should be applied by the reader in accordance with professional standards of care used in regard to the unique circumstances that may apply in each situation. The reader is advised always to check product information (package inserts) for changes and new information regarding dose and contraindications before administering any drug. Caution is especially urged when using new or infrequently ordered drugs.

Library of Congress Cataloging-in-Publication Data

Holloway, Brenda Walters, 1949-
Nurse's fast facts : your quick source for core clinical content / Brenda Walters Holloway.—3rd ed.
p. ; cm.
Includes index.
ISBN 0-8036-1161-7
1. Nursing—Handbooks, manuals, etc.
[DNLM: 1. Nursing Care—Handbooks. 2. Nursing Process—Handbooks. 3. Specialties, Nursing—methods—Handbooks. WY 49 H745n 2004] I. Title.
RT51.H65 2004
610.73—dc22

2004043215

This book is dedicated to my parents, Juanice and J. M. Walters, who provided me with the opportunity to obtain an education, and to Harry, Jason, Shanda, and Scott, who have provided me with many opportunities to use it.

Preface

Through years of clinical practice and teaching, I have observed that orientation to each major clinical nursing specialty usually leads the novice to ask a somewhat predictable set of questions ranging from specialty-related communication, to assessment and anatomy, physiology, and pathology involved in frequently seen conditions to questions related to the planning and implementation of patient care. Many excellent texts are available to provide in-depth information related to these topics. Although the use of such texts is essential to the acquisition of a thorough knowledge of comprehensive patient care, these texts are frequently too cumbersome to carry to the clinical area, where on-the-spot information may be needed.

My goal in writing this book has been to provide a portable and easy-to-use source for quick answers to questions I have frequently heard from students and practicing nurses. The sections of this book pertain to each major clinical nursing specialty and are identified by printed tabs to speed access to the information. At the end of each section are blank pages, which allow users to "customize" the book by adding information that they find helpful for each specialty.

It is hoped that the handy availability of information in this pocket-sized reference book not only will improve the accuracy and quality of patient care, but also will relieve some of the stress that students and graduate nurses experience when they must move from one clinical specialty area to another.

Acknowledgments

I would like to acknowledge the work of the professionals who contributed written information in this book. Their efforts have added greatly to the scope and quality of the reference material. I would also like to thank the faculty, staff, and students of the University of South Alabama as well as professionals from across the country who answered questions and provided me with information necessary to the completion of this work. In addition, I would like to thank the consultants to this book, who reviewed the manuscript in its early stages and provided many valuable insights and suggestions.

I would like to thank the F. A. Davis Company for its vote of confidence and support in the development and publication of this book. A very special thanks to Alan Sorkowitz, of Alan Sorkowitz Editorial Services, for the guidance and remarkable patience he exhibited during this endeavor.

Contributors to the 3rd edition

JUDITH AZOK, MSN, ARNP, GNP-BC
Assistant Clinical Professor of Nursing
University of South Alabama
Mobile, Alabama
Medical-Surgical Content

LISA BENFIELD, MSN, FNP-CNS, MATERNAL-CHILD CNS
Nurse Practitioner
Gulfport OB-GYN Clinic
Gulfport, Mississippi
Maternal-Infant Content

JASON BOX, MSN, FNP-BC, EMP-P
Family Nurse Practitioner
South Baldwin Regional Medical Center Emergency Department
Foley, Alabama
Emergency Content

KAREN HAMILTON, MSN, RNC
Assistant Clinical Professor of Nursing
University of South Alabama
Mobile, Alabama
Home Health Content

DEBORAH D. HYATT, FNP-C, PNP-C, GNP
Assistant Clinical Professor of Nursing
University of South Alabama
Family Nurse Practitioner
Providence Medical Group
Mobile, Alabama
Long-Term Care Content

PATRICIA NOONAN, MSN, PMH-NP, ANP
Assistant Clinical Professor of Nursing
University of South Alabama
Mobile, Alabama
Mental Health Content

MARTHA SURLINE, MS
Assistant Clinical Professor of Nursing
University of South Alabama
Mobile, Alabama
Nutrition Content

ELIZABETH A. VANDEWAA, B.A., PHD
Associate Professor
University of South Alabama
Mobile, Alabama
Pharmacology Content

Contributors to Previous Editions

JUDITH AZOK, MSN, RN, GNP, CS
Clinical Assistant Professor of Nursing
University of South Alabama
Mobile, Alabama
Medical-Surgical Content

THOMAS W. BARKLEY, JR., DSN, RN, CS, ACNP
Assistant Professor of Nursing
Program Coordinator, Advanced Adult Acute Care Nursing Specialty
University of South Alabama
Mobile, Alabama
Emergency and Critical Care Content

MARGARET DAHLBERG COLE, RN, DSN
Associate Professor
Spring Hill College
Mobile, Alabama
Maternal-Infant Content

VERA DOUGLAS, RN, MSN
Clinical Assistant Professor of Nursing
University of South Alabama
Mobile, Alabama
Mental Health Content

KATHERINE F. FREY, RN, MSN
Clinical Assistant Professor of Nursing
University of South Alabama
Mobile, Alabama
Medical-Surgical Content

SHEENA HOLMES, MSN, RNC
Clinical Assistant Professor of Nursing
University of South Alabama
Mobile, Alabama
Maternal-Infant Content

DEBORAH HYATT, RN, MSN, PNP, FNP, GNP
Family Nurse Practitioner
Three Notch Medical Center
Andalusia, Alabama
Gerontological Content

JASON JONES, RN, PHD
Assistant Professor of Nursing
University of South Alabama
Mobile, Alabama
Mental Health Content

CAROLYN MITCHELL, MT(ASCP), MA
Quality Assessment Specialist
Blood Systems, Inc.
Tupelo, Mississippi
Laboratory Tests Content

MONA L. NEWCOMB, RNC, MSN
Unit Manager, Adult Psychiatric Unit
Crestwood Hospital
Huntsville, Alabama
Mental Health Content

SHARON C. PRICE, RNC, MSN
Pensacola, Florida
Formerly Assistant Professor of Nursing
University of South Alabama
Mobile, Alabama
Physical Assessment Content

CHERIE REVERE, RN, MSN
Clinical Nurse Specialist
Emergency Department
University of South Alabama
Medical Center
Mobile, Alabama
Emergency Content

CANDY ROSS, RN, PHD
Professor of Nursing
University of South Alabama
Mobile, Alabama
Home Health Content

MARTHA NORRIS SURLINE, MS
Clinical Assistant Professor of Nursing
University of South Alabama
Mobile, Alabama
Nutrition Content

ELIZABETH VANDEWAA, PHD
Associate Professor of Nursing
University of South Alabama
Mobile, Alabama
Nutrition Content

JOSEPH F. WARD, RN, MSN, CPNP, CDE
Clinical Assistant Professor of Nursing
University of South Alabama
Mobile, Alabama
Child Health Content

STEPHANIE D. WIGGINS, RN, DSN
Assistant Professor of Nursing
University of South Alabama
Mobile, Alabama
Medical-Surgical Content

Contents

Medical-Surgical Fast Facts

Section 1

The Human Body

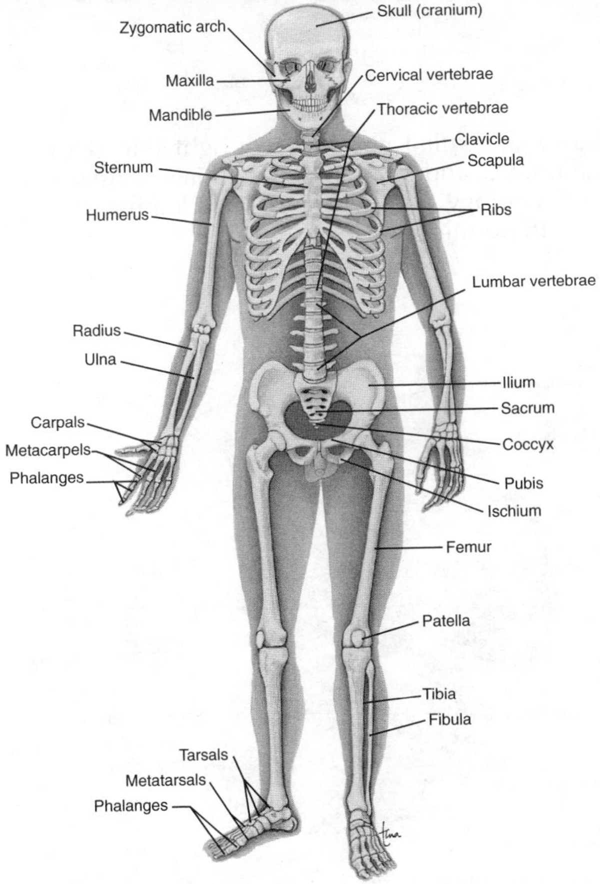

Figure 1–1. Skeleton. Anterior view. (From Scanlon, VC, and Sanders, T: Essentials of Anatomy and Physiology, ed 4. FA Davis, Philadelphia, 2003, p 108, with permission.)

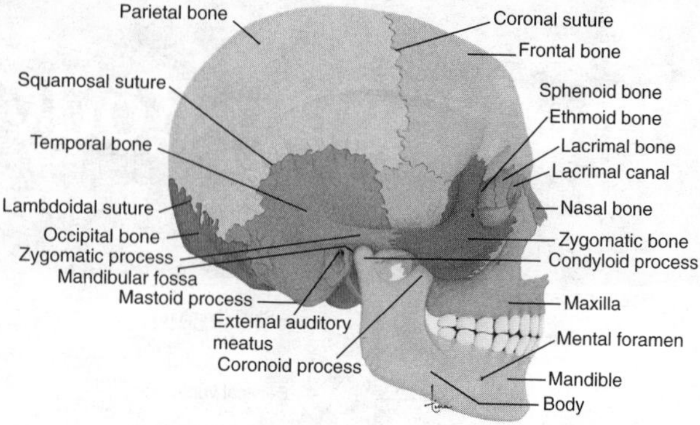

Figure 1–2. Skull. Lateral view of right side. (From Scanlon, VC, and Sanders, T: Essentials of Anatomy and Physiology, ed 4. FA Davis, Philadelphia, 2003, p 109, with permission.)

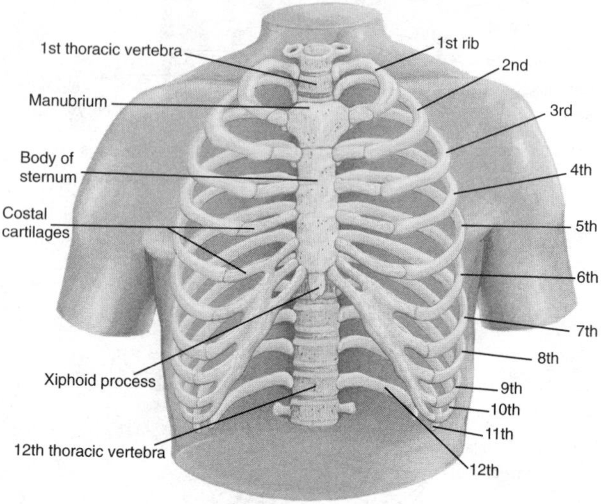

Figure 1–3. Rib cage. Anterior view. (From Scanlon, VC, and Sanders, T: Essentials of Anatomy and Physiology, ed 4. FA Davis, Philadelphia, 2003, p 116, with permission.)

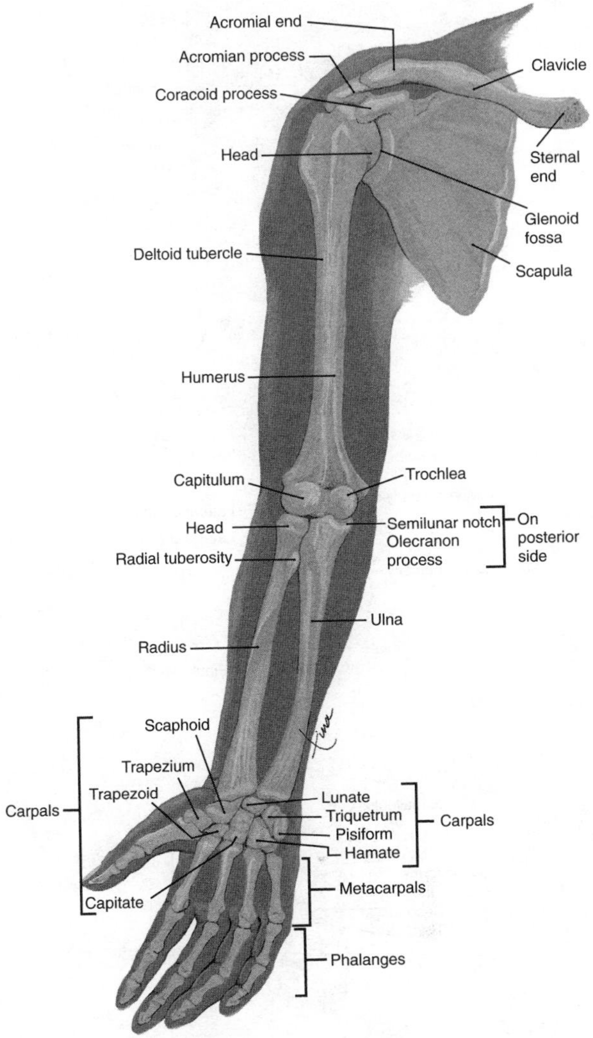

Figure 1–4. Bones of the arm and shoulder girdle. Anterior view of right arm. (From Scanlon, VC, and Sanders, T: Essentials of Anatomy and Physiology, ed 4. FA Davis, Philadelphia, 2003, p 117, with permission.)

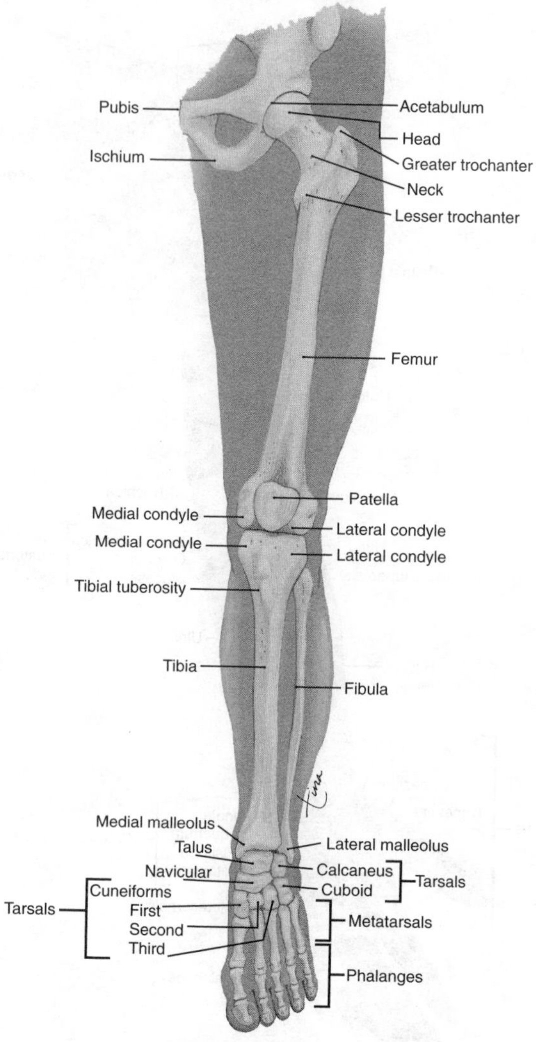

Figure 1–5. Bones of the leg and portion of hip bone. Anterior view of left leg. (From Scanlon, VC, and Sanders, T: Essentials of Anatomy and Physiology, ed 4. FA Davis, Philadelphia, 2003, p 121, with permission.)

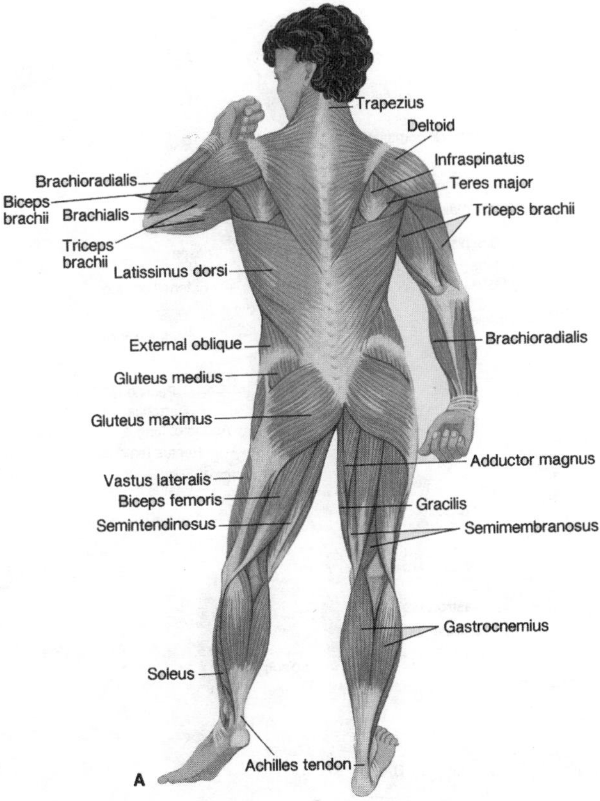

Figure 1–6. Major muscles of the body. (*A*) Posterior view. (From Scanlon, VC, and Sanders, T: Essentials of Anatomy and Physiology, ed 4. FA Davis, Philadelphia, 2003, p 142, with permission.)

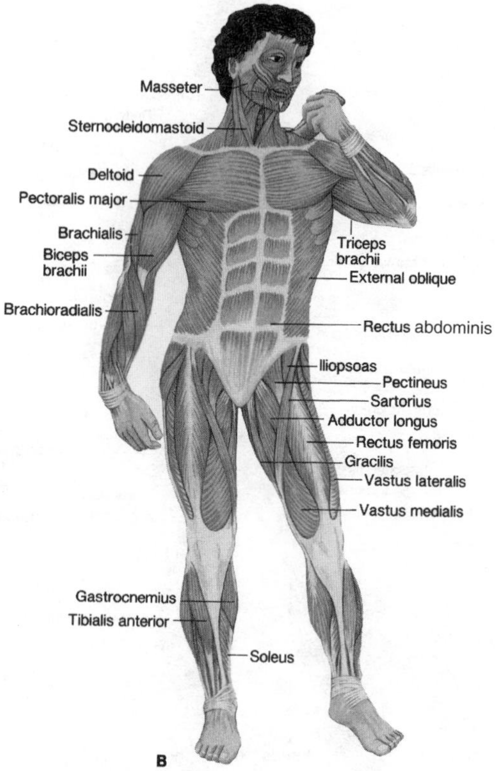

Figure 1–6. Major muscles of the body. (*B*) Anterior view. (From Scanlon, VC, and Sanders, T: Essentials of Anatomy and Physiology, ed 4. FA Davis, Philadelphia, 2003, p 143, with permission.)

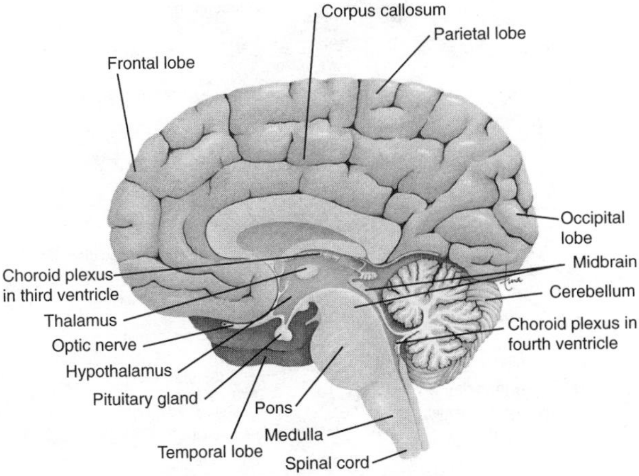

Figure 1–7. Midsagittal section of the brain as seen from the left side. (From Scanlon, VC, and Sanders, T: Essentials of Anatomy and Physiology, ed 4. FA Davis, Philadelphia, 2003, p 167, with permission.)

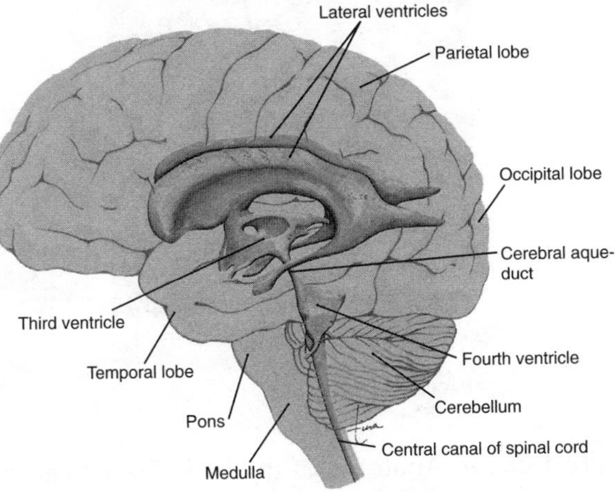

Figure 1–8. Ventricles of the brain as seen from the left side. (From Scanlon, VC, and Sanders, T: Essentials of Anatomy and Physiology, ed 4. FA Davis, Philadelphia, 2003, p 168, with permission.)

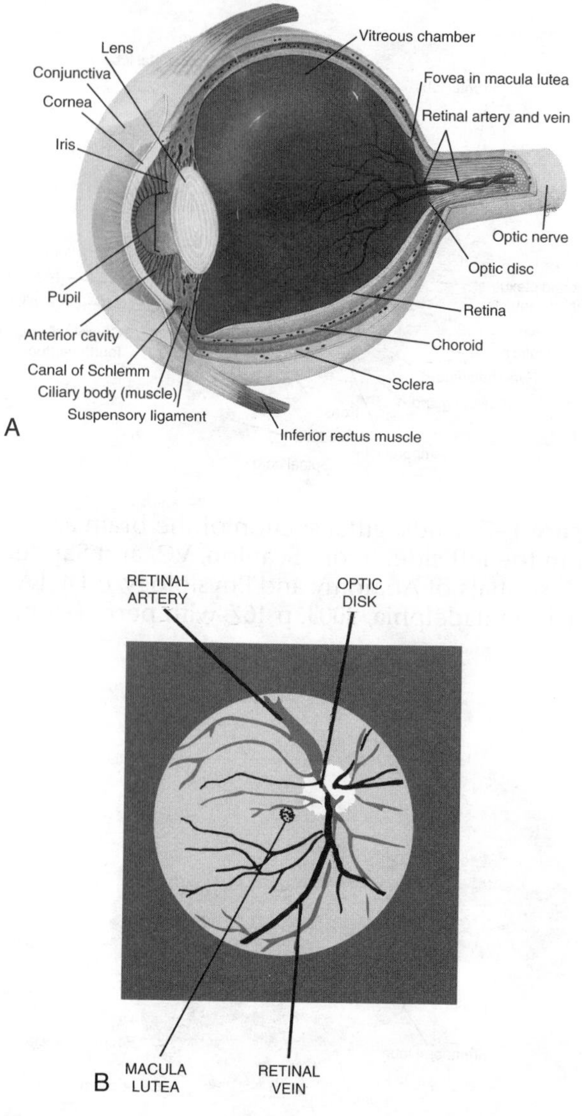

Figure 1–9. (*A*) Anatomy of the eye. (From Scanlon, VC, and Sanders, T: Essentials of Anatomy and Physiology, ed 4. FA Davis, Philadelphia, 2003, p 194, with permission.) (*B*) Retina of the right eye. (From Venes, D, and Thomas, CL [eds]: Taber's Cyclopedic Medical Dictionary, ed 19. FA Davis, Philadelphia, 2001, p 1874, with permission.)

A

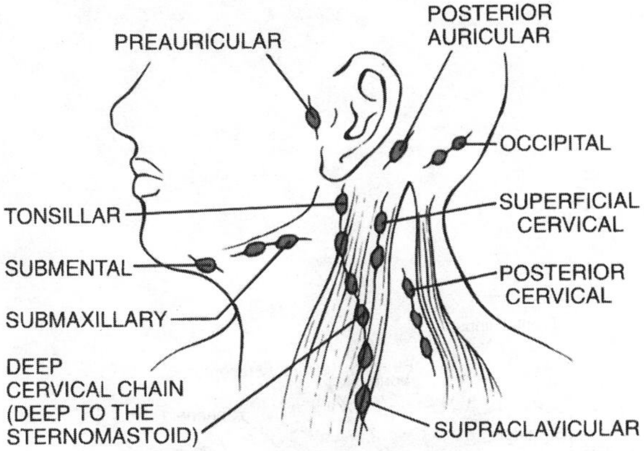

B

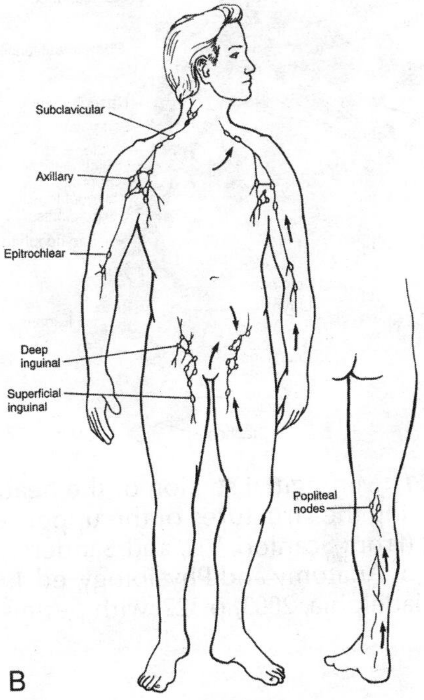

Figure 1–10. (*A*) Lymph nodes of the head and neck. (*B*) Lymph nodes of the body. ([*A*] From Hogstel, MO, and Curry, LC, Practical Guide to Health Assessment through the Lifespan, ed 3. FA Davis, Philadelphia, 2001, p 129, with permission.)

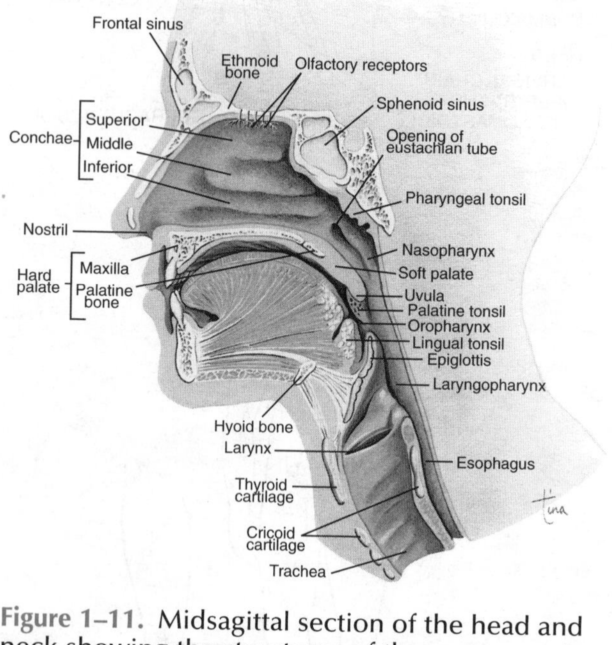

Figure 1–11. Midsagittal section of the head and neck showing the structures of the upper respiratory tract. (From Scanlon, VC, and Sanders, T: Essentials of Anatomy and Physiology, ed 4. FA Davis, Philadelphia, 2003, p 327, with permission.)

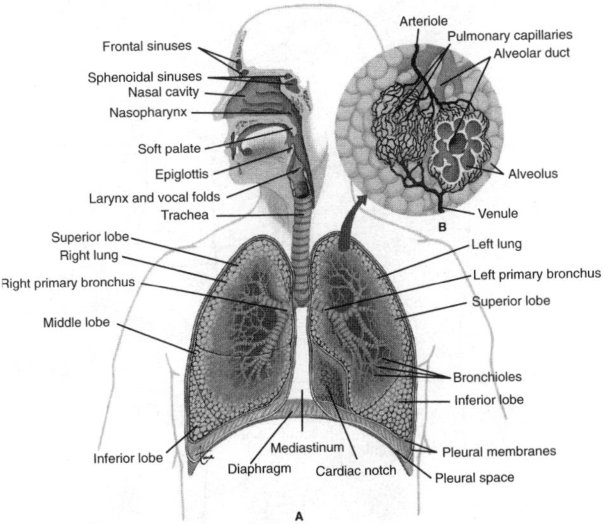

Figure 1–12. Respiratory system. (*A*) Anterior view of the upper and lower respiratory tracts. (*B*) Microscopic view of alveoli and pulmonary capillaries. (From Scanlon, VC, and Sanders, T: Essentials of Anatomy and Physiology, ed 4. FA Davis, Philadelphia, 2003, p 330, with permission.)

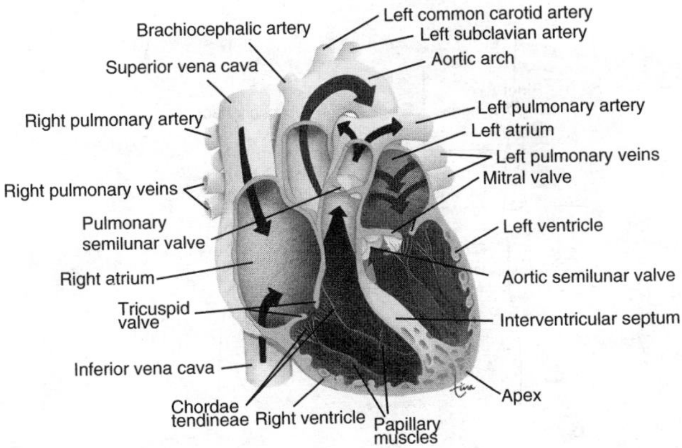

Figure 1–13. Frontal section of the heart in anterior view, showing internal structures. (From Scanlon, VC, and Sanders, T: Essentials of Anatomy and Physiology, ed 4. FA Davis, Philadelphia, 2003, p 262, with permission.)

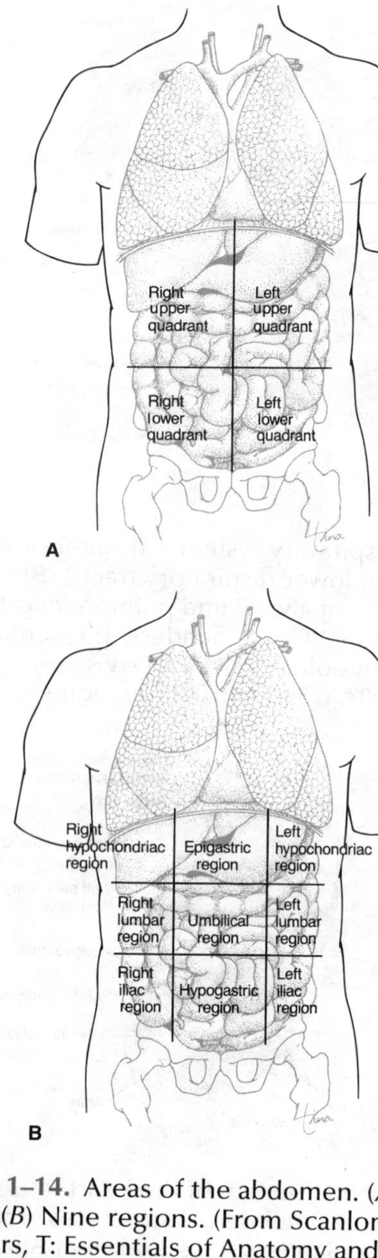

Figure 1–14. Areas of the abdomen. (*A*) Four quadrants. (*B*) Nine regions. (From Scanlon, VC, and Sanders, T: Essentials of Anatomy and Physiology, ed 4. FA Davis, Philadelphia, 2003, p 16, with permission.)

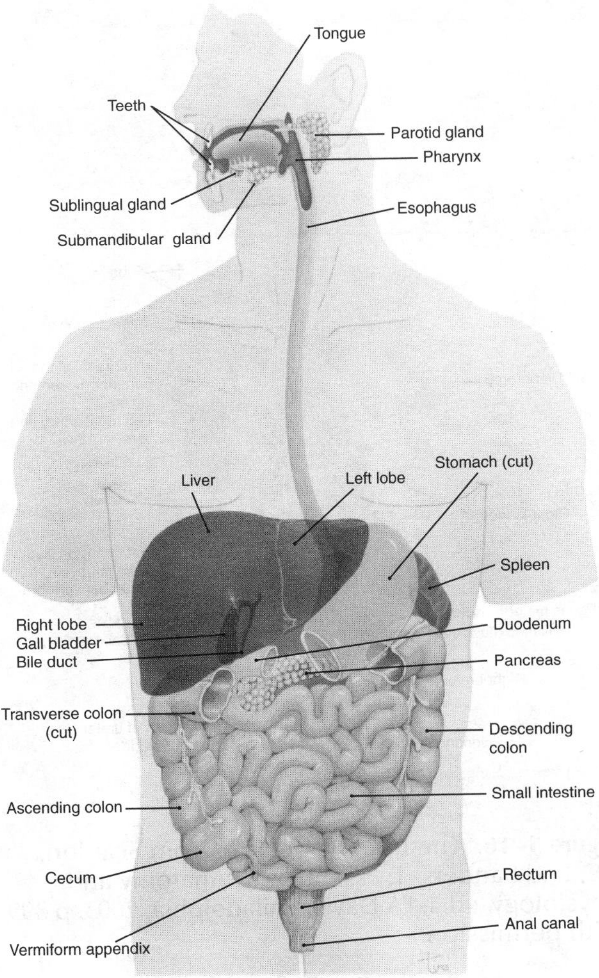

Figure 1–15. The digestive organs. (From Scanlon, VC, and Sanders, T: Essentials of Anatomy and Physiology, ed 4. FA Davis, Philadelphia, 2003, p 351, with permission.)

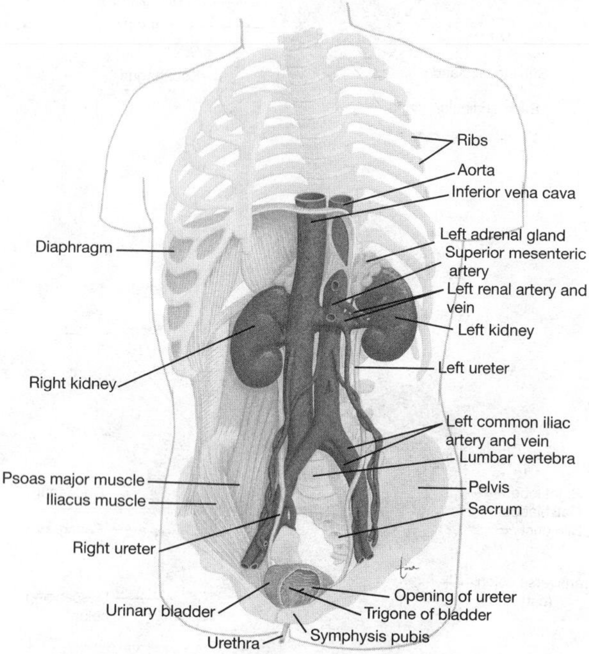

Figure 1–16. The urinary system. (From Scanlon, VC, and Sanders, T: Essentials of Anatomy and Physiology, ed 4. FA Davis, Philadelphia, 2003, p 399, with permission.)

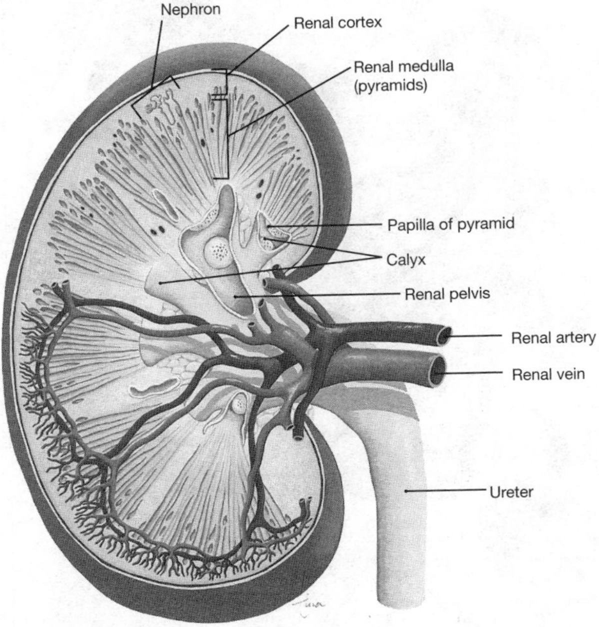

Figure 1–17. Frontal section of the right kidney. (From Scanlon, VC, and Sanders, T: Essentials of Anatomy and Physiology, ed 4. FA Davis, Philadelphia, 2003, p 401, with permission.)

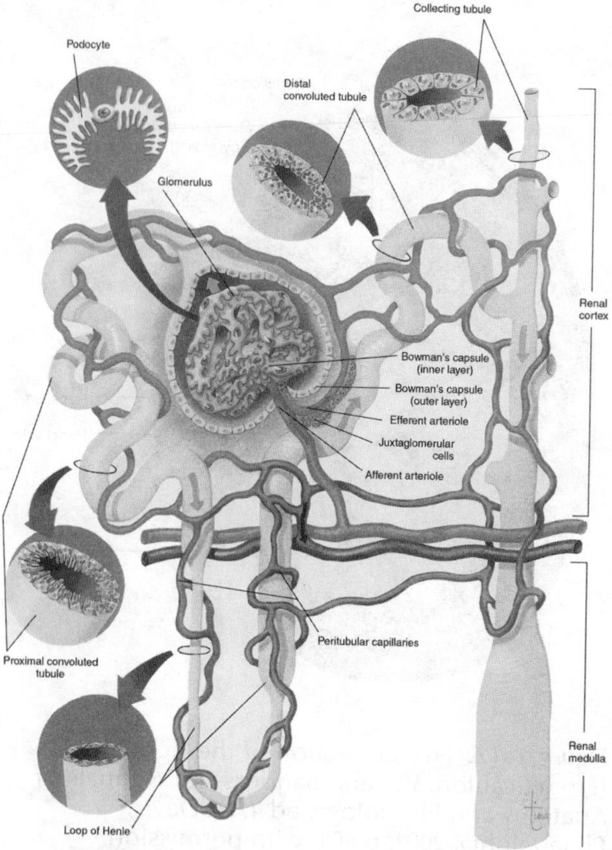

Figure 1–18. A nephron with its associated blood vessels. Portions of the nephron have been magnified. The arrows indicate the direction of blood flow and flow of renal filtrate. (From Scanlon, VC, and Sanders, T: Essentials of Anatomy and Physiology, ed 4. FA Davis, Philadelphia, 2003, p 402, with permission.)

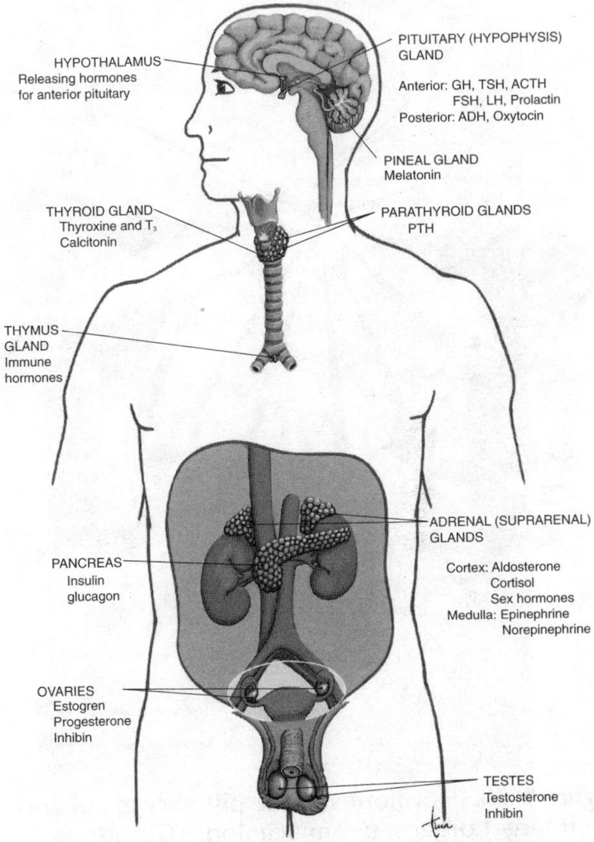

Figure 1–19. The endocrine system. Both male and female gonads (testes and ovaries) are shown. (From Scanlon, VC, and Sanders, T: Essentials of Anatomy and Physiology, ed 4. FA Davis, Philadelphia, 2003, p 213, with permission.)

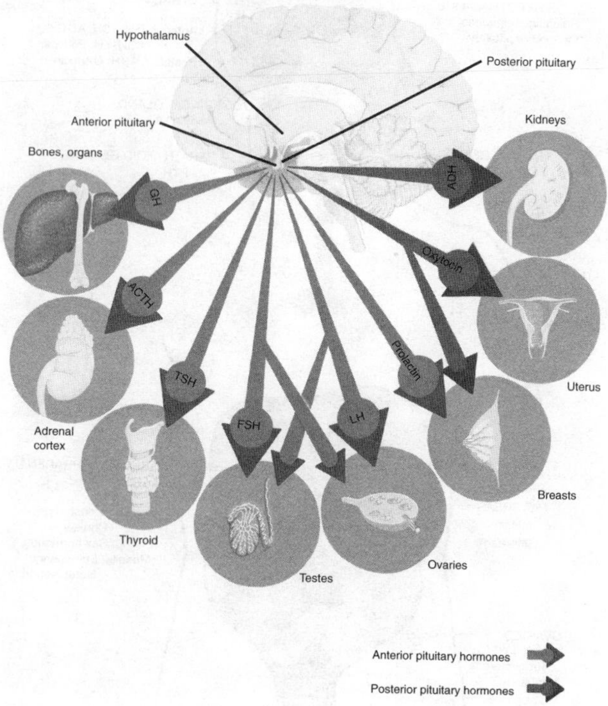

Figure 1–20. Hormones of the pituitary gland and their target organs. (From Scanlon, VC, and Sanders, T: Essentials of Anatomy and Physiology, ed 4. FA Davis, Philadelphia, 2003, p 218, with permission.)

Table 1–1. PRINCIPAL ENDOCRINE GLANDS

Name	Position	Function	Endocrine Disorders
Adrenal cortex	Outer portion of gland on top of each kidney	Steroid hormones regulate carbohydrate and fat metabolism and salt and water balance	Hypofunction: Addison's disease Hyperfunction: Adrenogenital syndrome; Cushing's syndrome
Adrenal medulla	Inner portion of adrenal gland; surrounded by adrenal cortex	Effects mimic those of sympathetic nervous system; increases carbohydrate use of energy	Hypofunction: Almost unknown Hyperfunction: Pheochromocytoma
Pancreas (endocrine portion)	Abdominal cavity; head adjacent to duodenum; tail close to spleen and kidney	Secretes insulin and glucagon, which regulate carbohydrate metabolism	Hypofunction: Diabetes mellitus Hyperfunction: If a tumor produces excess insulin, hypoglycemia

(continued on the following page)

Table 1–1. PRINCIPAL ENDOCRINE GLANDS (continued)

Name	Position	Function	Endocrine Disorders
Parathyroid	Four or more small glands on back of thyroid	Calcium and phosphorus metabolism; indirectly affects muscular irritability	Hypofunction: Tetany Hyperfunction: Resorption of bone; renal calculi
Pituitary, anterior	Front portion of small gland below hypothalamus	Influences growth, sexual development, skin pigmentation, thyroid function, adrenocortical function through effects on other endocrine glands (except for growth hormone, which acts directly on cells)	Hypofunction: Dwarfism in child; decrease in all other endocrine gland functions except parathyroids Hyperfunction; Acromegaly in adult; gigantism in child

Pituitary, posterior	Back portion of small gland below hypothalamus	Oxytocin increases uterine contraction Antidiuretic hormone increases absorption of water by kidney tubule	Unknown Hypofunction: Diabetes insipidus
Testes and ovaries	Testes—in the scrotum Ovaries—in the pelvic cavity	Development of secondary sex characteristics; some effects on growth	Hypofunction: Lack of sexual development or regression in adult Hyperfunction: Abnormal sexual development
Thyroid	Two lobes in anterior portion of neck	Increases metabolic rate; indirectly influences growth and nutrition	Hypofunction: Cretinism in young; myxedema in adult; goiter Hyperfunction: Goiter, thyrotoxicosis

Source: Thomas, CL (ed): Taber's Cyclopedic Medical Dictionary, ed 18. FA Davis, Philadelphia, 1997, p 637, with permission.

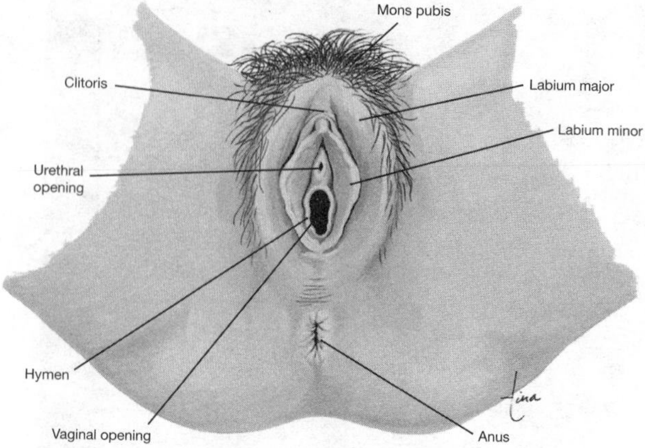

Figure 1–21. Female external genitalia (vulva). (From Scanlon, VC, and Sanders, T: Essentials of Anatomy and Physiology, ed 4. FA Davis, Philadelphia, 2003, p 444, with permission.)

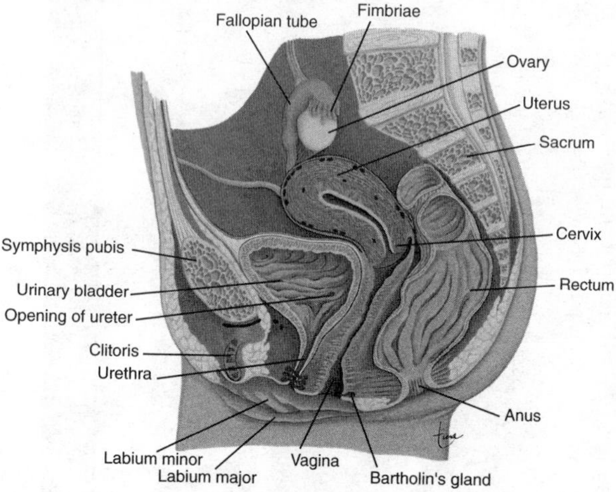

Figure 1–22. Female reproductive system. Midsagittal section. (From Scanlon, VC, and Sanders, T: Essentials of Anatomy and Physiology, ed 4. FA Davis, Philadelphia, 2003, p 441, with permission.)

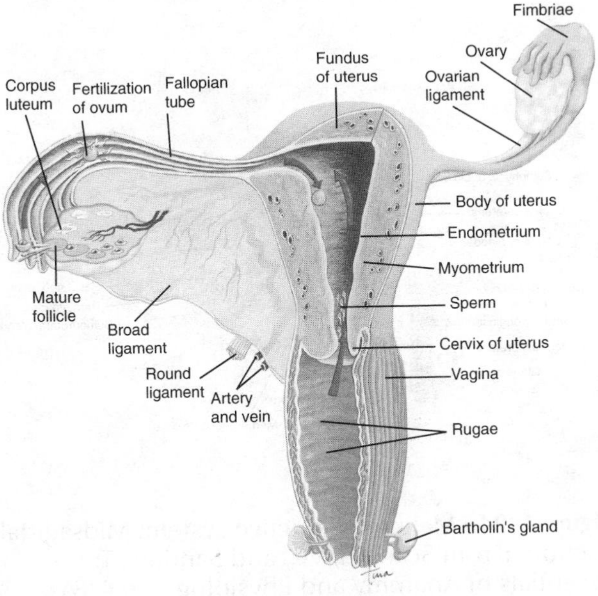

Figure 1–23. Female reproductive system. Anterior view. (From Scanlon, VC, and Sanders, T: Essentials of Anatomy and Physiology, ed 4. FA Davis, Philadelphia, 2003, p 442, with permission.)

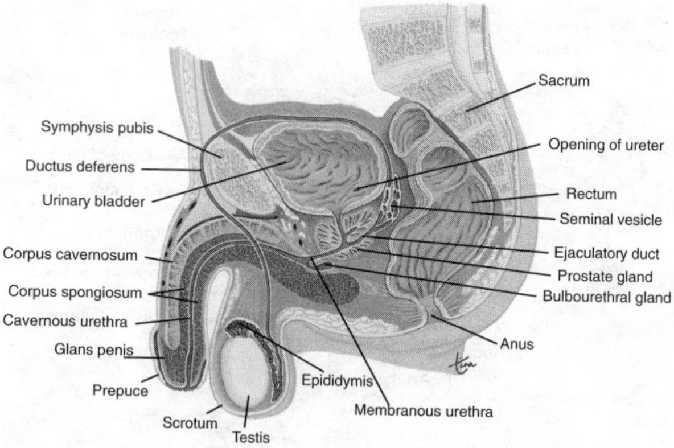

Figure 1–24. Male reproductive system. Midsagittal section. (From Scanlon, VC, and Sanders, T: Essentials of Anatomy and Physiology, ed 4. FA Davis, Philadelphia, 2003, p 438, with permission.)

Table 1–2. ORGAN SYSTEMS AND THEIR FUNCTIONS		
System	**Functions**	**Organs***
Integumentary	Is a barrier to pathogens and chemicals Prevents excessive water loss	Skin, hair, subcutaneous tissue
Skeletal	Supports the body Protects internal organs Provides a framework to be moved by muscles	Bones, ligaments
Muscular	Moves the skeleton Produces heat	Muscles, tendons
Nervous	Interprets sensory information Regulates body functions such as movement by means of electrochemical impulses	Brain, nerves, eyes, ears
Endocrine	Regulates body functions by means of hormones	Thyroid gland, pituitary gland
Circulatory	Transports oxygen and nutrients to tissues and removes waste products	Heart, blood, arteries
Lymphatic	Returns tissue fluid to the blood Destroys pathogens that enter the body	Spleen, lymph nodes

(continued on the following page)

Table 1–2. ORGAN SYSTEMS AND THEIR FUNCTIONS (continued)

System	Functions	Organs*
Respiratory	Exchanges oxygen and carbon dioxide between the air and blood	Lungs, trachea, larynx
Digestive	Changes food to simple chemicals that can be absorbed and used by the body	Stomach, colon, liver
Urinary	Removes waste products from the blood Regulates volume and pH of blood	Kidney, urinary bladder, urethra
Reproductive	Produces eggs or sperm *In women,* provides a site for the developing embryo-fetus	*Female:* Ovaries, uterus *Male:* Testes, prostate gland

* The organs listed here are representative, not all-inclusive.
Source: Scanlon, VC, and Sanders, T: Essentials of Anatomy and Physiology, ed 4. FA Davis, Philadelphia, 2003, p 7, with permission.

Terminology and Symbols

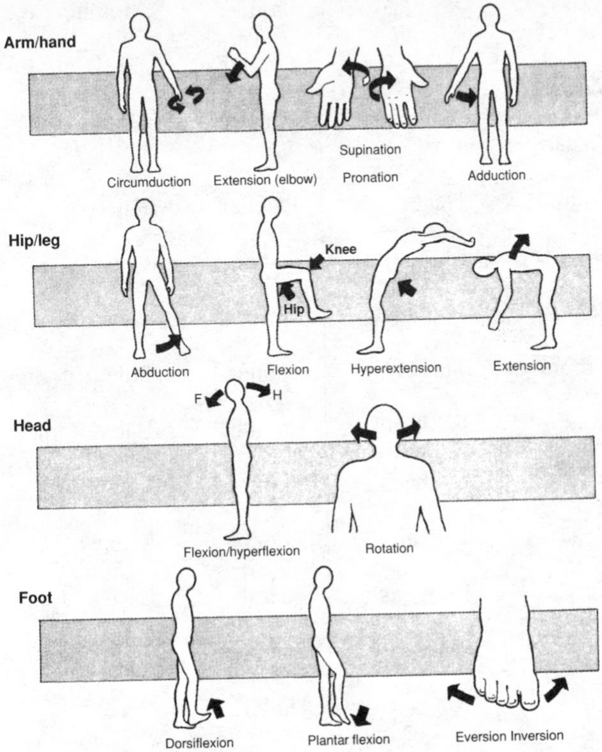

Figure 1–25. Movements of body parts. (From McCance, KL, and Huether, SE: Pathophysiology: The Biologic Basis for Disease in Adults and Children, ed 3. Mosby, St. Louis, 1994, p 1421, with permission.)

Table 1–3.	DESCRIPTIVE TERMS FOR BODY PARTS AND AREAS		
Term	**Body Area**	**Term**	**Body Area**
Antecubital	In front of elbow	Mammary	Breast
Axillary	Armpit	Nasal	Nose
Brachial	Upper arm	Occipital	Back of head
Buccal	Mouth	Oral	Mouth
Cardiac	Heart	Orbital	Eye
Costal	Rib	Parietal	Crown of head
Cranial	Head	Patellar	Kneecap
Cutaneous	Skin	Pectoral	Chest
Deltoid	Shoulder	Perineal	Pelvic floor
Femoral	Thigh	Plantar	Sole of foot
Frontal	Forehead	Popliteal	Back of knee
Gastric	Stomach	Pulmonary	Lungs
Glossal	Tongue	Renal	Kidney
Gluteal	Buttocks	Sacral	Base of spine
Hepatic	Liver	Temporal	Side of head
Iliac	Hip	Umbilical	Navel
Inguinal	Groin	Volar	Palm
Lumbar	Small of back		

Source: Adapted from Scanlon, VC, and Sanders, T: Essentials of Anatomy and Physiology, ed 4, FA Davis, Philadelphia, 2003, p 10, with permission.

Table 1–4.	TERMS OF LOCATION AND POSITION	
Term	**Definition**	**Example**
Superior	Above, or higher	The heart is superior to the liver.
Inferior	Below, or lower	The liver is inferior to the lungs.
Anterior	Toward the front	The chest is on the anterior side of the body.
Posterior	Toward the back	The lumbar area is posterior to the umbilical area.
Ventral	Toward the front	The mammary area is on the ventral side of the body.
Dorsal	Toward the back	The buttocks are on the dorsal side of the body.
Medial	Toward the midline	The heart is medial to the lungs.
Lateral	Away from the midline	The shoulders are lateral to the neck.
Internal	Within, or interior to	The brain is internal to the skull.
External	Outside, or exterior to	The ribs are external to the lungs.
Superficial	Toward the surface	The skin is the most superficial organ.
Deep	Within, or interior to	The deep veins of the legs are surrounded by muscles.

(continued on the following page)

Table 1–4. TERMS OF LOCATION AND POSITION (continued)

Term	Definition	Example
Central	The main part	The brain is part of the central nervous system.
Peripheral	Extending from the main part	Nerves in the arm are part of the peripheral nervous system.
Proximal	Closer to the origin	The knee is proximal to the foot.
Distal	Farther from the origin	The palm is distal to the elbow.
Parietal	Pertaining to the wall of a cavity	The parietal pleura lines the chest cavity.
Visceral	Pertaining to the organs within a cavity	The visceral pleura covers the lungs.

Source: Scanlon, VC, and Sanders, T: Essentials of Anatomy and Physiology, ed 4, FA Davis, Philadelphia, 2003, p 12, with permission.

WORD ELEMENTS AND MEANINGS

Word Element	*Meaning*
a-	without; not
ab-	from; away from
-ac	pertaining to
acr-	extremities
ad-	to; toward
aden-	gland
adip-	fat
-al	pertaining to
-algia	pain
ambi-	both
amph-	on both sides
an-	without; not
andr-	male

Word Element	*Meaning*
angi-	vessel
ante-	before
anti-	against
arteri-	artery
arthr-	joint
-ary	pertaining to
ather-	fat
audi-	hearing
auto-	self
bi-	two
blast-	embryonic; germ
blephar-	eyelid
brady-	slow
calc-	stone; heel
capit-	head
carcin-	cancer
cardi-	heart
caud-	tail
-cele	tumor; hernia
cente-	puncture
cephal-	head
cheil-	lip
chol-	bile; gall
chondr-	cartilage
circum-	around
contra-	against
cost-	rib
crani-	cranium; skull
cune-	wedge
cut-	skin
cyst-	bladder
cyt-	cell
de-	down; from
derm-	skin
-desis	a binding
dextr-	right
di-	two
digit-	finger; toe
dipl-	double

(continued on the following page)

Word Element	*Meaning*
dors-	back
dys-	bad; painful
ec-	out from
-ectomy	removal
ede-	swell
encephal-	brain
endo-	in
enter-	intestine
epi-	upon
erythr-	red
eu-	good
ex-	out from
febr-	fever
fiss-	split
flect-	bend
flux	flow
gastr-	stomach
gest-	bear; carry
gloss-	tongue
gluc-	sugar
gyn-	female
hem-	blood
hemi-	half; partial
hepat-	liver
heter-	different
hist-	tissue
homo-	same
hydr-	water
hyper-	over, above
hypo-	below
hyster-	uterus
-ia	unhealthy state
-ic	pertaining to
-icle	small
im-	not
immun-	protected
in-	not
infra-	below
inter-	between

Word Element	*Meaning*
intra-	in
iso-	equal
-itis	inflammation
karat-	cornea; hornlike
-kinesis	movement
later-	to the side of
leuc-; leuk-	white
lig-	tie; bind
lip-	fat
-lithiasis	condition of stones
macro-	large
mal-	ill; bad; poor
mamma-	breast
mani-	mental aberration
mast-	breast
medi-	in the middle of
mega-	great; large
melan-	black
mes-	middle
meta-	after; over; change
micr-	small
mon-	one
morph-	shape
multi-	many
myc-	fungus
myel-	bone marrow; spinal cord
myring-	tympanic membrane
my-	muscle
narc-	sleep
nas-	nose
neo-	new; young
nephr-	kidney
neur-	nerve
noct-	night
-ole	small
olig-	small
-oma	tumor

(continued on the following page)

Word Element	*Meaning*
onc-	tumor
oo-	egg; ovum
ophthalm-	eye
-opia	vision
-optysis	spitting
orchi-	testes
orth-	straight
os-	bone
-ostomy	forming an opening
ot-	ear
-otomy	incision
pan-	all
par-	near
-paresis	slight paralysis
ped-	foot
pend-	hang down
per-	across
peri-	around
phag-	swallow; eat
phil-	have an affinity for
phleb-	vein
phob-	fear; dread
phot-	light
-phylaxis	protection
-pnea	breathing
pneum-	air; lung
pod-	foot
poikilo-	varied; irregular
poly-	many
-porosis	cavities; backward
post-	after
-prandial	pertaining to a meal
pre-	before
primi-	first
pro-	before
proct-	anus
pseudo-	false
pulmon-	lung
py-	pus
pyel-	renal pelvis
quad-	four

Word Element	*Meaning*
ren-	kidney
retro-	after; backward
rhin-	nose
-rrhage	excessive flow
-rrhea	flow; discharge
salping-	eustachian or fallopian tubes
sanguin-	blood
scler-	hard
sect-	cut
semi-	half; partial
ser-	watery substance
spher-	round
-stalsis	contraction
-stasis	not moving
sten-	narrow
steth-	chest
stoma-	small opening
sub-	below
super-	above
supra-	above
sym-	union
syn-	union
tachy-	rapid
-taxia	muscle coordination
tetra-	four
thorac-	chest
thromb-	clot
-tic	pertaining to
tox-	poison
trans-	across
tri-	three
-trophy	nourishment; development
-tropia	turning
-ule	little
ultra-	excess
uni-	one
ur-	urine
uter-	uterus
vas-	vessel
ven-	vein

SELECTED SYMBOLS USED IN MEDICINE

−	Minus or negative	∞	Infinity
±	Plus or minus	:	Ratio or "is to"
#	Number or pounds	°	Degree
÷	Divided by	%	Percent
/	Divided by	□, ♂	Male
×	Multiplied by	○, ♀	Female
=	Equals	α	Alpha
≈	Approximately equals	β	Beta
>	Greater than or from which is derived	↑	Increase
<	Less than or derived from	↓	Decrease
≮	Not less than	1°	Primary
≯	Not greater than	2°	Secondary (to)
≥	Equal to or greater than	♏	Minim
≤	Equal to or less than	ʒ	Dram
≠	Not equal to	fʒ	Fluid dram
√	Square root	℥	Ounce

f℥	Fluid ounce	Ⓛ	Left
℞	recipe or take	mμ	Millimicron or nanometer
c̄	With	μg	Microgram
s̄	Without	p̄	After
Ⓡ	Right	s̈s̄	One half
		△	Change or heat

SELECTED MEDICAL ABBREVIATIONS

Abbreviations may be seen in practice with or without punctuation and may be found written in capital or lowercase letters. Punctuation has been omitted in this list.

Abbreviation	*Meaning*
a	Before
aa	Of each
ab	Abortion; antibiotic
abd	Abdomen
ABGs	Arterial blood gases
ac	Before meals; abdominal circumference
accel	(FHR) acceleration
ACE	Angiotensin-converting enzyme
ACTH	Adrenocorticotropic hormone
AD	Right ear
ADA	American Diabetes Association
ADD	Attention deficit disorder
ADH	Antidiuretic hormone
ADHD	Attention deficit hyperactive disorder
ADL	Activities of daily living
ad lib	As desired
AFB	Acid-fast bacilli
AFP	Alpha-fetoprotein
AFV	Amniotic fluid volume
AGA	Appropriate for gestational age
AGN	Acute glomerulonephritis
AID	Artificial insemination by donor

(continued on the following page)

Abbreviation	*Meaning*
AIDS	Acquired immunodeficiency syndrome
AIH	Artificial insemination by husband
AKA	Also known as
ALL	Acute lymphocytic leukemia
ALT	Same as SGOT
alt noc	Every other night
AM	Midnight to all times before noon
AMA	Against medical advice
amb	Ambulate
AMI	Acute myocardial infarction
ANA	Antinuclear antibodies
ANLL	Acute nonlymphoid leukemia
ant	Anterior
AOM	Acute otitis media
A/P	Anteroposterior
aq	Water
ARB	Angiotensin receptor blocker
ARC	AIDS-related complex
ARF	Acute rheumatic fever
AROM	Artificial rupture of membranes; active range of motion
ASA	Aspirin
ASAP	As soon as possible
ASD	Atrial septal defect
ASHD	Arteriosclerotic heart disease
ASO	Antistreptolysin O
AV	Atrioventricular
Ax	Axillary
Az	2-hour pregnancy test
BA	Barium enema
BAL	Blood alcohol level
BAT	Brown adipose tissue
BBB	Bundle branch block
BE	Barium enema
bid	Twice daily
BK	Below the knee
BM	Bowel movement
BMA	Bone marrow aspiration
BMR	Basal metabolic rate
BOW	Bag of waters

Abbreviation	*Meaning*
BP	Blood pressure
BPD	Biparietal diameter of fetal head; bronchopulmonary dysplasia
BPH	Benign prostatic hypertrophy
BPM	Beats per minute
BS	Blood sugar
BSA	Body surface area
BSST	Breast self-stimulation test
BUN	Blood urea nitrogen
Bx	Biopsy
C	Celsius or centigrade; calorie
CA	Cancer
Ca+	Calcium
CABG	Coronary artery bypass graft
CAD	Coronary artery disease
cal	Calorie
cap	Capsule
CAT	Computed axial tomography
CBC	Complete blood count
CC	Chief complaint; cubic centimeter
cc	Cubic centimeter; chief complaint
CCB	Calcium channel blocker
CCU	Coronary care unit
CDC	Centers for Disease Control (and Prevention)
CF	Cystic fibrosis
CFT	Capillary fill time
C-H	Crown-heel (length)
CHD	Congenital heart disease
CHF	Congestive heart failure
CID	Cytomegalic inclusion disease
circ	Circumcision
Cl	Chloride
CLL	Chronic lymphocytic leukemia
cm	Centimeter
CMV	Cytomegalovirus
CN	Cranial nerve
CNM	Certified nurse-midwife

(continued on the following page)

Abbreviation	*Meaning*
CNS	Central nervous system (brain and spinal column)
C/O	Complains of
CO_2	Carbon dioxide
COA	Coarctation of the aorta
COLD	Chronic obstructive lung disease
COM	Chronic otitis media
comp	Compound
COPD	Chronic obstructive pulmonary disease
CP	Cerebral palsy
CPAP	Continuous positive airway pressure
CPD	Cephalopelvic disproportion
CPK	Creatine phosphokinase
CPP	Cerebral perfusion pressure
CPR	Cardiopulmonary resuscitation
CPT	Chest physiotherapy
CR	Controlled release
C-R	Crown-rump (length)
CRNA	Certified registered nurse anesthetist
CS	Cesarean section
C&S	Culture and sensitivity
CSF	Cerebrospinal fluid
CST	Contraction stress test
CT	Computed tomography
CTA	Clear to auscultation
CUG	Cystourethrogram
CV	Cardiovascular
CVA	Cerebrovascular accident
CVD	Cardiovascular disease
CVP	Central venous pressure
CVTC	Central venous tunneled catheter
CXR	Chest x-ray
d	Day
DASH	Dietary approach to stop hypertension
D/C	Discontinue; discharge
D&C	Dilatation and curettage
DDST	Denver Developmental Standardized Test

Abbreviation	*Meaning*
ICF	Intracellular fluid
ICN	Intensive care nursery
ICP	Intracranial pressure
ICU	Intensive care unit
I&D	Incision and drainage
IDDM	Insulin-dependent diabetes mellitus
IDM	Infant of diabetic mother
I/E	Inspiratory/expiratory
IG	Immune globulin
IM	Intramuscular
incl	Including
inf	Infusion
inhal	Inhalation
inj	Injection
I&O	Intake and output
IOP	Intraocular pressure
IPPB	Intermittent positive-pressure breathing
IPPV	Intermittent positive-pressure ventilation
IQ	Intelligence quotient
SADH	Inappropriate secretion of antidiuretic hormone
E	Internal scalp electrode
P	Idiopathic thrombocytopenic purpura
	International unit
)	Intrauterine device
D	Intrauterine fetal demise
R	Intrauterine growth retardation
	Intrauterine pregnancy
	Intrauterine pressure catheter
	Intravenous
	In vitro fertilization
	Intravenous pyelogram;
	IV push
	IV piggyback
	Juvenile rheumatoid arthritis
	Jugular vein distention
	Potassium

Abbreviation	*Meaning*
del	(FHR) deceleration; delivery
DEXA (scan)	Dual energy x-ray absorptiometry
DHR	Department of Human Resources
DIC	Disseminated intravascular coagulation
dig	Digitalis
dL	Deciliter
DM	Diabetes mellitus
DO	Doctor of Osteopathy
DOA	Dead on arrival
DOB	Date of birth
DPT	Diphtheria; pertussis; tetanus
dr	Dram
DRG	Diagnosis-related group
DS	Double strength
dsg	Dressing
DTR	Deep tendon reflex
DVT	deep vein thrombosis
D_5W	5% dextrose in water
Dx	Diagnosis
ECF	Extracellular fluid
ECG	Electrocardiogram (*also* EKG)
ECT	Electroconvulsive therapy
ED	Emergency department
EDC	Estimated date of confinement
EEG	Electroencephalogram
EENT	Ear, eye, nose, and throat
EFM	External fetal monitor
EKG	Electrocardiogram (*also* ECG)
elix	Elixir
EMG	Electromyogram
ENT	Ear, nose, and throat
EOM	Extraocular movements
epis	Episiotomy
esp	Especially
ER	Emergency room
ESR	Erythrocyte sedimentation rate (sed rate)
EST	Electroshock therapy

(continued on the following page)

Abbreviation	Meaning
ET	Endotracheal
et	And
EUG	Excretory urogram
F	Fundus; Fahrenheit; female
FAD	Fetal activity diary
FAS	Fetal alcohol syndrome
FBM	Fetal breathing movements
FBS	Fasting blood sugar; fetal blood (scalp) sample
FDA	Food and Drug Administration
Fe	Iron
F&E	Fluids and electrolytes
FEV	Forced expiratory volume
FH	Fundal height
FHR	Fetal heart rate
FHT	Fetal heart tones
FiO_2	Fractional inspired O_2 concentration
fl dr	Fluid dram
fl oz	Fluid ounce
FM	Fetal movement
FOC	Fronto-occipital circumference (head circumference)
FSH	Follicle-stimulating hormone
FSHRH	Follicle stimulating hormone–releasing hormone
FTND	Full-term normal delivery
FTP	Full-term pregnancy
FTT	Failure to thrive
FUO	Fever of undetermined origin
fx	Fracture
G	Gravida (*also* grav)
g	Gram (*also* gm)
GB	Gallbladder
GC	Gonorrhea
GDM	Gestational diabetes mellitus
G&D	Growth and development
GER	Gastroesophageal reflux
GFR	Glomerular filtration rate
GH	Growth hormone
GI	Gastrointestinal
Gm	Gram (*also* g)

Abbreviation	Meaning
gr	Grain
grav	Gravida (*also* G)
GTT	Glucose tolerance test
gtt	Drop
GU	Genitourinary
GYN	Gynecology
H	Hypodermic
h	Hour (*also* hr)
HA	Headache
HAV	Hepatitis A
Hb	Hemoglobin (*also* hgb)
HBV	Hepatitis B
HC	Head circumference
HCG	Human chorionic gonadotropir
hct	Hematocrit
HCTZ	Hydrochlorothiazide
HDL	High-density lipoprotein
H-flu	*Haemophilus influenzae*
hgb	Hemoglobin (*also* Hb)
H&H	Hematocrit and hemoglo
HHNK	Hyperglycemic, hyperos nonketotic coma
Hib	*Haemophilus influenz* bacteria
HIV	Human immunodefi
HMD	Hyaline membrane
HMO	Health maintenanc tion
H_2O	Water
H_2O_2	Hydrogen perox
HOB	Head of bed
HPI	History of pre
HPF	High-powere scope)
HR	Heart rate
hr	Hour (*als*
hs	Hour of s
ht	Height
HTN	Hyperte
HVH	Herpe
Hx	Histo
hypo	Hyp

(continued o

IVF
IVP
IVPB
JRA
JVD
K+

Abbreviation	*Meaning*
kcal	Kilocalorie
KCl	Potassium chloride
kg	Kilogram
KUB	Kidney, ureter, bladder
L	Liter; left
LA	Long-acting
lat	Lateral
lb	Pound
LBW	Low birth weight
L&D	Labor and delivery
LDH	Lactase dehydrogenase
LDL	Low-density lipoprotein
LE	Lupus erythematosus
LFD	Low forceps delivery
lg	Large
LGA	Large for gestational age
LH	Luteinizing hormone
liq	Liquid
LLQ	Left lower quadrant
LMA	Left mentum anterior
LMLE	Left mediolateral episiotomy
LMP	Last menstrual period
LMT	Left mentotransverse (fetal position)
LOA	left occipitoanterior (fetal position)
LOC	Level of consciousness
LOF	Low outlet forceps
LOM	Left otitis media
LOP	Left occipitoposterior (fetal position)
LOT	Left occipitotransverse (fetal position)
lot	Lotion
LP	Lumbar puncture
LPN	Licensed practical nurse
LR	Lactated Ringer's
L/S	Lecithin/sphingomyelin
LSA	Left sacroanterior (fetal position)
LScA	Left scapuloanterior (fetal position)

(continued on the following page)

Abbreviation	*Meaning*
LScP	Left scapuloposterior (fetal position)
LSP	Left sacroposterior (fetal position)
LST	Left sacrotransverse (fetal position)
LUQ	Left upper quadrant
M	Male; minim
m	Meter; minute (*also* min)
m^2	Meter square
MAEW	Moves all extremities well
Mag	Magnesium sulfate (*also* $MgSO_4$)
MAO	Monoamine oxidase
MAOI	Monoamine oxidase inhibitor
MAP	Mean arterial pressure
MAS	Meconium aspiration syndrome
mcg	Microgram (*also* μg)
MCH	Mean corpuscular hemoglobin
MCHC	Mean corpuscular hemoglobin concentration
MCV	Mean corpuscular volume
MD	Doctor of medicine
mec	Meconium
mec st	Meconium stain
med	Medicine
mEq	Milliequivalent
MeSH	Medical subject heading
Mg	Magnesium
mg	Milligram
$MgSO_4$	Magnesium sulfate (*also* mag)
MI	Myocardial infarction
min	Minute (*also* m)
mL	Milliliter
MLE	Midline episiotomy
mm	Millimeter
μm	Microgram (*also* mcg)
mm^3	Cubic millimeter
MMR	Measles, mumps, rubella (vaccine)
mo	Month
mod	Moderate
MRI	Magnetic resonance imaging

Abbreviation	*Meaning*
MS	Multiple sclerosis; mitral stenosis; musculoskeletal
MTX	Methotrexate
MVA	Motor vehicle accident
Na+	Sodium
NaCl	Sodium chloride
NAD	No acute distress
$NaHCO_3$	Sodium bicarbonate
NB	Newborn; non–hepatitis B
NBN	Newborn nursery
NC	Nasal cannula
NEC	Necrotizing enterocolitis
NG	Nasogastric
NICU	Nursery intensive care unit
NIDDM	Non–insulin-dependent diabetes mellitus
NIH	National Institutes of Health
NKA	No known allergies
NMS	Neuroleptic malignant syndrome
no	Number
noc	Night
NPO	Nothing by mouth
NS	Normal saline (0.9% NaCl)
NSAIA	Nonsteroidal anti-inflammatory analgesics
NSAID	Nonsteroidal anti-inflammatory drug
NST	Non-stress test
NSVD	Normal sterile vaginal delivery
NTD	Neural tube defect
NTG	Nitroglycerin
N/V/D	Nausea/vomiting/diarrhea
O_2	Oxygen
OA	Occiput anterior (fetal position)
OB	Obstetrics
OBS	Organic brain syndrome
OC	Oral contraceptive
OCT	Oxytocin challenge test
OD	Overdose; right eye

(continued on the following page)

Abbreviation	*Meaning*
OFC	Occipitofrontal circumference (head circumference)
OL	Left eye
OM	Otitis media
OME	Otitis media with effusion
OOB	Out of bed
OP	Occiput posterior (fetal position)
OPV	Oral poliovirus vaccine
OR	Operating room
ORIF	Open reduction with internal fixation
OS	Left eye
os	Mouth
OTC	Over-the-counter
OU	Each eye
OV	Both eyes
oz	Ounce
P	Para; phosphorus; phosphate (*also* PO_4); pulse, wave on ECG complex
$\bar{p}$	After
pa	Posteroanterior
PAC	Premature atrial contraction
PaO_2	Partial arterial oxygen tension
paren	Parenterally
PAT	Paroxysmal atrial tachycardia
PCTA	Percutaneous transluminal angioplasty
Pb	Phenobarbital
PBI	Protein-bound iodine
pc	After meals
PCA	Patient-controlled analgesia
PCN	Penicillin
PCWP	Pulmonary capillary wedge pressure
PDA	Patent ductus arteriosus
PE	Physical exam
PE tubes	Pressure-equalizing tubes
PEEP	Positive end expiratory pressure
PEG tube	Percutaneous gastrostomy
PERL	Pupils equal, react to light

Abbreviation	*Meaning*
del	(FHR) deceleration; delivery
DEXA (scan)	Dual energy x-ray absorptiometry
DHR	Department of Human Resources
DIC	Disseminated intravascular coagulation
dig	Digitalis
dL	Deciliter
DM	Diabetes mellitus
DO	Doctor of Osteopathy
DOA	Dead on arrival
DOB	Date of birth
DPT	Diphtheria; pertussis; tetanus
dr	Dram
DRG	Diagnosis-related group
DS	Double strength
dsg	Dressing
DTR	Deep tendon reflex
DVT	deep vein thrombosis
D_5W	5% dextrose in water
Dx	Diagnosis
ECF	Extracellular fluid
ECG	Electrocardiogram (*also* EKG)
ECT	Electroconvulsive therapy
ED	Emergency department
EDC	Estimated date of confinement
EEG	Electroencephalogram
EENT	Ear, eye, nose, and throat
EFM	External fetal monitor
EKG	Electrocardiogram (*also* ECG)
elix	Elixir
EMG	Electromyogram
ENT	Ear, nose, and throat
EOM	Extraocular movements
epis	Episiotomy
esp	Especially
ER	Emergency room
ESR	Erythrocyte sedimentation rate (sed rate)
EST	Electroshock therapy

(continued on the following page)

Abbreviation	*Meaning*
ET	Endotracheal
et	And
EUG	Excretory urogram
F	Fundus; Fahrenheit; female
FAD	Fetal activity diary
FAS	Fetal alcohol syndrome
FBM	Fetal breathing movements
FBS	Fasting blood sugar; fetal blood (scalp) sample
FDA	Food and Drug Administration
Fe	Iron
F&E	Fluids and electrolytes
FEV	Forced expiratory volume
FH	Fundal height
FHR	Fetal heart rate
FHT	Fetal heart tones
FiO_2	Fractional inspired O_2 concentration
fl dr	Fluid dram
fl oz	Fluid ounce
FM	Fetal movement
FOC	Fronto-occipital circumference (head circumference)
FSH	Follicle-stimulating hormone
FSHRH	Follicle stimulating hormone–releasing hormone
FTND	Full-term normal delivery
FTP	Full-term pregnancy
FTT	Failure to thrive
FUO	Fever of undetermined origin
fx	Fracture
G	Gravida (*also* grav)
g	Gram (*also* gm)
GB	Gallbladder
GC	Gonorrhea
GDM	Gestational diabetes mellitus
G&D	Growth and development
GER	Gastroesophageal reflux
GFR	Glomerular filtration rate
GH	Growth hormone
GI	Gastrointestinal
Gm	Gram (*also* g)

Abbreviation	*Meaning*
gr	Grain
grav	Gravida (*also* G)
GTT	Glucose tolerance test
gtt	Drop
GU	Genitourinary
GYN	Gynecology
H	Hypodermic
h	Hour (*also* hr)
HA	Headache
HAV	Hepatitis A
Hb	Hemoglobin (*also* hgb)
HBV	Hepatitis B
HC	Head circumference
HCG	Human chorionic gonadotropin
hct	Hematocrit
HCTZ	Hydrochlorothiazide
HDL	High-density lipoprotein
H-flu	*Haemophilus influenzae*
hgb	Hemoglobin (*also* Hb)
H&H	Hematocrit and hemoglobin
HHNK	Hyperglycemic, hyperosmolar, nonketotic coma
Hib	*Haemophilus influenzae* bacteria
HIV	Human immunodeficiency virus
HMD	Hyaline membrane disease
HMO	Health maintenance organization
H_2O	Water
H_2O_2	Hydrogen peroxide
HOB	Head of bed
HPI	History of present illness
HPF	High-powered field (of microscope)
HR	Heart rate
hr	Hour (*also* h)
hs	Hour of sleep
ht	Height
HTN	Hypertension
HVH	Herpes virus hominis
Hx	History
hypo	Hypodermic

(continued on the following page)

Abbreviation	*Meaning*
ICF	Intracellular fluid
ICN	Intensive care nursery
ICP	Intracranial pressure
ICU	Intensive care unit
I&D	Incision and drainage
IDDM	Insulin-dependent diabetes mellitus
IDM	Infant of diabetic mother
I/E	Inspiratory/expiratory
IG	Immune globulin
IM	Intramuscular
incl	Including
inf	Infusion
inhal	Inhalation
inj	Injection
I&O	Intake and output
IOP	Intraocular pressure
IPPB	Intermittent positive-pressure breathing
IPPV	Intermittent positive-pressure ventilation
IQ	Intelligence quotient
ISADH	Inappropriate secretion of antidiuretic hormone
ISE	Internal scalp electrode
ITP	Idiopathic thrombocytopenic purpura
IU	International unit
IUD	Intrauterine device
IUFD	Intrauterine fetal demise
IUGR	Intrauterine growth retardation
IUP	Intrauterine pregnancy
IUPC	Intrauterine pressure catheter
IV	Intravenous
IVF	In vitro fertilization
IVP	Intravenous pyelogram; IV push
IVPB	IV piggyback
JRA	Juvenile rheumatoid arthritis
JVD	Jugular vein distention
K+	Potassium

Abbreviation	*Meaning*
kcal	Kilocalorie
KCl	Potassium chloride
kg	Kilogram
KUB	Kidney, ureter, bladder
L	Liter; left
LA	Long-acting
lat	Lateral
lb	Pound
LBW	Low birth weight
L&D	Labor and delivery
LDH	Lactase dehydrogenase
LDL	Low-density lipoprotein
LE	Lupus erythematosus
LFD	Low forceps delivery
lg	Large
LGA	Large for gestational age
LH	Luteinizing hormone
liq	Liquid
LLQ	Left lower quadrant
LMA	Left mentum anterior
LMLE	Left mediolateral episiotomy
LMP	Last menstrual period
LMT	Left mentotransverse (fetal position)
LOA	left occipitoanterior (fetal position)
LOC	Level of consciousness
LOF	Low outlet forceps
LOM	Left otitis media
LOP	Left occipitoposterior (fetal position)
LOT	Left occipitotransverse (fetal position)
lot	Lotion
LP	Lumbar puncture
LPN	Licensed practical nurse
LR	Lactated Ringer's
L/S	Lecithin/sphingomyelin
LSA	Left sacroanterior (fetal position)
LScA	Left scapuloanterior (fetal position)

(continued on the following page)

Abbreviation	*Meaning*
LScP	Left scapuloposterior (fetal position)
LSP	Left sacroposterior (fetal position)
LST	Left sacrotransverse (fetal position)
LUQ	Left upper quadrant
M	Male; minim
m	Meter; minute (*also* min)
m^2	Meter square
MAEW	Moves all extremities well
Mag	Magnesium sulfate (*also* $MgSO_4$)
MAO	Monoamine oxidase
MAOI	Monoamine oxidase inhibitor
MAP	Mean arterial pressure
MAS	Meconium aspiration syndrome
mcg	Microgram (*also* μg)
MCH	Mean corpuscular hemoglobin
MCHC	Mean corpuscular hemoglobin concentration
MCV	Mean corpuscular volume
MD	Doctor of medicine
mec	Meconium
mec st	Meconium stain
med	Medicine
mEq	Milliequivalent
MeSH	Medical subject heading
Mg	Magnesium
mg	Milligram
$MgSO_4$	Magnesium sulfate (*also* mag)
MI	Myocardial infarction
min	Minute (*also* m)
mL	Milliliter
MLE	Midline episiotomy
mm	Millimeter
μm	Microgram (*also* mcg)
mm^3	Cubic millimeter
MMR	Measles, mumps, rubella (vaccine)
mo	Month
mod	Moderate
MRI	Magnetic resonance imaging

Abbreviation	*Meaning*
MS	Multiple sclerosis; mitral stenosis; musculoskeletal
MTX	Methotrexate
MVA	Motor vehicle accident
Na+	Sodium
NaCl	Sodium chloride
NAD	No acute distress
$NaHCO_3$	Sodium bicarbonate
NB	Newborn; non–hepatitis B
NBN	Newborn nursery
NC	Nasal cannula
NEC	Necrotizing enterocolitis
NG	Nasogastric
NICU	Nursery intensive care unit
NIDDM	Non–insulin-dependent diabetes mellitus
NIH	National Institutes of Health
NKA	No known allergies
NMS	Neuroleptic malignant syndrome
no	Number
noc	Night
NPO	Nothing by mouth
NS	Normal saline (0.9% NaCl)
NSAIA	Nonsteroidal anti-inflammatory analgesics
NSAID	Nonsteroidal anti-inflammatory drug
NST	Non-stress test
NSVD	Normal sterile vaginal delivery
NTD	Neural tube defect
NTG	Nitroglycerin
N/V/D	Nausea/vomiting/diarrhea
O_2	Oxygen
OA	Occiput anterior (fetal position)
OB	Obstetrics
OBS	Organic brain syndrome
OC	Oral contraceptive
OCT	Oxytocin challenge test
OD	Overdose; right eye

(continued on the following page)

Abbreviation	*Meaning*
OFC	Occipitofrontal circumference (head circumference)
OL	Left eye
OM	Otitis media
OME	Otitis media with effusion
OOB	Out of bed
OP	Occiput posterior (fetal position)
OPV	Oral poliovirus vaccine
OR	Operating room
ORIF	Open reduction with internal fixation
OS	Left eye
os	Mouth
OTC	Over-the-counter
OU	Each eye
OV	Both eyes
oz	Ounce
P	Para; phosphorus; phosphate (*also* PO_4); pulse, wave on ECG complex
p̄	After
pa	Posteroanterior
PAC	Premature atrial contraction
PaO_2	Partial arterial oxygen tension
paren	Parenterally
PAT	Paroxysmal atrial tachycardia
PCTA	Percutaneous transluminal angioplasty
Pb	Phenobarbital
PBI	Protein-bound iodine
pc	After meals
PCA	Patient-controlled analgesia
PCN	Penicillin
PCWP	Pulmonary capillary wedge pressure
PDA	Patent ductus arteriosus
PE	Physical exam
PE tubes	Pressure-equalizing tubes
PEEP	Positive end expiratory pressure
PEG tube	Percutaneous gastrostomy
PERL	Pupils equal, react to light

Abbreviation	*Meaning*
PERLA	Pupils equal, react to light and accommodation
PERRLA	Pupils equal, regular, react to light and accommodation
PET	Positron emission tomography
PG	Prostaglandin
pH	Refers to acidity or alkalinity
PHN	Public health nurse
PICC	Peripherally inserted central catheter
PID	Pelvic inflammatory disease
PIH	Pregnancy-induced hypertension
pit	Pitocin
PKU	Phenylketonuria
PM	Noon to all times before midnight
PMH	Past medical history
PMI	Point of maximum impulse
PMN	Polymorphonuclear neutrophils
PMS	Premenstrual syndrome
PND	Paroxysmal nocturnal dyspnea; postnasal drip
PO	By mouth; phone order
PO_4	Phosphate (*also* P)
POHR	Problem-oriented health record
PP	Postpartum; postprandial
PPD	Purified protein derivative; percussion and postural drainage
PPN	Peripheral parenteral nutrition
PPTL	Postpartum tubal ligation
PR	Per rectum
primip	Primipara
prn	As needed
PROM	Passive range of motion; premature rupture of membranes
PSVT	Paroxysmal supraventricular tachycardia
PT	Prothrombin time; physical therapy
pt	Patient; pint
PTA	Prior to admission
PTT	Partial thromboplastin time

(continued on the following page)

Abbreviation	*Meaning*
PVC	Premature ventricular contraction
q	Every
qd	Every day
qh	Every hour
q 2 h	Every 2 hours
qid	Four times a day
qod	Every other day
QNS	Quantity not sufficient
QRS	Waves of electrocardiogram complex
qs	Quantity sufficient or as much as needed
qt	Quart
R	Respiration
RAIU	Radioactive iodine uptake
RBC	Red blood cell; red blood cell count
RDS	Respiratory distress syndrome
Rh	Rhesus (blood factor)
RL	Ringer's lactate
RLF	Retrolental fibroplasia
RLL	Right lower lobe (of lung)
RLQ	Right lower quadrant
RMA	Right mentoanterior presentation (fetal)
RMP	Right mentoposterior presentation (fetal)
RMT	Right mentotransverse (fetal position)
RNC	Registered nurse certified
R/O	Rule out
ROA	Right occipitoanterior (fetal position)
ROM	Right otitis media; range of motion; rupture of membranes
ROP	Right occipitoposterior (fetal presentation); retinopathy of prematurity
ROS	Review of systems
ROT	Right occipitotransverse (fetal position)

Abbreviation	*Meaning*
RR	Respiratory rate
RSA	Right sacroanterior (fetal position)
RSP	Right sacroposterior (fetal position)
RScA	Right scapuloanterior (fetal position)
RScP	Right sacroposterior (fetal position)
RST	Right sacrotransverse (fetal position)
RSV	Respiratory syncytial virus
R/T	Related to
RUL	Right upper lobe (of lung)
RUQ	Right upper quadrant
Rx	Prescription; therapy; recipe; take
rx	Reaction
SA	Sinoatrial
SaO_2	Oxygen saturation
SBS	Short-bowel syndrome
SC	Subcutaneous
SFB	Single footling breech
SGA	Small for gestational age
SGOT	Serum glutamic oxaloacetic transaminase (*also* ALT)
SGPT	Serum glutamic pyruvic transaminase
SIADH	Syndrome of inappropriate antidiuretic hormone secretion
SIDS	Sudden infant death syndrome
sig	Write or label
SL	Sublingual
SLE	Systemic lupus erythematosus
SOB	Shortness of breath
sol	Solution
SOM	Serous otitis media; suppurative otitis media
sos	If necessary
sp gr	Specific gravity
sq	Subcutaneous

(continued on the following page)

Abbreviation	*Meaning*
SR	Sustained release
SROM	Spontaneous rupture of membranes
SS	Serotonin syndrome
S&S	Signs and symptoms
SSRI	Selective serotonin reuptake inhibitor
stat	Immediately
STD	Sexually transmitted disease
STH	Somatotrophic hormone
suppos	Suppository
SVE	Sterile vaginal examination
Sx	Symptoms
syr	Syrup
Sz	Seizure
t	Teaspoon (*also* tsp)
T	Temperature; triiodothyronine; thyroxine; tablespoon (*also* tbsp)
T&A	Tonsillectomy and adenoidectomy
TAH	Total abdominal hysterectomy
TB	Tuberculosis
tbsp	Tablespoon (*also* T)
TCA	Tricyclic antidepressant
TCDB	Turn, cough, and deep breathe
TCM	Transcutaneous monitoring
TD	Tardive dyskinesia
tid	Three times a day
tinct	Tincture (*also* tr)
TOF	Tetralogy of Fallot
top	Topical
TOPV	Trivalent oral polio vaccine
TORCH	Toxoplasmosis, other, rubella, cytomegalovirus, herpes
TPN	Total parenteral nutrition
TPR	Temperature, pulse, respiration
TPUR	Transperineal urethral resection
tr	Tincture (*also* tinct)
TSH	Thyroid-stimulating hormone
tsp	Teaspoon (*also* t)
TTN	Transient tachypnea of the newborn

Abbreviation	*Meaning*
tr	Tincture (*also* tinct)
TUR	Transurethral resection
Tx	Treat or treatment
U	Unit
UA	Urinalysis
UC	Uterine contraction
UGI	Upper gastrointestinal
ung	Ointment
UOQ	Upper outer quadrant
UPI	Uterine placental insufficiency
URI	Upper respiratory infection
U/S	Ultrasound
UTI	Urinary tract infection
UV	Ultraviolet
vag	Vaginal
VBAC	Vaginal birth after cesarean birth
VD	Venereal disease
VF	Ventricular fibrillation
VHD	Ventricular heart disease
VLDL	Very low density lipoprotein
VMA	Vanillylmandelic acid
VNA	Visiting Nurses' Association
VO	Verbal order
vol	Volume
VS	Vital signs
VSD	Ventricular septal defect
VT	Ventricular tachycardia
WBC	White blood cell; white blood cell count
WIC	Supplemental food program for women, infants, and children
wk	Week
WNL	Within normal limits
wt	Weight
y/o	Years old
yr	Year

NANDA Nursing Diagnoses

Diagnoses* represent all nursing diagnoses developed by NANDA (North American Nursing Diagnosis Association) (2003–2004).† Definitions of diagnoses have in some instances been shortened and others have been omitted when the diagnostic name is easily associated with its meaning.

For more information on NANDA diagnoses, call 1-800-847-9002 or visit their Website at *www.nanda.org.*

ACTIVITY/REST

Activity Intolerance—insufficient physiologic or psychologic energy to endure or complete required or desired daily activities.

Activity Intolerance, risk for

Disuse Syndrome, risk for—at risk for deterioration of body systems as the result of prescribed or unavoidable musculoskeletal inactivity.

Diversional Activity Deficit

Fatigue

Mobility, Impaired Bed—limitation of independent movement from one bed position to another.

Mobility, Impaired Physical—limitation in independent, purposeful physical movement of the body or of one or more extremities.

---

*The diagnostic divisions used here were developed by Doenges, M, and Moorhouse, M: as presented in Venes, D, and Thomas, CL (eds): Taber's Cyclopedic Medical Dictionary. FA Davis, Philadelphia, 2001, pp. 2643–2645, with permission.

† Nursing diagnosis developed by and used with permission of NANDA. Philadelphia, 2003–2004.

Mobility, Impaired Wheelchair—limitation of independent operation of wheelchair within environment.

Sleep Deprivation

Sleep Pattern, Disturbed—time-limited disruption of sleep (natural, periodic suspension of consciousness) amount and quality

Sleep, Readiness for Enhanced—pattern of natural, periodic suspension of consciousness that provides adequate rest, sustains a desired lifestyle, and can be strengthened.

Transfer Ability, Impaired—limitation of independent movement between two nearby surfaces.

Walking, Impaired—limitation of independent movement within the environment on foot.

CIRCULATION

Autonomic Dysreflexia—life-threatening, uninhibited sympathetic response of the nervous system to a noxious stimulus after spinal cord injury at T7 or above.

Autonomic Dysreflexia, risk for

Cardiac Output, Decreased—inadequate blood is pumped by the heart to meet metabolic demands of the body.

Gastrointestinal, Peripheral—decrease in nutrition and oxygenation at the cellular level that is due to deficit in capillary blood supply.

Intracranial Adaptive Capacity, Decreased—intracranial fluid dynamic mechanisms that normally compensate for increases in intracranial volumes are compromised, resulting in repeated disproportionate increases in intracranial pressure (ICP).

Tissue Perfusion, Altered (specify): Renal, Cerebral, Cardiopulmonary, Gastrointestinal, Peripheral

EGO INTEGRITY

Adjustment, Impaired—inability to modify lifestyle/behavior in a manner consistent with a change in health status.

Anxiety—vague, uneasy feeling, the source of which is often nonspecific or unknown to the individual.

Anxiety, Death—apprehension related to death.

Body Image, Disturbed—disruption in the way one perceives one's physical appearance.

Coping, Defensive—projection of positive self-evaluation based on a self-protective pattern that defends against underlying perceived threats to positive self-regard.

Coping, Ineffective—inability to form a valid appraisal of the stressors, inadequate choices of practiced responses, and/or inability to use available resources.

Coping, Readiness for Enhanced—pattern of cognitive and behavioral efforts to manage demands that is sufficient for well-being and can be strengthened.

Decisional Conflict—uncertainty about course of action to be taken when choice among competing actions involves risk, loss, or challenge to personal life values.

Denial, ineffective—conscious or unconscious attempt to disavow knowledge or meaning of an event to reduce anxiety/fear to the detriment of health.

Energy Field Disturbance—disruption of the flow of energy surrounding a person's being that results in a disharmony of the body, mind, and/or spirit.

Fear

Grieving, Anticipatory—response to loss before it occurs.

Grieving, Dysfunctional—extended or exaggerated response to loss.

Hopelessness—person sees limited or no alternatives and is unable to mobilize energy on own behalf.

Personal Identity Disturbance—inability to distinguish between self and nonself.

Post-Trauma Syndrome—sustained, maladaptive response to an overwhelming traumatic event.

Post-Trauma Syndrome, risk for

Powerlessness—perceived lack of control over a current situation and/or ability to significantly affect an outcome.

Powerlessness, risk for

Protection, Ineffective—decrease in the ability to guard self from internal or external threats such as illness or injury.

Rape-Trauma Syndrome—sustained maladaptive

response to a forced, violent sexual penetration against the victim's will and consent.

Rape-Trauma Syndrome; Compound Reaction—reactivation of symptoms of rape-trauma syndrome.

Rape-Trauma Syndrome; Silent Reaction—no verbalization of occurrence of rape; sudden onset of phobic reactions with marked changes in sexual behavior.

Relocation Stress Syndrome—physiologic and/or psychologic disturbances as a result of transfer from one environment to another.

Relocation Stress Syndrome, risk for

Self-Esteem, Chronic Low—long-standing negative self-evaluation.

Self-Esteem, Situational Low—negative self-evaluation in response to loss or change in a person who previously had positive self-evaluation.

Self-Esteem, Situational Low, risk for

Sorrow, Chronic—cyclical, recurring, and potentially progressive pattern of pervasive sadness experienced (by a parent, caregiver, individual with chronic illness or disability) in response to continual loss throughout the trajectory of an illness or disability.

Spiritual Distress—impaired ability to experience and integrate meaning and purpose in life through a person's connectedness with self, others, art, music, literature, nature, or a power greater than oneself.

Spiritual Distress, risk for

Spiritual Well-Being, Readiness for Enhanced—ability to experience and integrate meaning and purpose in life through connectedness with self, other, art, music, literature, nature, or a power greater than oneself.

ELIMINATION

Bowel Incontinence—involuntary passage of stool.

Constipation—decrease in frequency and/or passage of hard, dry stools.

Constipation, Perceived—self-diagnosis of constipation and abuse of laxative, enemas, and suppositories.

Constipation, risk for

Diarrhea—frequent passage of loose, fluid, unformed stools.

Urinary Elimination, Impaired—disturbance in urine elimination.

Urinary Elimination, Readiness for Enhanced—a pattern of urinary functions that is sufficient for meeting eliminatory needs and can be strengthened.

Urinary Incontinence, Functional—inability of usually continent person to reach toilet in time to avoid unintentional loss of urine.

Urinary Incontinence, Reflex—involuntary loss of urine occurring at somewhat predictable intervals when a specific bladder volume is reached.

Urinary Incontinence, Stress—loss of less than 50 mL urine occurring with increased abdominal pressure.

Urinary Incontinence, Total—continuous and unpredictable loss of urine.

Urinary Incontinence, Urge—involuntary passage of urine occurring soon after a strong sense of urgency to void.

Urinary Incontinence, Urge, risk for

Urinary Retention—incomplete emptying of the bladder.

FOOD/FLUID

Breast-feeding, Effective—mother-infant dyad/family exhibits adequate proficiency and satisfaction with breast-feeding process.

Breast-feeding, Ineffective—mother or child experiences dissatisfaction or difficulty with breast-feeding process.

Breast-feeding, Interrupted—break in continuity of breast-feeding process as a result of inability or inadvisability to put baby to breast.

Dentition, Impaired—disruption in tooth development/eruption patterns or structural integrity of individual teeth.

Failure to Thrive, Adult—progressive functional deterioration of a physical and cognitive nature; ability to live with multisystem diseases, cope with ensuing problems, and manage his or her care are remarkably diminished.

Fluid Balance, Readiness for Enhanced—pattern of equilibrium between fluid volume and chemical composition of body fluids that is sufficient for meeting physical needs and can be strengthened.

Fluid Volume Deficit, risk for

Fluid Volume Excess—increased isotonic fluid retention

Infant Feeding Pattern, Ineffective—infant demonstrates impaired ability to suck or coordinate suck-swallow response.

Nutrition, Imbalanced, More than Body Requirements

Nutrition, Imbalanced, Risk for More than Body Requirements

Nutrition, Readiness for Enhanced—pattern of nutrient intake that is sufficient for meeting metabolic needs and can be strengthened.

Oral Mucous Membrane, Impaired

Swallowing, Impaired

HYGIENE

Self-Care Deficit (specify): Feeding, Bathing/Hygiene, Dressing/Grooming, Toileting—inability to perform any of aforementioned activities.

NEUROSENSORY

Confusion, Acute—abrupt onset

Confusion, Chronic—irreversible, long-standing, and/or progressive

Infant Behavior, Disorganized—disintegrated physiological and neurobehavioral responses to the environment.

Infant Behavior, Disorganized, risk for

Infant Behavior, Readiness for Enhanced Organized—pattern of modulation of the physiologic and behavioral systems of functioning (i.e., autonomic, motor, state-organizational, self-regulatory, and attentional-interactional systems) in an infant that is satisfactory but than can be improved resulting in higher levels of integration in response to environmental stimuli.

Memory, Impaired

Peripheral Neurovascular Dysfunction, Risk For—at risk for experiencing disruption in circulation, sensation, or motion of an extremity.

Sensory/Perception, Disturbed—change in amount or patterning of incoming stimuli accompanied by diminished, exaggerated, distorted, or impaired response to such stimuli.

Thought Processes, Disturbed—disruption in cognitive operations.

Unilateral Neglect—lack of awareness and attention to one side of body.

PAIN/COMFORT

Nausea

Pain, Acute

Pain, Chronic—constant or recurring pain without an anticipated or predictable end and a duration of greater than 6 mos.

RESPIRATION

Airway Clearance, Ineffective—inability to clear secretions or obstructions from respiratory tract to maintain airway patency.

Aspiration, risk for—at risk for entry of gastric secretions, oropharyngeal secretions, solids, or fluids into tracheobronchial passages.

Breathing Pattern, Ineffective—inhalation and/or exhalation pattern does not provide adequate ventilation.

Gas Exchange, Impaired—excess or deficit in oxygenation and/or carbon dioxide elimination at the alveolar-capillary membrane.

Ventilation, Impaired Spontaneous—decreased energy reserves result in an individual's inability to maintain breathing adequate to support life.

Ventilatory Weaning Response, Dysfunctional (DVWR)—inability to adjust to lowered levels of mechanical ventilator support.

SAFETY

Body Temperature, Risk for Imbalance—at risk for failure to maintain body temperature within normal range.

Environmental Interpretation Syndrome, Impaired—consistent lack of orientation to person, place, time, or circumstances over more than 3 to 6 months necessitating a protective environment.

Falls, risk for—increased susceptibility to falling.

Health Maintenance, Ineffective—inability to identify, manage, and/or seek help to maintain health.

Home Maintenance, Impaired—inability to independently maintain a safe, growth-promoting, immediate environment.

Hyperthermia—body temperature elevated above normal range.

Hypothermia—body temperature reduced below normal range.

Infection, risk for—at increased risk for being infected by pathogenic organisms.

Injury, risk for—at risk for injury as a result of environmental conditions interacting with individual's adaptive and defensive resources.

Perioperative Positioning Injury, risk for—at risk for injury as a result of the environmental conditions found in the perioperative setting.

Poisoning, risk for

Protection, Ineffective—decrease in ability to guard self from internal or external threats, such as illness or injury (as may occur with age extremes or alcohol abuse).

Self-Mutilation—deliberate, self-injurious behavior causing tissue damage with the intent of causing nonfatal injury to attain relief of tension.

Self-Mutilation, risk for

Skin Integrity, Impaired

Skin Integrity, Impaired, risk for

Sudden Infant Death Syndrome, risk for—presence of risk factors for sudden death of an infant under 1 yr of age.

Suffocation, risk for

Suicide, risk for

Surgical Recovery, Delayed

Thermoregulation, Ineffective—temperature fluctuates between hypothermia and hyperthermia.

Tissue Integrity, Impaired—damage to mucous membrane or corneal, integumentary, or subcutaneous tissues.

Trauma, risk for—accentuated risk of accidental tissue injury; for example, wound, burn, fracture.

Violence, risk for, Directed at Self

Violence, risk for, Directed at Others

Wandering—meandering, aimless, or repetitive locomotion that exposes the individual to harm; frequently incongruent with boundaries, limits, or obstacles.

SEXUALITY

Sexual Dysfunction—change in sexual function that is viewed as unsatisfying.

Sexuality Patterns, Ineffective—expressions of concern regarding own sexuality.

SOCIAL INTERACTION

Attachment, risk for Impaired Parent/Infant/Child—disruption of the interactive process between parent/significant other, child, and infant that fosters the development of a protective and nurturing reciprocal relationship.

Caregiver Role Strain—difficulty in performing family caregiver role.

Caregiver Role Strain, risk for

Communication, Impaired, Verbal

Communication, Readiness for Enhanced—pattern of exchanging information and ideas with another that is sufficient for meeting one's needs and life's goals.

Community Coping, Ineffective—pattern of community activities (for adaptation and problem solving) that is unsatisfactory for meeting the demands or needs of the community.

Community Coping, Readiness for Enhanced—pattern of community activities for adaptation and problem solving that is satisfactory for meeting the demands or needs of the community but can be improved for management of current and future problems/stressors.

Family Coping, Compromised—significant other who is usually supportive is providing insufficient support to the patient.

Family Coping, Disabled—significant other disables own and patient's capacities to effectively address tasks essential to either's adaptation to the health challenge.

Family Coping, Readiness for Enhanced—pattern of family functioning that is sufficient to support the well-being of family members and can be strengthened.

Family Process, Dysfunctional; Alcoholism—psychosocial, spiritual, and physiologic functions of the family are chronically disorganized, leading to conflict, denial of problems, resistance to change, ineffective problem solving, and a series of self-perpetuating crises.

Family Processes, Interrupted—change in family relationships and/or functioning.

Loneliness, risk for—at risk for experiencing vague dysphoria.

Parent-Infant Attachment, Insecure, risk for—risk for disruption of the interactive process between parent (or significant other) and infant that fosters the development of a protective and nurturing reciprocal environment.

Parental Role Conflict—parent experiences role confusion and conflict in response to crisis.

Parenting, Enhanced Readiness for—pattern of providing an environment for children or other dependent person(s) that is sufficient to nurture growth and development and can be strengthened.

Parenting, Impaired—inability of primary caretaker to create, maintain, or regain an environment that promotes the optimum growth and development of the child.

Parenting, Risk for Impaired—risk for inability of the primary caretaker to create, maintain, or regain an environment that promotes the optimum growth and development of the child.

Relocation Stress Syndrome—physiologic and/or psychosocial disturbances as result of transfer from one environment to another.

Relocation Stress Syndrome, risk for

Role Performance, Ineffective—patterns of behavior and self-expression that do not match the environmental context, norms, and expectations.

Social Interaction, Impaired—insufficient or excessive quantity or ineffective quality of social exchange.

Social Isolation—aloneness perceived as imposed by another and as a negative state.

TEACHING/LEARNING

Development, Risk for Delayed—at risk for delay of 25% or more in one or more of the areas of social or self-regulatory behavior, or in cognitive, language, gross or fine motor skills.

Growth, Risk for Disproportionate—at risk for growth above the 97th percentile or below the 3rd percentile for age, crossing two percentile channels.

Growth and Development, Delayed—deviation from norms for age group.

Health-Seeking Behaviors—active seeking (by person in stable health) of ways to alter personal health habits and/or the environment in order to move toward a higher level of health.

Knowledge, Readiness for Enhanced (specify)—presence of acquisition of cognitive information related to a specific topic is sufficient for meeting health-related goals and can be strengthened.

Knowledge Deficit (specify)—lack of information necessary for patient/significant others related to a specific topic.

Noncompliance (specify)—behavior of person and/or caregiver that fails to coincide with health-promoting or therapeutic plan agreed on by the person (and/or family and/or community) and health-care professional.

Therapeutic Regimen: Community, Ineffective Management—pattern of regulating and integrating into community processes programs for treatment of illness and the sequelae of illness that are unsatisfactory for meeting specific health-related goals.

Therapeutic Regimen: Families, Ineffective Management—pattern of regulating and integrating into family processes a program for treatment of illness and the sequelae of illness that are unsatisfactory for meeting specific health goals.

Therapeutic Regimen, Effective Management—pattern of regulating and integrating into daily living a program for treatment of illness and its sequelae that is satisfactory for meeting specific health goals.

Therapeutic Regimen, Ineffective Management—see definition above.

Therapeutic Regimen Management, Readiness for Enhanced—pattern of regulating and integrating into daily living a program(s) for treatment of illness and its sequelae that is sufficient for meeting health-related goals and can be strengthened.

Documentation and Reporting

IN-HOSPITAL ASSESSMENT

Each patient should have a comprehensive assessment on admission to the hospital. After this, patients are generally assessed at the beginning of each shift and thereafter as ordered or indicated. **Even though doctor's orders and hospital policies must be followed regarding assessment, the nurse must also be aware that many times a patient's condition necessitates more frequent assessment than required by order or policy.** The following are guidelines for the minimal elements of assessment and documentation pertinent to the patient with a physical illness. Individual patients may need more thorough assessment.

1. Assess level of consciousness.
2. Assess mood and comfort.
3. Assess vital signs.
4. Assess tissue perfusion.
5. Validate movement of all extremities.
6. If the patient has altered consciousness or is unable to turn and move freely, inspect the *entire* body for pressure areas.
7. If patient is attending his or her own personal needs, question regarding urinary and bowel elimination (constipation is a frequent complication of hospitalization). If patient cannot supply this information, the record must be checked to ensure that elimination is adequate.
8. Question regarding appetite and acceptability of food provided.
9. Auscultate heart, lungs, and bowel sounds.

10. Inspect surgical wounds (or wound dressing if dressing is not to be removed).
11. Inspect any previously documented injuries or lesions.
12. Inspect IV site. If IV site is covered with a dressing that makes visualization of the site impossible, the dressing should be removed and the site assessed for leakage, swelling, or redness.
13. Check labels on any fluids being administered to be sure the proper fluids are being infused. Check actual infusion rate.
14. Inspect all drains, including catheters, nasogastric (NG) tubes, and wound drains to validate patency. Note amount, color, and consistency of drainage.
15. Assess function of and readings from any monitors in use.
16. Inspect all equipment to be sure that it is functioning properly. Check settings on all equipment such as IV pumps and suction equipment to be sure settings match physician's orders.
17. If urinary "intake and output" (I&O) has been ordered or is indicated based on patient condition, use patient's record to assess status of I&O for past 24 hours.
18. Make further assessments based on doctor's orders and patient's condition (such as neurologic checks on a patient with a head injury or an SaO_2 measurement on a patient with impaired gas exchange).

In addition:

- **Be sure to leave call bell within patient's reach before leaving bedside.**
- **Document findings in patient's record.**
- **Alert physician to abnormal or unexpected findings.**

WRITTEN DOCUMENTATION

Written documentation, "nurse's notes," or "charting" provides legal documentation and communication of information to other health care providers.

DOCUMENTATION GUIDELINES

DO

1. Be factual.
2. Chart nursing actions (including teaching) and outcomes.
3. Chart everything that is clinically significant.
4. Note the site of injections to provide for patient safety (adequate rotation of sites).
5. At the end of every shift, check all charting for legibility and accuracy.
6. Correct errors by drawing one line through the incorrect data, then initialing.
7. If you must chart out of sequence, write the current date followed by "addition to nurse's notes of (date)," followed by the omitted data.

DO NOT

1. Do not chart opinions.
2. Do not chart an action before it occurs (including medication administration).
3. Do not erase or destroy a record.
4. Do not leave blank spaces.
5. Do not chart medications given by someone else. It is not possible to be certain about the identity or amount of medication administered by another.

CHARTING FORMATS

Documentation or charting format is determined by agency policy and personal preference, if policy allows. Common formats used for charting are SOAP, DAR, narrative, and exception.

SOAP Charting

SOAP charting is based on a problem or nursing diagnosis list. Each diagnosis has its own number that never changes. When a SOAP entry is made, it is preceded by the problem or diagnosis number and/or name to which it refers. Following diagnosis identification, information related to the diagnosis is charted in the following manner:

S (subjective). Anything the patient says; also may include statements made by family members.

O (objective). Observed data; avoid stating opinions: "Just the facts."

A (analysis) (also known as "assessment"). This is the recorder's chance to state what he or she "thinks" about what he or she has seen and heard. This is usually done in the form of a diagnosis (nurses use nursing diagnoses).

P (plan). Includes nursing actions implemented or to be implemented. Therapy, teaching, and plans for further assessment are included regarding the diagnosis in A (analysis). The plan states *who* will implement and *when* implementation is to take place. (It is important to remember that the reason many things don't go "according to plan" is that there never was a *specific* plan.)

The following three categories are sometimes added to the SOAP entry:

I (intervention). Documents implementation if not covered in Plan.

E (evaluation). Documents the effects of the Plan (and intervention if category is used) on the Analysis (diagnosis). It may be entered at a different time from the initial SOAP entry.

R (revisions). Nursing diagnoses, interventions, goals, or outcome dates may be revised in this section.

NOTE: Some institutions have modified SOAP charting significantly. Policies and documentation format acceptable to the institution should be assessed before charting is begun.

DAR Charting

DAR is the initial letter abbreviation for "data, action, response." It is also known as FOCUS charting. DAR charting may be begun in a manner similar to SOAP charting with identification of a nursing diagnosis or an identification of a *subject* (focus) to be addressed (such as "fever" or "transfer"). Information related to the identified "focus" is recorded in the following manner:

D (data). Any significant observation can be included. Unlike documentation in SOAP format, subjective data are not separated from objective data.

A (action). Documents actual and planned interventions.

R (response). Documents the patient's response to Action.

Narrative Charting

Narrative (also known as *source-oriented*) charting is the oldest and most traditional form of charting. It is a less rigid form of charting that allows the nurse to document observations, actions, and reactions without the use of a prescribed format. This form of charting makes a chronologic record of the nurse's observations and events that take place during the course of care.

Exception Charting

Exception charting means it is assumed that a customary activity was performed unless the nurse charts otherwise. This type of charting may be used in conjunction with a checklist for documenting certain activities. A checklist is also frequently used for the physical assessment. The "exceptions" may be charted using SOAP or another system of documentation.

NURSING CHANGE-OF-SHIFT REPORT

Report the following	***Example***
Room number, name, age, diagnosis, and physician	"In room 414 is Mr. Jones, a 58-year-old with rheumatoid arthritis. He is a patient of Dr. Smith."
Abnormalities/changes inassessment findings	"Robert developed cyanosis this AM." or "Martha's ankle edema has resolved."
Diagnostic procedures and results	"Robert's oxygen saturation is 92% on 2 L of oxygen. Chest x-ray report is not back yet."
Variations from usual routine	"Robert was not out of bed this AM, but he was up for lunch and tolerated it well."
Activities not completed on your shift	"The walker is in Martha's room, but Physical Therapy has not been in to instruct her in its use."
Status of invasive treatments	"Robert's IV of D5 1/2 NS is infusing in the right fore-arm at 75 mL/h with 700 mL remaining."
Additions or changes to the plan of care (include evaluation of outcomes and status of problems)	"Robert's airway clearance problem has recurred, requiring aggressive pulmonary toilet q 2 h."

Source: Adapted from Doenges, ME, and Moorhouse, MF: Application of Nursing Process and Nursing Diagnosis: An Interactive Text for Diagnostic Reasoning, ed 4. FA Davis, Philadelphia, 2003, pp. 113, with permission.

GENERAL REPORTING GUIDELINES

- **Be brief.**
- **Be organized.**
- **Provide pertinent data.**
- **Report by exception.** Report only those occurrences that are out of the ordinary.

SURGICAL TERMS DEFINED

ablation—removal of a part, pathway, or function by surgery, chemical destruction, electrocautery, or radiofrequency.

anastomosis—connection of two tubular structures.

anesthesia, general—complete loss of consciousness and sensation in the entire body (given by inhalation or IV).

anesthesia, intrathecal—anesthesia injected within the spinal canal.

anesthesia, local—anesthesia affecting a local area only.

anesthesia, regional—nerve or field blocking, causing insensibility over a particular area.

anesthesia, spinal—anesthesia produced by injection of anesthetic into the subarachnoid space of the spinal cord.

anesthetic—agent that produces anesthesia (partial or complete loss of sensation).

anesthesiologist—physician who administers anesthetics.

anesthetist—physician or nurse who administers anesthetics.

aneurysmectomy—excision of a widened area of the aortic wall.

angioplasty—altering the structure of a vessel.

antrostomy (antral window)—formation of an opening in an antrum (any nearly closed cavity or chamber) for drainage; may be performed on sinuses.

A and/or P repair (anterior and/or posterior colporrhaphy)—repair and reinforcement of structures that support the bladder and urethra (anterior) and/or the distal rectum (posterior).

---

*References: Goldman, MA: Pocket Guide to the Operating Room, ed. 2. FA Davis, Philadelphia, 1996; and Venes, D, and Thomas, CL (eds): Taber's Cyclopedic Medical Dictionary, ed 19, FA Davis, Philadelphia, 2001.

appendectomy—removal of the appendix.
arthrodesis—surgical immobilization of a joint.
arthroplasty—reshaping or reconstructing a diseased joint.
arthroscopy—joint visualization by means of an arthroscope.
arthrotomy—cutting into a joint.
augmentation—adding to or increasing.
autologous—indicates something that has its origin within an individual's body.
autotransfusion—returning the patient's own blood to the circulation.
banding—(pulmonary artery) constriction of the pulmonary artery to decrease blood flow to the lungs.
Billroth I—excision of the pylorus of the stomach with anastomosis of the upper portion of the stomach to the duodenum.
Billroth II—subtotal excision of the stomach with closure of the proximal end of the duodenum and side-to-side anastomosis of the jejunum to the stomach.
biopsy—excision of a small piece of tissue for microscopic examination.
Blalock-Taussig—end-to-end anastomosis between the proximal ends of the subclavian and pulmonary arteries.
blepharoplasty—plastic surgery upon the eyelid.
bypass—surgical creation of an alternate route to bypass an obstruction or disease area.
CABG (coronary artery bypass graft) (*see coronary artery bypass*)
cesarean section—delivery of a fetus through an abdominal incision.
cholecystectomy—removal of the gallbladder.
circulating nurse—nurse who works outside the sterile field of the operating room.
circumcision—surgical removal of the end of the prepuce of the penis.
colectomy—excision of part or all of the colon.
colostomy—opening of the colon through the abdominal wall to its outside surface.
colpotomy—incision into the wall of the vagina.
commissurotomy—surgical incision of a commissure (*commissure* is the connection of a dividing space of

two structures such as the lips, heart chambers, or brain areas). Examples of surgery are incision of adhesions that cause the leaves of the mitral valve to stick together or incision of the anterior commissure of the brain.

conization—excision of a cone of tissue (frequently performed on a diseased cervix).

cordotomy—cutting of the spinal cord lateral pathways to relieve pain.

coronary artery bypass—establishment of a shunt to allow blood to travel from the aorta to a branch of the coronary artery at a point past an obstruction.

craniotomy—incision through the cranium (skull).

cryosurgery—freezing of diseased tissue.

culdoscopy—endoscopic examination of the female pelvic cavity through the posterior vaginal wall.

curettage—scraping of a cavity or removal of tissue.

cutaneous ureterostomy—establishment of a ureteral stoma on the abdominal wall.

cystectomy—removal of a cyst, or removal of the cystic duct and the gallbladder or just the cystic duct, or removal of all or part of the urinary bladder.

cystocele repair—repair of a bladder hernia that protrudes into the vagina.

cystolithotomy—excision of a stone from the bladder.

cystoscopy—examination of the bladder with the cystoscope.

dilation—expansion of an organ, vessel, or orifice.

D&C (dilation and curettage)—enlargement of the cervical canal and scraping of endocervical or endometrial tissue.

dermabrasion—sanding or removal of skin to remove irregularities.

Duhamel—formation of a common lumen (inner space) between the normal colon and rectum by crushing the adjacent bowel walls with clamps.

-ectomy—word element that means "removal."

enucleation—removal of an eyeball.

excavation—formation of a cavity.

excision—cutting away or taking out.

fistula—an abnormal passage between two surfaces or cavities or between a surface and a cavity.

fixation—immobilization; fastening in a fixed position.
fulguration—destruction of tissue by means of electric sparks.
fundoplication—reducing the size of the fundal opening of the stomach and suturing the previously removed end of the esophagus to it.
fusion—joining together.
gastrectomy—removal of all or part of the stomach.
gastrojejunostomy—anastomosis between the stomach and jejunum.
gastrostomy—creation of an opening into stomach.
graft—moving tissue from a healthy site to an injured site.
herniorrhaphy—repair of hernia.
hypospadias repair—repair of an opening on the undersurface of the penis or the urethral opening into the vagina.
hysterectomy, total—removal of the entire uterus.
ileal conduit—attachment of one or both ureters to a loop of ileum with establishment of drainage through the abdominal wall.
implant—to transfer a part or to graft tissue.
labyrinthectomy—excision of the labyrinth of the ear.
laminectomy—excision of the vertebral posterior arch.
laparotomy—surgical opening of the abdomen.
laser—surgical instrument that converts light to intense heat and power.
ligation—tying or binding procedure.
lipectomy—removal of fatty tissue.
liposuction—removal of fatty tissue by suction.
lithotomy—incision for removal of a calculus (stone).
lithotripsy—crushing of a calculus (stone).
lobectomy—removal of a lobe of an organ or gland.
lobotomy—incision of a lobe of an organ or gland.
lumpectomy—removal of a tumor (usually from the breast) (tylectomy).
McDonald procedure—placement of a purse-string-type suture around the cervix to correct cervical incompetency.
malignant hyperpyrexia—high fever caused by the use of muscle relaxants or general inhalation anesthesia (results from an inherited trait).
mammoplasty—reconstruction of breast tissue.

Marshall-Marchetti-Krantz procedure—correction of urinary stress incontinence by suspending the bladder neck and proximal urethra to the symphysis pubis.

marsupialization—raising the borders of an evacuated tumor sac or cyst to the edges of the incision and stitching them there to form a pouch that gradually closes.

mastectomy—removal of a breast.

meniscectomy—removal of meniscus cartilage of the knee.

myectomy—excision of muscle.

myomectomy—removal of fibroid tumors from the uterus.

myotomy—division or dissection of muscle.

myringotomy with pressure-equalizing (PE) tubes—incision into tympanic membrane (eardrum) and placement of pressure-equalizing tubes in the membrane.

nailing—repair of bone fractures by use of a nail.

nephrectomy—removal of a kidney.

Nissen fundoplication—antireflux procedure in which the fundus of the stomach is wrapped around the distal esophagus.

oophorectomy—removal of an ovary.

orchiectomy—removal of a testicle.

orchiopexy—suturing of an undescended testicle in the scrotum.

-ostomy—word element that means "formation of an opening."

-otomy—word element that means "cutting."

otoplasty—correction of defects or deformities of the ear.

PARS—postanesthesia recovery score.

-plasty—word element that means "molding" or surgically forming.

pneumonectomy—removal of a lung.

polypectomy—removal of a polyp (polyps may be found in the nose, uterus, larynx, or colon).

Potts-Smith procedure—side-to-side anastomosis between the aorta and the left pulmonary artery.

prostatectomy—removal of the prostate gland.

prosthesis—an artificial organ or part.

pyeloplasty—incision made in the pylorus to enlarge the outlet of the stomach.

radial keratotomy—incision of the cornea to correct nearsightedness.

radical—surgery that attempts to remove all diseased tissue.
radical neck dissection—removal of lymph-node–bearing tissue as well as adjacent muscles and vessels of the neck.
Ramstedt-Fredet procedure—division of the pyloric muscle to correct pyloric stenosis.
Rashkind procedure—balloon atrial septostomy.
reduction—restoration to normal position.
resection—partial removal of a structure.
resection & pull through—diseased bowel is removed, and healthy bowel is anastomosed to the anus.
rhinoplasty—reshaping of the nose.
rhizotomy—cutting of a spinal nerve root for the relief of pain or spasticity.
rhytidectomy (facelift)—removal of loose skin from face and upper neck.
salpingo-oophorectomy—excision of a fallopian tube and ovary.
scleral buckling—reattachment of the retina.
scrub nurse—nurse who works inside the sterile field of the operating room.
section—cutting.
septoplasty—plastic surgery of the nasal septum.
Shirodkar's procedure—placement of tape around the cervical os to correct cervical incompetency.
shunt—procedure to divert flow from one route to another.
Soave procedure—removal of rectal mucosa and the formation of a sleeve through which normal colon is passed for anastomosis to the anus.
spinal fusion—immobilization of the spine by fusion (uniting) of two or more vertebrae.
spinal instrumentation—placement of metal rods to support the spine (used to treat abnormal spine curvature).
squint repair—correction of strabismus (malalignment of eyes, or "cross eye").
stenosis—narrowing of a passage.
submucous resection of nasal septum (SMR)—removal of a portion of the nasal septum.
sympathectomy—excision of a portion of the sympathetic nervous system.
T&A—removal of tonsils and adenoids.

thoracotomy—incision of the chest wall.
transurethral resection (TUR), (TURP)—removal of the prostate through the urethra with use of a scope.
trephination—cutting of a piece of bone with a cylindrical saw.
tylectomy—local removal of a lesion (lumpectomy).
tympanoplasty—reconstruction of the tympanic membrane and middle ear structure.
UPJ repair or ureteropelvioplasty—repair of the junction of the ureter and pelvis of the kidney.
ureterolithotomy—removal of a stone from the ureter.
ureteroneocystostomy—formation of a new passage between a ureter and the bladder.
vagotomy—cutting of the vagus nerve.
vasectomy—excision of a section of the vas deferens.
vitrectomy—removal of the contents of the vitreous chamber of the eye.
Waterson shunt—anastomosis of the ascending aorta and the right pulmonary artery.
xenograft—graft from one species to another.

AGENCY PHONE NUMBERS

ABUSE (child): 800-4-A-CHILD
AIDS: 800-342-AIDS
ALCOHOL: 800-ALCOHOL
ALZHEIMER'S: 800-272-3900
BLIND: 800-424-8666
CANCER: 800-4-CANCER
CLEFT PALATE FOUNDATION: 800-24-CLEFT
COCAINE: 800-662-HELP
COLITIS, CROHN'S, ILEITIS FOUNDATION: 212-679-1570
CYSTIC FIBROSIS: 800-FIGHT-CF
DEPRESSION: 800-969-NMHA
DIABETES, JUVENILE: 800-223-1138
DOWN'S SYNDROME: 800-221-4602
DRUG ABUSE (confidential referral): 800-662-HELP
HEART: 800-242-8721
HEMOPHILIA: 212-219-8180
HERPES: 800-227-8922

HOSPITAL EMERGENCY TELEPHONE (phone system for the elderly and handicapped): 800-451-0525

KIDNEY: 800-638-8299

LUPUS: 800-558-0121

MEDIC ALERT (provides ID tags and maintains records): 800-344-3226

MENTAL HEALTH ASSOCIATION: 800-969-NMHA

MENTAL HEALTH INSTITUTE: 800-421-4211

MENTALLY ILL (NATIONAL ALLIANCE): 800-950-NAMI

ORGAN DONATION: 800-528-2971

PARENTS ANONYMOUS (for abusive parents): 909-621-6184

PARKINSON'S DISEASE: 800-327-4545

POISON CONTROL CENTERS: The number of your state's poison control center should be recorded here: 800-___________________*

REHABILITATION: 800-34-NARIC

RESPIRATORY (asthma and lung diseases): 800-222-LUNG

SAFETY (products): 800-638-CPSC

SEXUALLY TRANSMITTED DISEASES: 800-227-8922

SICKLE CELL ANEMIA: 800-421-8453

SPINA BIFIDA: 800-621-3141

SUDDEN INFANT DEATH SYNDROME: 800-221-SIDS

SUICIDE PREVENTION: 800-SUICIDE

U.S. CONSUMER PRODUCT SAFETY COMMISSION: 800-638-CPSC

VENEREAL DISEASES: 800-227-8922

---

*Additional agency numbers, including *Poison Control Center* numbers, can be found in the appendix of Taber's Cyclopedic Medical Dictionary. The number of your state's poison control center should be recorded on this page.

Calculation and Medication Administration

MEASUREMENT ABBREVIATIONS

Symbol	*Unit*	*Symbol*	*Unit*
c	cup	M*	meter
cc	cubic centimeter	µg	microgram
cm	centimeter	mg	milligram
dL	deciliter	mL	milliliter (*preferred to* cc)
ft	foot	mm	millimeter
g (*also* gm)	gram	ng	nanogram
gr	grain	oz	ounce
gtt	drop	pt	pint
in	inch	qt	quart
kg	kilogram	T (*also* tbsp)	tablespoon
L	liter	t (*also* tsp)	teaspoon
lb	pound	yd	yard
m*	minim		

*In clinical practice, both *minim* and *meter* may be abbreviated by a capital or lowercase *m.*

ROMAN NUMERALS

Arabic	*Roman*	*Arabic*	*Roman*	*Arabic*	*Roman*
1	I	8	VIII	16	XVI
2	II	9	IX	20	XX
3	III	10	X	40	XL
4	IV	11	XI	50	L
5	V	12	XII	80	LXXX
6	VI	14	XIV	90	XC
7	VII	15	XV	100	C

APPROXIMATE LIQUID EQUIVALENTS

1 m = 1 gtt = 0.07 mL

1 gtt = 1 m = 0.07 mL

1 mL = 1 cc = 15 m = 15 gtt = 1 g

1 dL = 100 mL = 0.1 L

4 mL = 1 dr = 60 gr

1 L = 1000 mL = 2 pt = 1 qt = 1 kg

1 t = 5 mL

1 T = 15 mL = 3 t = 1/2 oz

1 oz = 30 mL = 8 dr = 6 t = 2 T

1 c = 240 mL = 8 oz = 1/2 pt

1 pt = 480 mL = 16 oz = 1/2 qt

1 qt = 950 mL = 32 oz = 2 pt = 1 L

NOTE: For purposes of home use, a teaspoon is equal to a dram (dr) or 4 milliliters (4 mL) or 60 grains (gr).

APPROXIMATE WEIGHT EQUIVALENTS

1 mcg = 0.001 mg

1 mg = 1000 mcg (μg) = 0.001 g = 0.017 gr

1 gr = 60 mg = 0.06 g

1 g = 1000 mg = 15 gr

1 ng = one billionth (10^{-9}) of 1 g

1 dr = 60 gr

1 oz = 31 g = 0.06 lb = 0.03 kg

1 lb = 16 oz = 454 g = 0.45 kg

1 kg = 1000 g = 2.2 lb = 34 oz

APPROXIMATE LENGTH EQUIVALENTS

1 mm = 0.1 cm = 0.04 in

1 cm = 10 mm = 0.4 in

1 in = 25 mm = 2.54 cm

1 ft = 305 mm = 30.5 cm = 12 in

1 M = 1000 mm = 100 cm = 39.37 in = 3.2 ft

1 yd = 91.44 cm = 36 in = 3 ft

Long lines = 1 cm

Short lines = 1 mm

APPROXIMATE TEMPERATURE EQUIVALENTS

Fahrenheit	*Centigrade*
212°	100°(water boils)
105°	40.56°
104°	40°
103°	39.44°
102°	38.89°
101°	38.33°
100°	37.78°
99°	37.22°
98.6°	**37°**
98°	36.67°
97°	36.11°
96°	35.56°
32°	0°(water freezes)

Fahrenheit–Centigrade Conversions

$$F = (C \times {}^{9}/_{5}) + 32$$
$$C = (F - 32) \times {}^{5}/_{9}$$

APPROXIMATE EQUIVALENTS FOR GRAINS AND MILLIGRAMS

Grains, gr	*Milligrams,* mg	*Grains,* gr	*Milligrams,* mg
1/300	0.2	1/60	1
1/200	0.3	1/4	15

Grains, gr	*Milligrams,* mg	*Grains,* gr	*Milligrams,* mg
1/150	0.4	1/2	30
1/120	0.5	1	60
1/100	0.6		

FRACTION–DECIMAL EQUIVALENTS

1/10 = 0.1

1/100 = 0.01

1/5 = 0.2

1/4 = 0.25

1/3 = 0.33

1/2 = 0.5

2/3 = 0.66

3/4 = 0.75

HOW TO MAKE CONVERSIONS

To Convert	*Do This*
c to mL	multiply c by 240
cm to mm	multiply cm by 10
cm to in	multiply cm by 0.394
dr to mL	multiply dr by 4
g to gr	multiply g by 15
g to lb	divide g by 454

(continued on the following page)

To Convert	*Do This*
g to mg	multiply g by 1000
gr to g	multiply gr by 0.06
gr to mg	multiply gr by 60
in to cm	multiply in by 2.54
in to mm	multiply in by 25.4
kg to g	multiply kg by 1000
kg to lb	multiply kg by 2.2
L to mL	multiply L by 1000
lb to g	multiply lb by 454
lb to kg	multiply lb by 0.45 *or* divide lb by 2.2 *or* divide lb by 2 and subtract 10% of the answer
lb to oz	multiply lb by 16
m to mL	divide m by 15
mcg (μg) to mg	divide mcg by 1000
mg to mcg (μg)	multiply mg by 1000
mg to g	divide mg by 1000
mL to m	multiply mL by 15
mL to oz	divide mL by 30
mL to dr	divide mL by 4
mL to t	divide mL by 5
mm to cm	divide mm by 10

To Convert	*Do This*
oz to mL	multiply oz by 30
t to mL	multiply t by 5
T to mL	multiply T by 15

TIME CONVERSIONS

12-h Time	*24-h* Time	12-h Time	*24-h* Time
12:00 AM (midnight)	2400	12:00 PM (noon)	1200
12:01 AM	0001	1:00 PM	1300
12:59 AM	0059	2:00 PM	1400
1:00 AM	0100	3:00 PM	1500
2:00 AM	0200	4:00 PM	1600
3:00 AM	0300	5:00 PM	1700
4:00 AM	0400	6:00 PM	1800
5:00 AM	0500	7:00 PM	1900
6:00 AM	0600	8:00 PM	2000
7:00 AM	0700	9:00 PM	2100
8:00 AM	0800	10:00 PM	2200
9:00 AM	0900	11:00 PM	2300
10:00 AM	1000	12:00 AM (midnight)	2400
11:00 AM	1100		

NOTE: 12:01 AM to 12:00 PM are identical in both systems except that all 24-h times have four places; i.e. 8:00 AM = 0800.

To change 12-h time to 24-h time, add 12 to PM time.

MEDICATION ADMINISTRATION

MEDICATIONS ARE GIVEN ACCORDING TO THE "FIVE RIGHTS"

1. Right patient
2. Right drug
3. Right dose
4. Right time
5. Right route

"Right documentation" is sometimes referred to as the "sixth right."

Medications Are Checked at Least Three Times According to the Five Rights

1. When the medication container is removed from storage
2. When the medication dose is removed from the container
3. Before returning the medication container to storage

Common Routes of Medication Administration

1. *PO*: by mouth
2. *Sublingual*: under the tongue
3. *Topical*: on the skin
4. *Subcutaneous*: into adipose tissue (usually given at a 45-degree angle, with a 1/2- to 1-inch–long needle)
5. *Intramuscular*: into the muscle (given at a 90-degree angle, with a needle long enough to pass through adipose tissue and enter the muscle)
6. *Intravenous*: into the vein
7. *Rectal*: into the rectum
8. *Intrathecal*: into the spinal canal (not usually administered by nurse)

CALCULATION OF DOSAGES

METHOD 1: SOLVING FOR X

This particular formula is set up on two lines. It is *essential* that the same symbols, letters, or words used in the first line of the formula be used again in the *same order* in the second line of the formula.

Step 1: Write the known—that is, the drug dosage available in the volume available—on the first line.
Step 2: Write the unknown—that is, the dosage ordered by the doctor—*directly under* the dosage available, and write X *directly under* the volume available.
Step 3: Cross multiply in a diagonal fashion, and write the products on the third line.
Step 4: Divide the number in front of X into the other number on the third line to determine the answer.

Example: The physician has ordered 35 mg of Demerol. On hand you have Demerol 50 mg = 2 mL

50 mg = 2 mL	(The known; dosage [50 mg] in volume [2 mL] available.)
35 mg = X mL	(The unknown; *note* that it is *essential* to place the mg *under* mg and the mL *under* mL.)
50X = 70	(Derived by cross, or diagonal, multiplying; 50 times X and 2 times 35.)
X = 1.4 mL	(The number in front of X is divided into the other number on the third line.)

NOTE: Because only identical terms can be used (as explained) in the first two lines of the formula, a drug ordered in grains and supplied in milligrams cannot be calculated by the formula until both the ordered and available drugs are converted to like forms (both to grains or both to milligrams).

METHOD 2: FRACTION FORMAT

$$\frac{\text{Dose ordered}}{\text{Dose on hand}} \times \text{volume of dose on hand} = \text{amount to administer}$$

Example:

$$\frac{\text{35 mg (ordered)}}{\text{50 mg (on hand)}} \times \text{2 mL (volume of 50 mg)} = \text{1.4 mL}$$

METHOD 3: RATIO AND PROPORTIONS

Although this formula seems to yield more errors than other calculation methods, it is used by many nurses. The information used in the *solving for* X example is set up in the following fashion:

$$50 \text{ mg} : 2 \text{ mL} = 35 \text{ mg} : X \text{ mL}$$
$$50X = 70$$
$$X = 1.4 \text{ mL}$$

The extremes ("outside" by "outside" and "inside" by "inside") are multiplied on the first line to determine the numbers on the second line. Note that dosage and volume must be in the same order on each side of the "equals" sign on the first line.

NOMOGRAM FOR ESTIMATING BODY SURFACE AREA OF INFANTS AND YOUNG CHILDREN

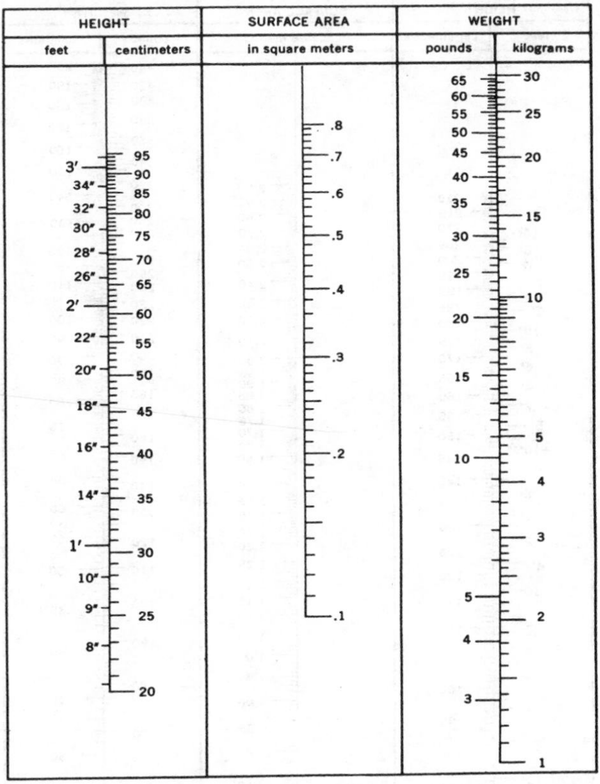

Figure 1–26. Nomogram for estimating surface area of infants and young children. To determine the surface area of the patient, draw a straight line between the point representing the patient's height on the left vertical scale to the point representing the patient's weight on the right vertical scale. The point at which this line intersects the middle vertical scale represents the surface area in square meters. (Reprinted with permission of Ross Laboratories, Columbus, OH 43216. From Dietetic Currents, Vol 16 (No 2), 1989, Ross Laboratories.)

NOMOGRAM FOR ESTIMATING BODY SURFACE AREA OF OLDER CHILDREN AND ADULTS

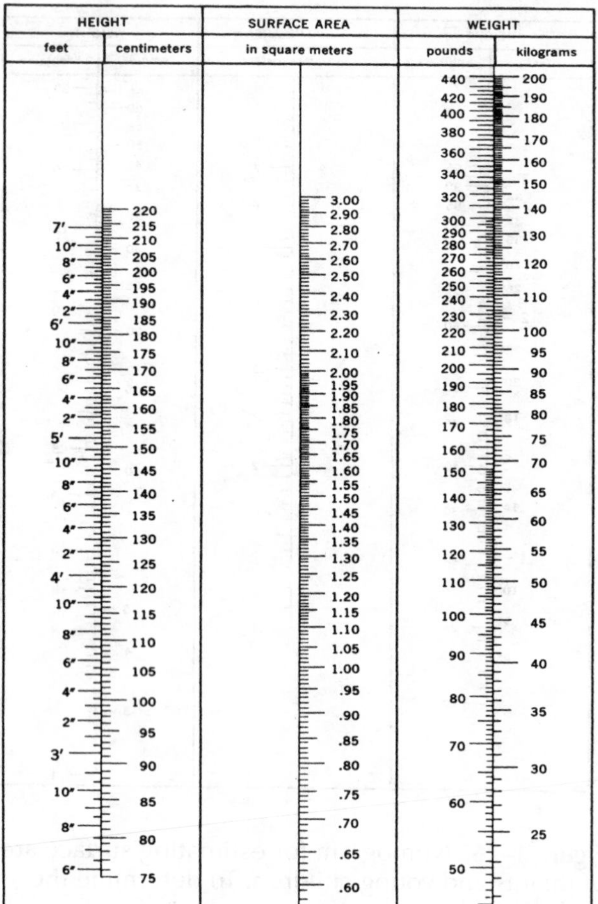

Figure 1–27. Nomogram for estimating surface area of older children and adults. See Nomogram for Estimating Surface Area of Infants and Young Children for instructions on use. (Reprinted with permission of Ross Laboratories, Columbus, OH 43216. From Dietetic Currents, Vol 16 (No 2), 1989, Ross Laboratories.)

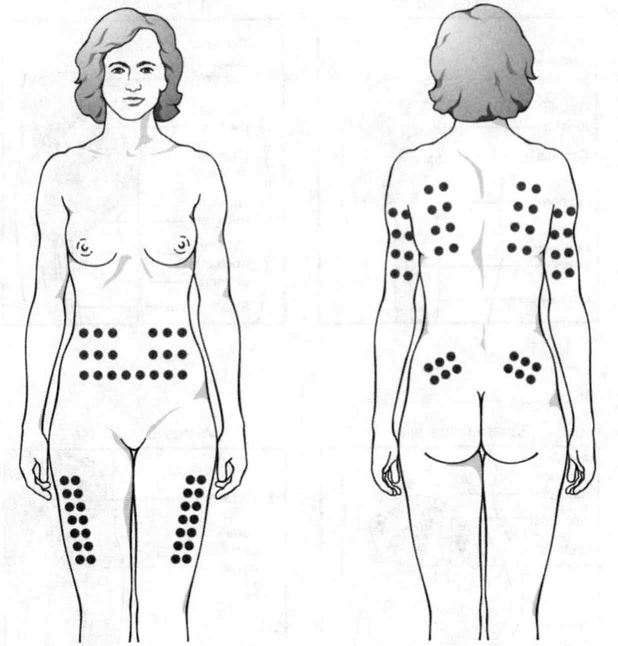

Figure 1–28. Subcutaneous injection sites. (From Deglin, JH, and Vallerand, AH: Davis's Drug Guide for Nurses, ed 8. FA Davis, Philadelphia, 2003, p. 1142, with permission.)

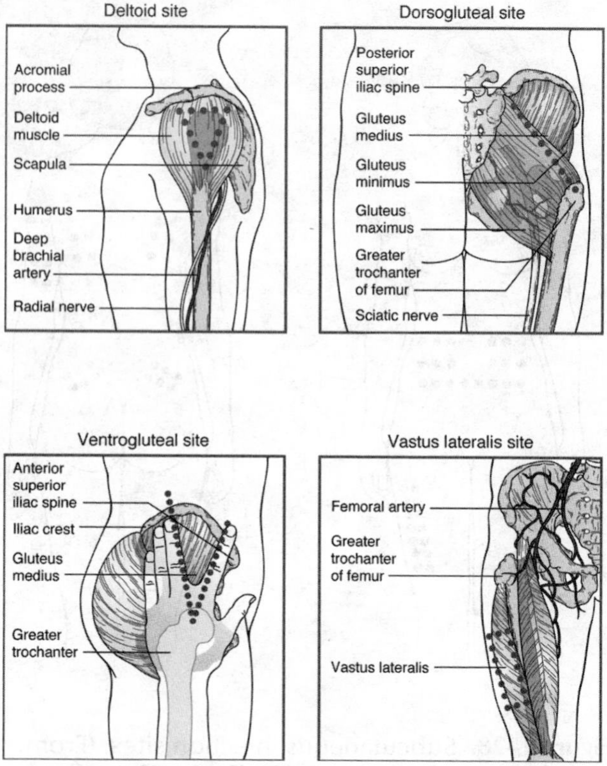

Figure 1–29. Intramuscular injection sites. (From Deglin, JH, and Vallerand, AH: Davis's Drug Guide for Nurses, ed 8. FA Davis, Philadelphia, 2003, p. 1144, with permission.)

Table 1–5. TIME/ACTION PROFILE OF INSULINS

Type	Onset	Peak	Duration
Insulin aspart SC	15 min	1–3h	3–5 h
Insulin lispro SC	15 min	30–90 min	6–8 h
Regular IV	10–30 min	15–30 min	30–60 min
Regular SC	0.5–1 h	2–4 h	8–12 h
NPH SC	1–1.5 h	4–12 h	24 h
Lente SC	1–2.5 h	7–15 h	24 h
Insulin glargine SC	1.1 h	5 h	24 h*
Ultralente SC	8 h	10–30 h	>36 h

*Small amts. of insulin glargine slowly released resulting in a relatively constant effect over time.
Source: Adapted from Deglin, JH, and Vallerand, AH: Davis's Drug Guide for Nurses, ed 8. FA Davis, Philadelphia, 2003, p 523, with permission.

Table 1–6. BLOOD LEVELS OF DRUGS

Drug	Peak Time	Duration of Action	Therapeutic Level	Toxic Level
ANTIBIOTICS				
Amikacin	IM: 1/2 h IV: 15 min	2 d	20–25 μg/mL	35 μg/mL
SI units*			34–43 μmol/L	60 μmol/L
Gentamicin	IM: 1/2 h IV: 15 min	2 d	4–8 μg/mL	12 μg/mL
SI units			8.4–16.8 μmol/L	25.1 μmol/L
Kanamycin	1/2 h	2 d	20–25 μg/mL	35 μg/mL
SI units			42–52 μmol/L	73 μmol/L
Streptomycin	1/2–1 1/2 h	5 d	25–30 μg/mL	>30 μg/mL
SI units				

Tobramycin	IV: 15 min	2 d	2–8 µg/mL	12 µg/mL
SI units			4–17 µmol/L	25 µmol/L
ANTICONVULSANTS				
Barbiturates and barbiturate-related				
Amobarbital	IV: 30 sec	10–20 h	7 µg/mL	30 µg/mL
SI units			30 µmol/L	132 µmol/L
Pentobarbital	IV: 30 sec	15 h	4 µg/mL	15 µg/mL
SI units			18 µmol/L	66 µmol/L
Phenobarbital	15 min	80 h	10 µg/mL	>55 µg/mL
SI units			43 µmol/L	>230 µmol/L
Primidone	PO: 3 h	7–14 h	1 µg/mL	>10 µg/mL
SI units			4 µmol/L	>45 µmol/L

(continued on the following page)

Table 1–6. **BLOOD LEVELS OF DRUGS** (continued)

Drug	Peak Time	Duration of Action	Therapeutic Level	Toxic Level
Benzodiazepines				
Clonazepam (Klonopin)	1–4 h	60 h	5–70 ng/ml	>70 ng/mL
SI units			55–222 µmol/L	>222 µmol/L
Diazepan (Valium)	1–4 h	1–2 d	5–70 ng/mL	>70 ng/mL
SI units			0.01–0.25 µmol/L	>0.25 µmol/L
Hydantoins				
Phenytoin (Dilantin)	3–12 h	7–42 h	10–20 µg/mL	>20 µg/mL
SI units			40–80 µmol/L	>80 µmol/L
Succinimides				
Ethosuximide (Zarontin)	1 h	8 d	40–80 µg/mL	100 µg/mL
SI units			283–566 µmol/L	708 µmol/L

Miscellaneous				
Carbamazepine (Tegretol)	4 h	2 d	2–10 μg/mL	12 μg/mL
SI units			8–42 μmol/L	50 μmol/L
Valproic acid (Depakene)	1–4 h	24 h	50–100 μg/mL	>100 μg/mL
SI units			350–700 μmol/L	>700 μmol/L
BRONCHODILATORS				
Aminophylline/theophyline	PO: 2 h IV: 15 min	8–9 h	10–18 μg/mL	>20 μg/mL
CARDIAC DRUGS				
Disopyramide (Norpace)	PO: 2 h	25–30 h	2–4.5 μg/mL	>9 μg/mL
SI units			5.9–13 μmol/L	>6 μmol/L
Quinidine	PO: 1 h IV: immediate	20–30 h	2.4–5 μg/mL	>6 μg/mL
SI units			7–15 μmol/L	>18 μmol/L

(continued on the following page)

Table 1–6. BLOOD LEVELS OF DRUGS (continued)

Drug	Peak Time	Duration of Action	Therapeutic Level	Toxic Level
Procainamide (Pronestyl)	PO: 1 h IV: 1/2 h	10–20 h	4–8 μg/mL	>12 μg/mL
SI units			17–35 μmol/L	>50 μmol/L
NAPA (*N*-acetyl procainamide, a procainamide metabolite)	—	—	2–8 μg/mL	>30 μg/mL
SI units			7–29 μmol/L	108 μmol/L
Lidocaine	IV: immediate	5–10 h	2–6 μg/mL	>9 μg/mL
SI units			8–25 μmol/L	>38 μmol/L
Bretylium	15–30 min	6–8 h	5–10 mg/kg	30 mg/kg
Verapamil	PO: 5 h IV: 3–5 min	8–10 h IV: 1/2–1 h	5–10 mg/kg	>15 mg/kg

Diltiazem	PO: 2–3 h	3–4 h	50–200 ng/mL	>200 ng/mL
Nifedipine	1–3 h	3–4 h	5–10 mg	90 mg
Digitoxin	4 h	30 d	10–25 ng/mL	30 ng/mL
SI units			13–33 nmol/L	39 nmol/L
Digoxin	2 h	7 d	0.5–2 ng/mL	>2.5 ng/mL
SI units			0.6–2.5 nmol/L	>3.0 nmol/L
Phenytoin (Dilantin)	PO: 2 h	96 h	10–18 µg/mL	>20 µg/mL
SI units			40–71 µmol/L	>80 µmol/L
Quinidine	IV: 1 h			
	—	—	2.3–5 µg/mL	>5 µg/mL
SI units			7–15 µmol/L	>15 µmol/L

(continued on the following page)

Table 1–6. BLOOD LEVELS OF DRUGS (continued)

Drug	Peak Time	Duration of Action	Therapeutic Level	Toxic Level
SALICYLATES				
Aspirin	15 min	12–30 h	2–20 mg/dL	>30 mg/dL
SI units			0.1–1.4 mmol/L	>2.1 mmol/L
			2–30 mg/dL	40 mg/dL
SI units			0.1–2.1 mmol/L	2.8 mmol/L
NARCOTICS				
Codeine	—	—	—	>0.005 mg/dL
SI units				>17 nmol/L
Hydromorphone (Dilaudid)	—	—	—	>0.1 mg/dL
SI units				>350 nmol/L
Methadone	—	—	—	>0.2 mg/dL
SI units				6.46 µmol/L

Meperidine (Demerol)	—	—	—	>0.5 mg/dL
SI units				>20 µmol/L
Morphine	—	—	—	>0.005 mg/dL
BARBITURATES				
Phenobarbital	—	—	10 µg/mL	55 µg/mL
SI units			43 µmol/L	230 µmol/L
Amobarbital	—	—	7 µg/mL	30 µg/mL
SI units			30 µmol/L	130 µmol/L
Pentobarbital	—	—	4 µg/mL	15 µg/mL
SI units			17 µmol/L	66 µmol/L
Secobarbital	—	—	3 µg/mL	10 µg/mL
SI units			12 µmol/L	42 µmol/L

(continued on the following page)

Table 1–6. BLOOD LEVELS OF DRUGS (continued)

Drug	Peak Time	Duration of Action	Therapeutic Level	Toxic Level
ALCOHOLS				
Ethanol	—	—	0.1 g/dL (legal level for intoxication)	100 mg/dL
Methanol	—	—	—	20 mg/dL
PSYCHIATRIC DRUGS				
Amitriptyline (Elavil) SI units	—	—	100–250 ng/mL 361–902 nmol/L	>300 ng/mL >1083 nmol/L
Imipramine (Tofranil) SI units	—	—	100–250 ng/mL 357–898 nmol/L	>300 ng/mL >1071 nmol/L

Lithium (Lithonate)	1–4 h	—	0.8–1.4 mEq/L	1.5 mEq/L
SI units			0.8–1.4 µmol/L	1.5 µmol/L
MISCELLANEOUS				
Acetaminophen	—	—	0–25 µg/mL	>150 µg/mL
SI units			0–170 µmol/L	>1000 µmol/L 4 hr after ingestion
Prochlorperazine	—	—	0.5 µg/mL	1.0 µg/mL
Bromides	—	—	75–150 mg/dL	>150 mg/dL
SI units			7–15 mmol/L	>15 mmol/L

*The first units given are the conventional units.

Source: Adapted from Cavanaugh, BM: Nurse's Manual of Laboratory and Diagnostic Tests, ed 4. FA Davis, Philadelphia, 2003, pp. 214–217, with permission.

DRUG COMPATIBILITY CHART (SYRINGE)

(From Deglin, JH, and Vallerand, AH: Davis's Drug Guide for Nurses, ed 8. FA Davis, Philadelphia, 2003, Insert, with permission.)

Syringe Compatibility

KEY

- C =Compatible
- L =Compatible for a limited period
- I =Incompatible
- * =Conflicting data
- – =Data unavailable
- ■ =Identical drug

	1. atropine	2. benzquinamide	3. buprenorphine	4. butorphanol	5. chlorpromazine	6. diazepam	7. diphenhydramine
1. atropine	■	C	–	L	L	–	L
2. benzquinamide	C	■	–	–	–	I	–
3. buprenorphine	–	–	■	–	–	–	–
4. butorphanol	L	–	–	■	L	–	L
5. chlorpromazine	L	–	–	L	■	–	L
6. diazepam	–	I	–	–	–	■	–
7. diphenhydramine	L	–	–	L	L	–	■
8. droperidol	L	–	–	L	L	–	L
9. glycopyrrolate	C	C	–	–	C	I	C
10. hydromorphone	L	–	–	–	L	–	L
11. hydroxyzine	L	C	–	C	L	–	L
12. meperidine	L	C	–	L	L	–	L
13. metoclopramide	L	–	–	L	L	–	L
14. midazolam	L	L	L	L	L	–	L
15. morphine	L	C	–	L	L	–	L
16. nalbuphine	C	–	–	–	–	I	C
17. pentazocine	L	C	–	L	L	–	L
18. pentobarbital	*	I	–	I	I	–	I
19. prochlorperazine	L	–	–	L	L	–	L
20. promethazine	L	–	–	L	L	–	L
21. scopolamine	L	C	–	L	L	–	L

	8. droperidol	9. glycopyrrolate	10. hydromorphone	11. hydroxyzine	12. meperidine	13. metoclopramide	14. midazolam	15. morphine	16. nalbuphine	17. pentazocine	18. pentobarbital	19. prochlorperazine	20. promethazine	21. scopolamine
1.	L	C	L	L	L	L	L	L	C	L	*	L	L	L
2.	–	C	–	C	C	–	L	C	–	C	I	–	–	C
3.	–	–	–	–	–	–	L	–	–	–	–	–	–	–
4.	L	–	–	C	L	L	L	L	–	L	I	L	L	L
5.	L	C	L	L	L	L	L	L	–	L	I	L	L	L
6.	–	I	–	–	–	–	–	–	I	–	–	–	–	–
7.	L	C	L	L	L	L	L	L	C	L	I	L	L	L
8.		C	–	L	L	L	L	L	C	L	I	L	L	L
9.	C		C	C	C	–	L	C	C	I	I	C	C	C
10.	–	C		L	–	–	L	–	–	L	L	*	L	L
11.	L	C	L		L	L	L	L	C	L	I	L	L	L
12.	L	C	–	L		L	L	I	–	L	I	L	L	L
13.	L	–	–	L	L		L	*	–	L	–	L	L	L
14.	L	L	L	L	L	L		*	L	–	I	I	L	L
15.	L	C	–	L	I	*	*		–	L	*	*	*	L
16.	C	C	–	C	–	–	L	–		–	I	C	*	C
17.	L	I	L	L	L	L	–	L	–		I	L	L	L
18.	I	I	L	I	I	–	I	*	I	I		I	I	L
19.	L	C	*	L	L	L	I	*	C	L	I		L	L
20.	L	C	L	L	L	L	L	*	*	L	I	L		L
21.	L	C	L	L	L	L	L	L	C	L	L	L	L	

IV ADMIXTURE COMPATIBILITY

(From Deglin, JH, and Vallerand, AH: Davis's Drug Guide for Nurses, ed 3. FA Davis, Philadelphia, 1993, pp 1258–1259, with permission.)

Drug Compatibility Charts

IV Admixture Compatibility

KEY
C =Compatible
L =Compatible for a limited period of time
I =Incompatible
* =Conflicting data
– =Data unavailable
■ =Identical drug

	1. amikacin	2. aminophylline	3. amphotericin B	4. ampicillin	5. calcium chloride	6. calcium gluconate	7. cefamandole	8. cefazolin	9. cefoxitin	10. chloramphenicol	11. cimetidine	12. clindamycin	13. dexamethasone	14. diphenhydramine	15. gentamicin
1. amikacin	■	*	I	I	C	C	–	I	C	C	C	C	*	C	–
2. aminophylline	*	■	–	–	–	C	–	–	–	C	I	I	C	C	–
3. amphotericin B	I	–	■	I	I	I	–	–	–	–	I	–	–	I	I
4. ampicillin	I	–	I	■	–	I	–	–	–	–	*	*	–	–	I
5. calcium chloride	C	–	I	–	■	–	–	–	–	C	–	–	–	–	–
6. calcium gluconate	C	C	I	I	–	■	I	I	–	C	–	I	C	C	I
7. cefamandole	–	–	–	–	–	I	■	–	–	–	*	C	–	–	I
8. cefazolin	I	–	–	–	–	I	–	■	–	L	I	C	C	–	I
9. cefoxitin	C	–	–	–	–	–	–	–	■	–	C	C	–	–	I
10. chloramphenicol	C	C	–	–	C	C	–	L	–	■	–	–	C	C	I
11. cimetidine	C	I	I	*	–	–	*	*	C	–	■	C	C	–	C
12. clindamycin	C	I	–	*	–	I	C	C	C	–	C	■	–	–	C
13. dexamethasone	*	C	–	–	–	C	–	C	–	C	C	–	■	I	I
14. diphenhydramine	C	C	I	–	–	C	–	–	–	C	–	–	I	■	I
15. gentamicin	–	–	I	I	–	I	I	I	I	I	C	C	I	I	■
16. heparin	I	C	C	*	–	C	–	–	L	C	–	C	L	–	I
17. hydrocortisone	C	C	C	*	C	C	–	–	–	C	–	C	L	I	I
18. insulin, regular	–	I	–	–	–	–	–	–	C	–	C	–	–	–	I
19. lidocaine	–	C	–	*	C	C	C	–	–	C	C	–	C	C	C
20. methicillin	I	C	–	I	C	C	–	–	–	I	–	–	C	C	I
21. methylprednisolone	–	*	–	–	–	I	–	–	–	C	–	C	–	–	–
22. metoclopramide	–	–	–	–	–	I	–	–	–	–	C	C	C	–	–
23. metronidazole	C	C	–	*	–	–	*	C	*	C	–	C	–	–	C
24. mezlocillin	–	–	–	–	–	–	–	–	–	–	–	–	–	–	I
25. multivitamin infusion	–	–	–	–	–	–	–	–	C	–	–	–	–	–	–
26. nafcillin	–	*	–	–	–	–	–	–	–	C	–	–	C	C	–
27. oxacillin	*	–	–	–	–	–	–	–	–	C	–	–	–	–	–
28. oxytocin	–	–	–	–	–	–	–	–	–	C	–	–	–	–	–
29. penicillin G	*	I	I	–	C	C	–	–	–	C	C	C	–	C	*
30. piperacillin	–	–	–	–	–	–	–	–	–	–	–	C	–	–	–
31. potassium chloride	*	C	I	–	–	C	–	–	–	C	C	C	–	–	–
32. procainamide	–	–	–	–	–	–	–	–	–	–	–	–	–	–	–
33. ranitidine	C	–	I	*	–	–	–	*	–	C	–	I	C	–	C
34. ticarcillin	–	–	–	–	–	–	–	–	–	–	–	–	–	–	–
35. tobramycin	–	–	–	–	–	C	I	–	C	–	–	*	–	–	–
36. vancomycin	C	*	–	–	–	C	–	–	–	I	C	–	I	–	–
37. verapmil	C	C	I	*	C	C	C	C	C	C	C	C	C	–	C

	16. heparin	17. hydrocortisone	18. insulin, regular	19. lidocaine	20. methicillin	21. methylprednisolone	22. metoclopramide	23. metronidazole	24. mezlocillin	25. multivitamin infusion	26. nafcillin	27. oxacillin	28. oxytocin	29. penicillin G	30. piperacillin	31. potassium chloride	32. procainamide	33. ranitidine	34. ticarcillin	35. tobramycin	36. vancomycin	37. verapmil
1.	I	C	–	–	I	–	–	C	–	–	–	*	–	*	–	*	–	C	–	–	C	C
2.	C	C	I	C	C	*	–	C	–	–	*	–	–	I	–	C	–	–	–	–	*	C
3.	C	C	–	–	–	–	–	–	–	–	–	–	–	I	–	I	–	I	–	–	–	I
4.	*	*	–	*	I	–	–	*	–	–	–	–	–	–	–	–	–	*	–	–	–	*
5.	–	C	–	C	I	–	–	–	–	–	–	–	–	C	–	–	–	–	–	–	–	C
6.	C	L	–	C	C	I	I	–	–	–	–	–	–	C	–	C	–	–	–	C	C	C
7.	–	–	–	C	–	–	–	*	–	–	–	–	–	–	–	–	–	–	–	I	–	C
8.	–	–	–	–	–	–	–	C	–	–	–	–	–	–	–	–	–	*	–	–	–	C
9.	L	C	–	–	–	–	–	*	–	C	–	–	–	–	–	–	–	–	–	C	–	C
10.	C	C	–	C	I	C	–	C	–	–	C	C	C	C	–	C	–	C	–	–	I	C
11.	–	–	C	C	–	C	C	–	–	–	–	–	–	C	–	C	–	–	–	–	C	C
12.	C	C	–	–	–	C	C	C	–	–	–	–	–	C	C	C	–	I	–	*	–	C
13.	L	L	–	C	C	–	C	–	–	–	C	–	–	–	–	–	–	C	–	–	I	C
14.	–	I	–	C	C	–	–	–	–	–	C	–	–	C	–	–	–	–	–	–	–	–
15.	I	I	I	C	I	–	–	C	I	–	–	–	–	*	–	–	–	C	–	–	–	C
16.		*	I	C	*	C	–	C	–	–	C	–	–	*	–	C	–	–	–	–	I	C
17.	*		L	C	*	–	–	*	–	–	I	–	–	C	C	C	–	–	–	–	C	C
18.	I	L		C	–	I	–	–	–	–	–	–	–	–	–	–	–	–	–	–	–	C
19.	C	C	C		–	–	–	–	–	–	–	–	–	C	–	C	C	–	–	–	–	C
20.	*	*	–	–		–	–	–	–	–	–	–	–	C	–	C	–	–	–	–	I	C
21.	C	–	I	–	–		C	–	–	–	I	–	–	*	–	–	–	–	–	–	–	C
22.	–	–	–	–	–	C		–	–	C	–	–	–	–	–	C	–	–	–	–	–	–
23.	C	*	–	–	–	–	–		–	C	–	–	–	C	–	–	–	–	–	C	–	–
24.	–	–	–	–	–	–	–	–		–	–	–	–	–	–	–	–	–	–	–	–	*
25.	–	–	–	–	–	–	C	C	–		–	–	–	L	–	–	–	–	–	–	–	C
26.	C	I	–	–	–	I	–	–	–	–		–	–	–	–	C	–	–	–	–	–	*
27.	–	–	–	–	–	–	–	–	–	–	–		–	–	–	C	–	–	–	–	–	*
28.	–	–	–	–	–	–	–	–	–	–	–	–		–	–	–	–	–	–	–	–	C
29.	*	C	–	C	C	*	–	*	–	L	–	–	–		–	*	–	C	–	–	–	C
30.	–	C	–	–	–	–	–	–	–	–	–	–	–	–		C	–	–	–	–	–	C
31.	C	C	–	C	C	–	C	–	–	–	C	C	–	*	C		–	–	–	–	C	C
32.	–	–	–	C	–	–	–	–	–	–	–	–	–	–	–	–		–	–	–	–	C
33.	–	–	–	–	–	–	–	–	–	–	–	–	–	C	–	–	–		C	C	C	–
34.	–	–	–	–	–	–	–	–	–	–	–	–	–	–	–	–	–	C		–	–	C
35.	–	–	–	–	–	–	–	C	–	–	–	–	–	–	–	–	–	C	–		–	C
36.	I	C	–	–	I	–	–	–	–	–	–	–	–	–	–	C	–	C	–	–		C
37.	C	C	C	C	C	C	–	–	*	C	*	*	C	C	C	C	C	–	C	C	C	

IV THERAPY, ADULT

DAILY MAINTENANCE FLUID REQUIREMENTS

Usually about 30 mL/kg/24 hr is needed to maintain hydration.

Each 1°C increase in patient's temperature above 37°C increases fluid requirements by 15%.

Other factors affecting requirements are patient's condition and age.

NORMAL DAILY ELECTROLYTE REQUIREMENTS

Sodium (Na^+):	1–2 mEq/kg/24 h
Potassium (K^+):	0.5–1 mEq/kg/24 h
Chloride (Cl^-):	1–2 mEq/kg/24 h

TONICITY OF FLUIDS

Isotonic fluids have an osmolality the same as that of blood; that is, about **310 mEq/L** of total electrolytes.

Hypotonic fluids have an electrolyte content below **250 mEq/L.**

Hypertonic fluids have an electrolyte content above **375 mEq/L.**

Table 1–7. COMMON IV FLUIDS AND THEIR USES

Product	Tonicity*	Osmolarity	pH	Nonelectrolyte: Dext. (g/L)	Nonelectrolyte: kcal/L	Cations/Liter: Na	Cations/Liter: K	Cations/Liter: Ca	Cations/Liter: Mg	Anions/Liter: Cl	Anions/Liter: Acetate	Anions/Liter: Lactate	Uses
DEXTROSE SOLUTIONS													
5% dextrose and water	Iso	252	4.8	50	170								Supplies calories as carbohydrates; prevents dehydration; maintains water balance; promotes sodium diuresis
10% dextrose and water	Hyper	505	4.7	100	340								
20% dextrose and water	Hyper	1010	4.8	200	680								
50% dextrose and water	Hyper	2525	4.6	500	1700								
SALINE SOLUTIONS													
0.45% NaCl	Hypo	154	5.9			77				77			Treats alkalosis; corrects fluid loss; treats sodium depletion
0.9% NaCl	Iso	308	6.0			154				154			
3% NaCl	Hyper	1026	6.0			513				513			

(continued on the following page)

Table 1–7. COMMON FLUIDS AND THEIR USES (continued)

Product	Tonicity*	Osmolarity	pH	Nonelectrolyte		Cations/Liter				Anions/Liter			Uses
				Dext. (g/L)	kcal/L	Na	K	Ca	Mg	Cl	Acetate	Lactate	
DEXTROSE AND SALINE SOLUTIONS													
5% dextrose/ 0.2% NaCl	Iso	320	4.6	50	170	34				34			Promotes diuresis; corrects moderate fluid loss; prevents alkalosis; provides calories and sodium chloride
5% dextrose/ 0.45% NaCl	Hyper	406	4.6	50	170	77				77			
5% dextrose/ 0.9% NaCl	Hyper	559	4.4	50	170	154				154			
10% dextrose/ 0.9% NaCl	Hyper	812	4.8	100	340	154				154			

MULTIPLE ELECTROLYTE SOLUTIONS

Ringer's solution	Iso	304	6.0		147	4	4	0	155	0	0	Replaces fluid lost through vomiting or gastrointestinal suctioning; treats dehydration; restores normal fluid balance
Lactated Ringer's	Iso	273	6.5		130	4	3	0	109	0	28	
Normosol R (Abbott)	Iso	295	6.4	18	140	5		3	98	27	0	
Plasma Lyte M with dextrose[†] (Baxter)	Hyper	383	5.2	18	40	16	5	3	40	12	12	

*Indicated tonicity for solutions containing dextrose is the tonicity *at the time* of administration. Within a short period of time, the dextrose is metabolized and the tonicity of the infused solution decreases in proportion to the tonicity of electrolytes within the water.

[†]The addition of dextrose to any multiple electrolyte solution renders the solution hypertonic *at the time of administration*; the dextrose is metabolized within a short time after administration, decreasing the tonicity of the solution to that of the nondextrose components (electrolytes) in water.

Source: Adapted from Phillips, LD: Manual of IV Therapeutics ed. 3. FA Davis, Philadelphia, 2001, pp. 206–209.

CALCULATION OF IV RATES

$$\text{Rate of flow} = \frac{\text{amount of fluid} \times \text{drop factor on tubing box}}{\text{running time stated in total number of minutes}}$$

To determine running time "stated in total number of minutes," multiply 60 by the number of hours that the infusion is to run.

Example:

$$\text{Rate of flow} = \frac{1000 \text{ mL} \times 15}{480} = 31 \text{ gtt/min}$$

The above example shows the flow rate (drops per minute) for 1000 mL of fluid to be infused over an 8-hour (480-minute) period using tubing that delivers 15 gtt/mL.

Table 1–8. HOURLY INFUSION RATES FOR 1000 MILLILITERS OF FLUID

Hours to Infuse	mL/hr	gtt Factor	gtt/min
6	167	10	28
6	167	12	33
6	167	15	42
6	167	60	167
8	125	10	21
8	125	12	25
8	125	15	31
8	125	60	125
10	100	10	17

Table 1–8. HOURLY INFUSION RATES FOR 1000 MILLILITERS OF FLUID (continued)

Hours to Infuse	mL/hr	gtt Factor	gtt/min
10	100	12	20
10	100	15	25
10	100	60	100
12	83	10	14
12	83	12	17
12	83	15	21
12	83	60	83

PARENTERAL NUTRITION

Parenteral nutrition is used when a patient is unable to take or adequately absorb sufficient nutrients via PO or enteral feedings to meet metabolic demands and/or achieve tissue synthesis and repair.

Peripheral parenteral nutrition (PPN) is designed to increase nutrient intake in mildly stressed patients who are expected to return to PO or enteral feedings alone within 1 to 2 weeks. PPN is delivered through a peripheral line or peripherally inserted central line (PICC); dextrose percentages of the infusion remain <20 percent with the addition of amino acids and lipids. PPN avoids the hazards associated with a central line and the metabolic complications of TPN but is not adequate for nutritionally depleted patients or those needing to gain weight.

Total parenteral nutrition (TPN) is delivered via a central venous catheter to reverse starvation and promote tissue synthesis, wound healing, and normal metabolic function. TPN solutions are nutritionally complete, based on the patient's weight and caloric/nutrient needs. The content of TPN is highly concentrated (hypertonic); a mixture of dextrose (20 to 70 percent), amino acids, multivitamins, electrolytes, and trace elements. Insulin is often added to the content as needed to control blood glucose. Five hundred milliliters of 10 or 20 percent fat emulsion (lipids) is also administered qd or qod to meet the patient's remaining nutritional needs.

BASIC GUIDELINES FOR TPN ADMINISTRATION

1. Verify central line placement after initial insertion via chest (radiograph) prior to beginning TPN infusion; pneumothorax or hemothorax is a risk with central line placement.
2. Check vital signs (including blood pressure) at least every 6 hours after initiating infusion.
3. Check central line insertion site frequently for signs of infection (infection is a common complication when a central line is used and may lead to sepsis).
4. Follow agency policy regarding frequency of dressing changes and procedure.
5. Change IV line setup every 24 hours. (TPN fluids are an excellent medium for bacterial growth.)
6. Do not administer IV piggyback or direct IV push medications through or draw blood samples from the TPN line. Only lipids may be "piggybacked" carefully through the TPN line beyond the in-line filter.
7. Monitor blood glucose every 6 hours; administer sliding scale insulin as ordered.
8. Weigh patient daily. (High glucose content of TPN can cause an osmotic diuresis and lead to dehydration.)
9. Order TPN solutions from the pharmacy in a timely manner; remove the next container from the refrigerator an hour before needed to prevent central infusion of cold solutions.
10. When a new container of TPN is needed, but is not available, follow agency policy to maintain the ordered fluid delivery rate with $D_{10}W$ until the TPN is available. (High glucose content of fluid stimu-

lates release of insulin, which may cause hypoglycemia if fluids are discontinued abruptly.)

11. Do not attempt to "catch up" on fluids if rate inadvertently slows.
12. Discontinue TPN solution gradually at the end of therapy to prevent hypoglycemia.
13. Monitor lab values. (Liver complications, electrolyte imbalances, and pH changes are possible.)

ADMINISTRATION OF BLOOD PRODUCTS

DO

1. Verify physician's order.
2. Check expiration date on product.
3. Verify accuracy of component with another licensed nurse or physician.
4. Check patient's ID band for proper identification.
5. Explain procedure to patient and tell him or her to report any unusual symptoms or sensations that may occur during infusion.
6. Check baseline vital signs (VS) and report any abnormal findings to the physician before beginning infusion of component.
7. Warm blood in approved blood warmer for use in rapid transfusions or for neonatal exchange transfusions.
8. Ascertain that the IV line is present and not infiltrated before beginning infusion.
9. Flush any solution from present IV line with 0.9% normal saline. (Flush again with saline after completion of product.)
10. Check manufacturer's information before using any pump to administer product. (Some pumps may cause hemolysis of red cells.)
11. Initiate infusion within 30 minutes from the time the product is released from the blood bank.
12. Remain with the patient for at least 5 minutes after transfusion has begun.
13. Check VS 15 minutes after product infusion has

begun, then 15 minutes later, and at least every 30 minutes until the infusion is completed.

14. Stop infusion of blood product, maintain IV access with 0.9% normal saline, and notify the physician if any of the following occurs:

    Burning at injection site
    Pain in any area
    Flushing or rash
    Itching
    Fever
    Chills
    Marked change in VS

15. Administer a maximum of 50 mL of product over the first 15 minutes of transfusion.
16. Complete the infusion within a 4-hour period.
17. Validate teaching, assessment (including VS), product ID check, procedure (including time infusion begun and completed), and reaction in the patient's record.

DO NOT

1. Do not store blood products in nursing unit refrigerators. (Blood must be stored at a temperature between 1° and 6°C.)
2. Do not use a blood filter for more than 6 hours nor administer more units than recommended by the manufacturer.
3. Do not heat blood products in a microwave oven. (Doing so could result in cellular damage.)
4. Do not discontinue IV access if an undesirable reaction occurs.
5. Do not save blood administration tubing for future use.

CENTRAL VENOUS TUNNELED CATHETERS (CVTCs)

CVTCs can be used for months or years if infection does not occur. They are available with single, double, or triple lumens and can be used for administering drugs, blood products, and total parenteral nutrition as well as for obtaining blood samples for lab tests. Breaks or tears in these catheters can be repaired without removal, and urokinase may be used to dissolve clots in the catheter. Names of some of these catheters are Hickman, Broviac, Groshong, Raal, Hemed, and Chemo Cath.

CARE OF THE PATIENT WITH A CVTC

1. Monitor the patient for infection.
2. Maintain patency by flushing catheter according to agency policy. Usually the catheter is flushed with twice the catheter volume of heparinized saline at specified intervals, and all medication dosages and blood sample withdrawals are followed by saline and heparin flushes.
3. The Groshong catheter is not flushed with heparin because it has a valve that restricts blood backflow. Clamps should not be used on the Groshong as they may damage the catheter. This catheter is flushed, according to agency policy, with 0.9% normal saline after medication administration and after withdrawal of blood samples.
4. Dressing changes are made on all catheters using sterile technique. (Both nurse and patient should wear a mask during the procedure.)

Procedures

CATHETERIZATION

1. Explain procedure to the patient.
2. Provide privacy.
3. Prepare trash receptacle.
4. Wash hands.
5. Position the female patient supine with knees flexed; male patient supine with legs slightly spread.
6. Place waterproof pad under buttocks.
7. Drape patient, diamond fashion, with sheet.
8. Arrange for adequate lighting.
9. Wash perineum with soap and water if soiled.
10. Open kit using sterile technique.
11. Don sterile gloves.
12. Set up sterile field (off bed if the patient may contaminate).
13. Test balloon if catheter will be indwelling.
14. With nondominant hand, spread labia (female) or retract foreskin (male). **This hand is no longer sterile.** Using provided antiseptic solution and cotton balls or swabs, cleanse perineum (female) from clitoris toward anus with top-to-bottom motion or retract foreskin (male) and use circular motion from meatus outward. Repeat this step at least three times.

    NOTE: Each swab is used only once and discarded into the trash receptacle, away from the sterile field.
15. Lubricate catheter.
16. Slowly insert catheter until urine is noted (2 to 3 inches for female or 7 to 8 inches for male)

(Fig. 1–30). For male patient, hold penis perpendicular to body and pull up gently during insertion.

17. Collect specimen if needed.
18. Remove catheter if it is not indwelling, and refer to step 23.

IF INDWELLING

19. Inflate balloon. If patient has sudden pain, deflate balloon, then advance catheter slightly and reinflate.
20. Pull catheter gently to check adequacy of balloon.
21. Attach catheter to collection tubing if not already connected by manufacturer.
22. Tape catheter to patient's inner thigh. Allow slack for patient movement.
23. Discard gloves and equipment.
24. Wash hands.
25. Document size and type of catheter inserted, amount and appearance of urine, and patient's tolerance of procedure.

> Example: Number 16 Foley catheter inserted, 520 mL clear yellow urine drained from bladder and discarded, catheter taped to R inner thigh and connected to drainage system, procedure tolerated well.

NOTE: Always keep drainage tubing coiled on the bed and drainage bag below level of the bladder.

PEDIATRIC ADAPTATIONS

- Use doll to demonstrate and explain procedure to child.
- Small (number 5, 8, or 10) feeding tube may be used for intermittent catheterization.
- Catheter is advanced 1 to 2 inches in young female child and 2 to 3 inches in young male.

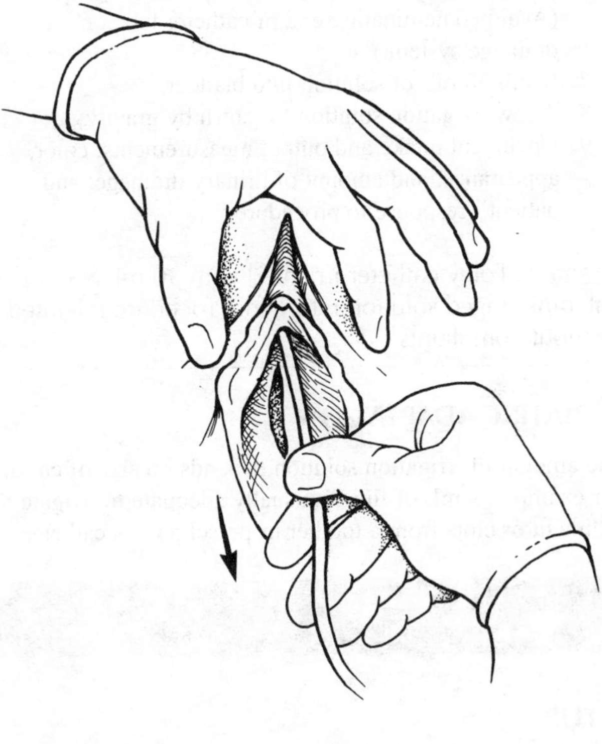

Figure 1–30. Female catheterization.

CATHETER IRRIGATION, OPEN METHOD

1. Gather equipment.
2. Explain procedure to the patient.
3. Wash hands and don gloves.
4. Place waterproof pad beneath the patient's hips.
5. Pour sterile normal saline into a sterile basin and draw into sterile irrigation syringe.
6. Using aseptic technique, disconnect drainage tubing. (Avoid contaminating end of catheter tube or drainage system.)
7. Instill 30 mL of solution into bladder.
8. Allow irrigation solution to return by gravity.
9. Document intake and output measurements; color, appearance, and amount of urinary drainage; and patient's response to procedure.

> Example: Foley catheter irrigated with 30 mL NS, 50 mL pink-tinged solution returned. Procedure tolerated without complaints.

PEDIATRIC ADAPTATION

The amount of irrigation solution depends on size of child. For example, 5 mL of fluid is usually adequate to irrigate sediment or clots from a toddler or preschooler's catheter.

CHEST TUBE SETUP AND MAINTENANCE

SETUP

1. Gather equipment and unwrap Pleur-Evac or other closed-chest drainage apparatus.
2. Fill the water-seal chamber to the 2-cm level according to manufacturer's instructions regardless of whether suction is to be used.
3. If suction is ordered, fill chamber to the ordered level; typically 20 cm H_2O.
4. Hang drainage unit from the bed frame.

5. After chest tube insertion (by the physician) and before tube clamp removal, attach drainage unit to the tube.
6. Attach long (drainage unit) tube to suction source, if ordered, and advance suction until gentle bubbling occurs in suction-control chamber. Amount of suction applied to the pleural space is determined by the height of fluid in the suction-control chamber and not the wall suction source.

MAINTENANCE

1. Note accumulated drainage in the collection chamber at the start of each shift or more frequently if warranted by patient condition, and mark the date and time of observation on the collection chamber.
2. Check the water-seal and suction-control fluid levels at the start of each shift and replace water as necessary; water will evaporate from the suction-control chamber, especially with vigorous bubbling. To check fluid levels, temporarily turn off the wall suction.
3. Observe the water-seal chamber for fluctuations (tidaling) that occur with the patient's ventilations; unless the patient is on a ventilator, the column of fluid rises with inhalation and falls with exhalation.
4. Observe the water-seal chamber for bubbling. Bubbling is normal on exhalation when the patient has a pneumothorax; continuous bubbling indicates an (abnormal) air leak in the system.
5. Maintain extra lengths of tubing by coiling it on the bed in order to prevent dependent loops that may slow/stop drainage.
6. If drainage slows or stops, gently "milk" the chest tube from proximity to the patient toward the collection chamber: to milk the tube, grasp and squeeze it between the fingers and palm of one hand; release and repeat with the other hand on the next lower portion of the tube; continue toward the collection chamber, squeezing the tube with only one hand at a time.

Do NOT strip the tube; stripping involves both hands with one holding the tube while the other squeezes and pulls toward the drainage chamber. (Stripping greatly increases the negative pressure applied to the pleural space and can cause tissue damage, bleeding, and pain.)

7. Document system function, including time initiated/ discontinued, type and amount of drainage, patient respiratory status, details related to chest dressing, and appearance of the tube insertion site.
8. Notes for safety:
   - Maintain all connections in the system to prevent inadvertent entrance of air into the patient's pleural space.
   - Keep drainage unit below chest level.
   - If drainage system is turned over or water seal disrupted: re-establish water seal, assess the patient's condition, and encourage coughing and deep breathing. If secretions were present in the disrupted system, obtain a new system.
   - If the drainage system is broken and no new drainage system is immediately available, place the end of the chest tube in a bottle of saline or water and place the bottle below chest level, encourage the patient to cough and deep breathe, obtain a new drainage system, and attach it to the patient's chest tube.
   - During system change, prevent tension pneumothorax (air enters the pleural space without a route to escape) by clamping tube for only a very brief period.

COLOSTOMY CARE

1. Gather equipment.
2. Place the patient in supine position.
3. Wash hands.
4. Don gloves.
5. Remove old pouch by grasping pouch and gently pulling away from skin. (You may use warm water or an adhesive solvent to loosen the seal.)

6. Discard gloves.
7. Wash hands and don new pair of gloves.
8. Gently wash stoma area with warm, soapy water.
9. Dry skin thoroughly.
10. Assess (and document after procedure):
    Stoma: Appearance
    Peristomal skin: Condition
    Feces: Amount, color, consistency, and presence of unusual odor
    Emotional status
11. Temporarily cover stoma with a gauze pad to absorb drainage during ostomy care.
12. Apply skin prep in a circular motion. (Allow to air dry for approximately 30 seconds.)
13. Apply skin barrier in a circular motion.
14. Measure stoma using a stoma guide.
15. Cut ring to size.
16. Moisten ring with warm water and rub it until sticky, or remove paper backing from adhesive-backed ring.
17. Center ring over the stoma, gently pressing it to the skin. (Smooth out any wrinkles to prevent seepage of effluent.)
18. Center faceplate of bag over stoma and gently press down until completely closed.
19. Document procedure and assessments from step 10 (above):

> Example: Colostomy bag changed, stoma pink, peristomal skin intact without signs of irritation. 70 mL of liquid greenish stool discarded with old colostomy bag. Patient looked away during procedure and appeared to ignore nurse's verbal communication.

COLOSTOMY IRRIGATION

1. Explain procedure to the patient and encourage participation.
2. Position in a side-lying position or sitting on the toilet in bathroom if bed rest is not necessary.
3. Place bedpan on top of a disposable pad beneath stoma (if patient is in bed).

4. Fill solution bag with prescribed type and amount of irrigating solution, expelling air from irrigating tube prior to insertion.
5. Hang solution bag 12 to 18 inches above the stoma.
6. Don gloves.
7. Remove stoma appliance.
8. Place irrigation drainage sleeve over the stoma, attaching it snugly to prevent seepage of fluid onto the skin.
9. Place opposite end of drainage sleeve into bedpan or toilet.
10. Dilate stoma, if ordered, by gently inserting the lubricated tip of gloved fifth finger into stoma (use a massaging motion to relax the intestinal muscle until maximum dilation is accomplished).
11. Lubricate tip of stoma cone or catheter.
12. Insert stoma cone or catheter by using a rotating motion until it fits snugly (about 3 inches). Do not insert against resistance.
13. Open tubing clamp, allowing irrigating solution to flow into the bowel slowly. (If cramping occurs, stop flow until cramps subside.)
14. After instillation of fluid, remove cone or catheter, and allow colon to empty.
15. Gently massage the abdomen to encourage emptying of colon (usually takes up to half an hour).
16. Empty and remove irrigation sleeve.
17. Discard old gloves and don new pair.
18. Clean area around stoma.
19. Apply colostomy appliance.
20. Wash hands.
21. Document type and amount of irrigation solution instilled; size, color, and consistency of returned solution; patient response; and complications.

Example: Colostomy irrigated with ——mL NS. Solution returned with moderate amount loose, greenish fecal material. No complaints during procedure. States she irrigates colostomy once a day at home.

DRESSING CHANGE, STERILE

1. Explain procedure to the patient.
2. Wash hands.
3. Place bedside table near the area to be dressed.
4. Gather supplies and place on bedside table.
5. Place a disposable cuffed bag within reach of the work area.
6. Position and drape the patient in a comfortable position, exposing the area to be dressed.
7. Open sterile gloves and retain the inside of the glove package for use as a sterile field.
8. Open sterile gauze pads and all supplies needed, and drop them onto the sterile field.
9. Open the prescribed cleansing agents and pour onto at least two gauze pads.
10. Don nonsterile gloves.
11. Place a towel or waterproof pad under wound area.
12. Remove tape and soiled dressing (soak dressing in sterile saline if it adheres to wound), noting the appearance of the wound, drain placement (if any), suture or skin closure integrity; and amount, color, and consistency of the drainage on the dressing.
13. Discard the dressing in a cuffed trash bag.
14. Remove and place gloves into the trash bag.
15. Wash hands.
16. Don sterile gloves.
17. Use gauze pads (which may be lifted with sterile forceps) to cleanse the wound with prescribed antiseptic solution. Cleanse the wound from the center outward, using a new gauze pad for each outward motion.

    NOTE: Iodine solutions may cause skin irritation if they are left on the skin between dressing changes.

18. Discard used gauze pads into the cuffed bag, away from the sterile field.
19. Apply sterile dressings to the incision or wound site one at a time. (If a drain is present, use a precut dressing to fit around the drain.)
20. Apply ABD pad if needed. (The blue line down the middle of the pad marks the outside surface.)

NOTE: "Wet-to-dry dressing change" describes the technique of applying several layers (the number of layers depends on the size of the wound area and the patient) of saline-soaked dressings next to the wound and covering these with dry dressings.

21. Apply tape over the dressing or secure it with Montgomery ties.
22. Discard supplies and used gloves into a trash bag.
23. Wash hands.
24. Document observations of the wound, dressing, drainage, dressing change, and patient response.

> _Example_: Abdominal dressing changed. Small amount serosanguineous drainage on old dressing. Wound cleansed with H_2O_2. Wound edges approximated well.

ENEMA ADMINISTRATION

1. Explain procedure to the patient.
2. Provide privacy.
3. Gather all equipment.
4. Position the patient in left side-lying position with the right knee flexed (dorsal recumbent position for infants and small children).
5. Place waterproof pad under the patient's hips and buttocks, and drape to expose anal area only.
6. Prepare the solution as ordered.
7. Lubricate 2 inches of rectal tube to facilitate insertion.
8. Open the clamp to allow solution to run through and expel air from tubing. Reclamp tubing.
9. Place a bedpan near the bedside.
10. Don gloves.
11. Instruct the patient to take slow deep breaths to facilitate relaxation.
12. Separate the buttocks and insert rectal tube, directing it toward the umbilicus about 3 to 4 inches.
13. Raise the enema container about 12 to 18 inches above the rectum and open the regulating clamp.
14. Administer the fluid slowly.
15. Lower the container or clamp the tubing if the patient experiences cramping.

16. After the solution is instilled, close the clamp and remove the rectal tube.
17. Instruct the patient to retain solution as long as possible (5 to 10 minutes for cleansing enema, 30 minutes for retention enema).
18. Assist the patient to the bathroom or position him or her on the bedpan.
19. Discard equipment.
20. Remove gloves and wash hands.
21. Document the type and amount of enema solution administered; approximate amount, color, and consistency of expelled material; and patient response.

> Example: Positioned on left side, NS enema, 500 mL given. Lg. amt. formed brown stool returned with enema solution. Complained of abdominal cramping during procedure. Quietly watching TV following procedure.

PEDIATRIC ADAPTATION

The amount of enema solution used for infants and small children ideally is ordered by the physician. Caution should be used if it is necessary to give an enema to a premature or low-birth-weight infant. A 5- to 10-mL syringe attached to a number 5 feeding tube can be used for the procedure. Solutions may usually be given to other children as follows:

Age	*Amount of Solution*	*Tube Insertion*
Infant	100 mL	1 in
2–4 yr	200 mL	2 in
4–10 yr	200–400 mL	3 in
Over 10 yr	500 mL	3 in

INFECTION CONTROL HIGHLIGHTS

Infection control highlights are based on the "universal precautions" issued by the Centers for Disease Control (CDC).

1. Wash hands thoroughly with warm water and soap:

- Immediately if contaminated with blood or other body fluids.
- Immediately after gloves are removed.
- Between patients.

2. Wear gloves:
   - When touching blood and body fluids.
   - If you have cuts, scratches, or other breaks in the skin.
   - When contamination with blood may occur.
   - During phlebotomy techniques.
3. Change gloves between patient contacts.
4. Wear a mask and protective eyewear or face shield to protect yourself during procedures likely to generate droplets of blood or other body fluids.
5. Wear a disposable gown during procedures likely to generate splatters of blood or other body fluids.
6. Equipment that may come in contact with body fluids should be discarded or, if reusable, thoroughly cleaned and disinfected after each use.
7. Discard used needle-syringes (uncapped and unbroken) and other sharp items in puncture-resistant containers for disposal.
8. Place all linen soiled with blood or other body fluids in leakage-resistant bags.
9. Place all specimens of blood and other body fluids in containers with secure lids to prevent leakage during transport. (Avoid contaminating the outside of the container when collecting specimens.)
10. Use a chemical germicide approved for use as a hospital disinfectant or a solution of household bleach (1 : 1000 dilution) to decontaminate work surfaces after blood or other body fluid spills.
11. Pour suctioned fluids, excretions containing blood, and secretions down a drain that is connected to a sanitary sewer.

NASOGASTRIC TUBE INSERTION

1. Gather the necessary equipment.
2. Explain procedure to the patient.
3. Wash hands.
4. Position the patient in a sitting position.

5. Check nostrils for patency by asking the patient to breathe through one naris while occluding the other.
6. Measure length of NG tubing to be inserted by measuring the distance from tip of nose to ear-lobe and from ear-lobe to about 1 inch beyond base of xiphoid process. Use a small strip of adhesive tape to mark the measured distance on the tube.
7. Don gloves and lubricate tube in water or a water-soluble lubricant. (*Never use mineral oil or petroleum jelly.*)
8. Ask the patient to tilt his or her head backward, and gently advance the NG tube into an unobstructed nostril; direct tube toward back of throat and down.
9. As the tube approaches the nasopharynx, ask the patient to flex head toward chest (to close the trachea) and allow him or her to swallow sips of water or ice chips as the tube is advanced into the esophagus (about 3 to 5 inches each time the patient swallows).

   NOTE: If the patient coughs or gags, check the mouth and oropharynx. If the tube is curled in the mouth or throat, withdraw the tube to the pharynx and repeat attempt to insert the tube.

10. Ask the patient to continue swallowing until the tube reaches the premeasured mark.
11. Check for proper tube placement in the stomach by aspirating with a syringe for gastric drainage or by instilling about 20 mL of air into the NG tube while listening with a stethoscope for a gurgling sound over the stomach.
12. Secure the tube after checking for proper placement by cutting a 3-inch strip of 1-inch tape and then splitting the tape lengthwise at one end, leaving 1 inch intact at the opposite end (Fig. 1–31).
13. Place the intact end of the tape on top of the patient's nose, and wrap one side of the split tape end around the tube and secure on a nostril. Repeat with the other split tape end.
14. Connect the NG tube to suction if ordered, or clamp.

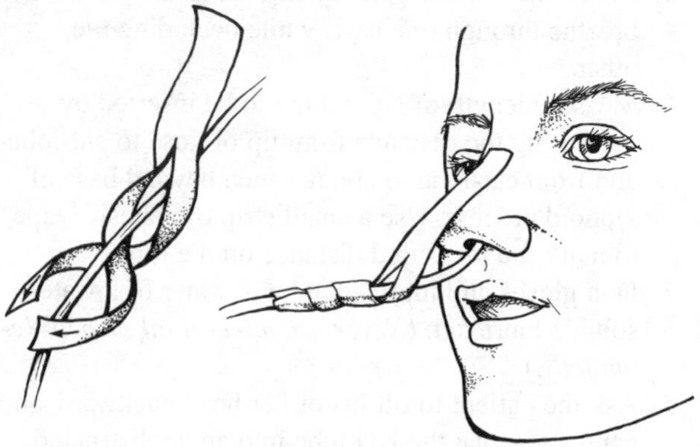

Figure 1–31. Nasogastric tube insertion; method of securing tube with tape.

15. Wrap adhesive tape around the distal end of the tubing and attach a safety pin through the tape tab to the patient's gown.
16. Document the size and type of tube inserted. Note the nostril used and the patient's tolerance of the procedure. Document how placement was validated and whether tubing was left clamped or attached to other equipment.

> _Example_: Number 10 NG tube placed per R naris and secured with tape. Procedure tolerated well. Tube placement validated by auscultation while instilling air into stomach. Distal tubing clamped.

PEDIATRIC ADAPTATION

Infant

Follow adult procedure with these adaptations:

1. Sharply bend NG tube about 1/4 to 1/2 inch from tip. (There is a sharp bend "downward" almost immediately after insertion of tube into the nostril.)
2. Flex the infant's head gently onto the chest with your nondominant hand.

3. With the dominant hand, insert the tube using a downward motion almost immediately after the tube enters the nostril.
4. Because the infant's chest is small and sounds are conducted throughout the chest and abdomen, auscultation of sounds may give a false impression of placement. Other standard methods of placement validation may be used. A sensitive method of placement validation for the infant is to place your hand flat over the stomach area while forcing 2 to 3 mL of air through the tube. Vibrations that reveal the location of the tube tip can usually be felt through the abdominal wall.

Toddler or Preschooler

1. Demonstrate the procedure on a doll.
2. One or two additional people are usually needed to help restrain the child. The parent should not be asked to assist with child restraint.

TUBE FEEDING: NASOGASTRIC, NASODUODENAL, OR GASTROSTOMY (INCLUDING PEG)

INTERMITTENT (BOLUS) TUBE FEEDING

1. Explain procedure to the patient.
2. Assist the patient to a normal position for eating; if patient cannot tolerate this position or it is contraindicated, raise head of bed at least 30 degrees.
3. Wash hands, don gloves, and organize supplies.
4. Verify gastric tube placement by aspirating gastric contents and checking its pH level (this may be difficult with small-bore duodenal tubes); or quickly instill 20 ml air into the tube while auscultating for gurgling sound over the gastric area. See pediatric adaptation above for information regarding validation of pediatric tube placement.
5. Aspirate and measure gastric residual and reinstill contents through tube; check physician's orders or follow unit policy regarding residual as the

determinant of whether to administer or avoid feeding (commonly held if residual greater than 100 mL); if feeding held due to excess gastric residual, turn patient on right side and recheck residual in 30 to 60 minutes.

6. Prepare dietary formula; formula should be at room temperature to prevent gastrointestinal muscle cramping.
7. Place syringe barrel (with plunger removed) into the end of the tube and slowly pour formula into the barrel until it is almost full; regulate formula administration rate by adjusting the height of the syringe (typically held 6 to 8 inches above tube insertion site). **Allow formula to flow slowly by gravity.** Continue to add formula to the syringe barrel until feeding is complete; to prevent entrance of air into the stomach, do not allow the syringe to completely empty.
8. Follow the feeding with water as ordered or 30 to 50 ml to flush the tube.
9. Clamp the tube and maintain elevation of the head of the bed at least 30 degrees for 30 to 60 minutes following feeding to prevent aspiration.
10. Clean or dispose of equipment appropriately.
11. Wash hands.
12. Related Care:
    - After checking residual between bolus feedings, follow by using water to clear the tubing unless contraindicated (i.e., patient on restricted fluids or with electrolyte imbalance).
    - Monitor bowel sounds, bowel regularity, and hydration on any patient receiving tube feedings.
13. Document tube placement, gastric residual check, type and amount of feeding, and patient tolerance.

> Example: 30 mL cloudy white liquid aspirated and returned through NG tube. Ensure 240 mL given by gravity feeding over 10 minutes, followed by 50 mL water. No movement or other response noted during feeding. Remained with head of bed elevated 30 degrees for 45 minutes after feeding.

CONTINUOUS TUBE FEEDING

The feeding bag is hung on an IV pole about 12 inches above the patient's head if dietary formula is delivered by gravity; the drop factor is regulated to deliver the ordered rate of flow. If using a pump designed for tube feedings, simply hang the bag above the pump.

1. For bolus feeding, follow steps 1 to 6 above.
2. Pour no more than 1 can (240 mL) or approximately 4 hours' volume into the bag (bacterial growth is promoted when formula hangs for prolonged periods at room temperature).
3. Prime the tubing by allowing the formula to run through and expel air; clamp the tube and attach it to the patient's feeding tube.
4. Insert the bag's tubing into the pump mechanism and set pump to deliver appropriate volume; unclamp the tubing and start the pump.
   If using gravity delivery method, calculate the drip rate and regulate manually with the tubing clamp.
5. Maintain elevation of head of bed at least 30 degrees while dietary formula infuses and for 30 to 60 minutes thereafter, if feedings are stopped.
6. Related care:
   - Monitor bowel sounds, bowel regularity, and hydration on any patient receiving tube feedings.
   - Check tube placement at least once per shift.
   - Check gastric residuals every four hours during continuous tube feedings; flush tube with water after checking residuals.
   - Replace bag and tubing every 24 hours or according to agency policy to decrease chance of organism growth and contamination of feeding.

POSITIONING

DORSAL RECUMBENT

- Flat on back with legs flexed at hips and knees
- Feet flat on mattress

FOWLER'S

- Head of bed up 30 to 90 degrees
  - High Fowler's: sitting upright at 90 degrees

    - Semi-Fowler's: head and torso elevated 45 to 60 degrees
    - Low Fowler's: head and torso elevated to 30 degrees
- Knees slightly flexed

KNEE-CHEST
- Prone with weight of upper body supported on flat surface by chest
- Hips and knees flexed to elevate buttocks

LITHOTOMY
- Flat on back with legs flexed 90 degrees at hips and knees
- Feet up in stirrups

PRONE
- Flat on abdomen with knees slightly flexed
- Head turned to side
- Arms flexed at side

SIMS
- Halfway between side lying and prone with bottom knee slightly flexed
- Lower arm behind back
- Upper arm flexed, hand near head

TRENDELENBURG'S
- Head is low with body and legs elevated on an inclined plane

TRENDELENBURG (MODIFIED)
- Head and torso flat with legs elevated

LATERAL RECUMBENT
- Side lying with upper leg flexed at hip and knee
- Lower arm flexed with shoulder positioned to avoid weight of body on shoulder

SUPINE
- Flat on back with body in anatomic alignment

(See Fig. 1–32 for illustrations of these positions.)

POSTOPERATIVE CARE

1. Have all necessary equipment available e.g., IV pole, emesis basin, vital signs monitoring equipment, suction).
2. Assess and maintain patency of airway.
3. Read postoperative orders.

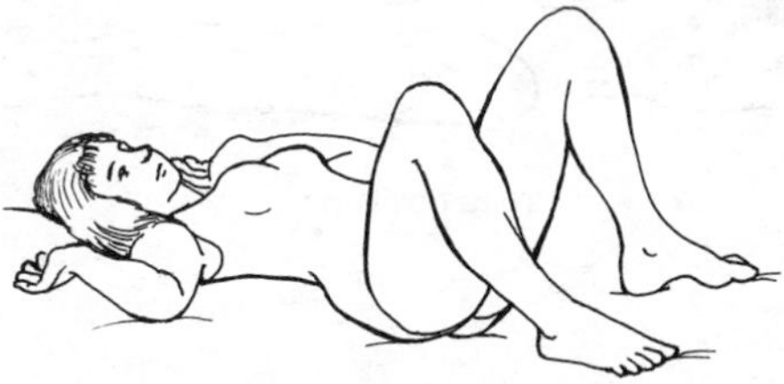

Dorsal recumbent position

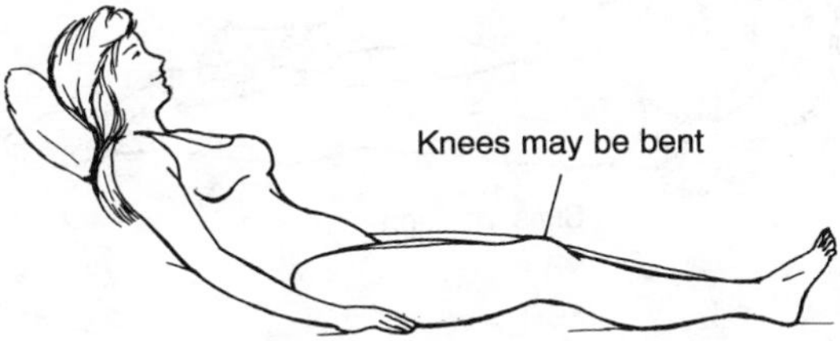

Fowler's position

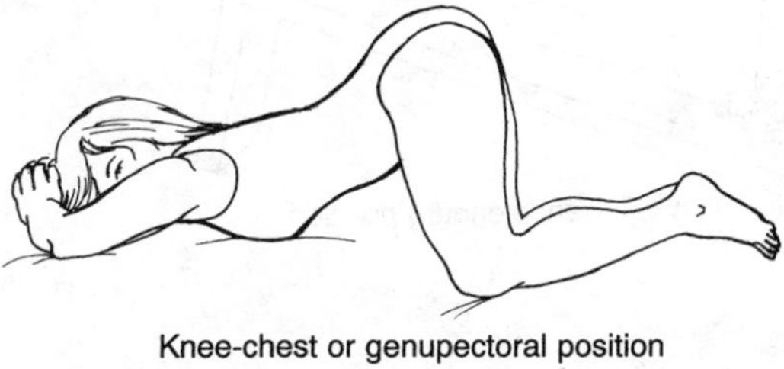

Knee-chest or genupectoral position

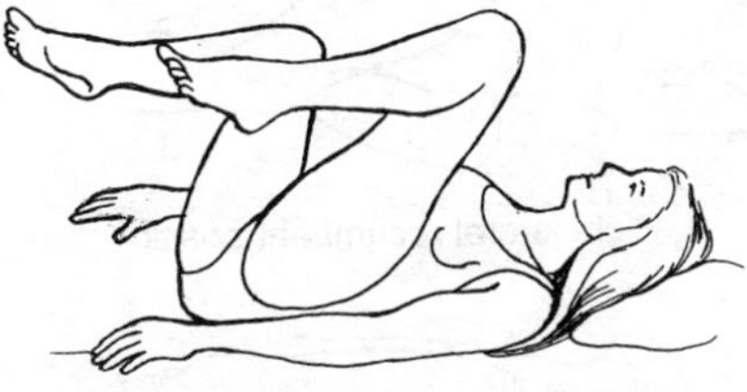

Lithotomy or dorsosacral position

Figure 1–32. Positioning.

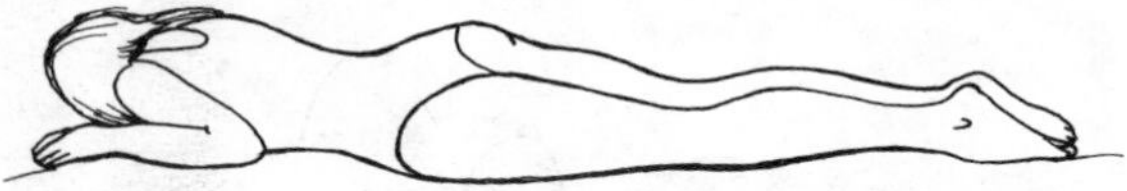

Prone position

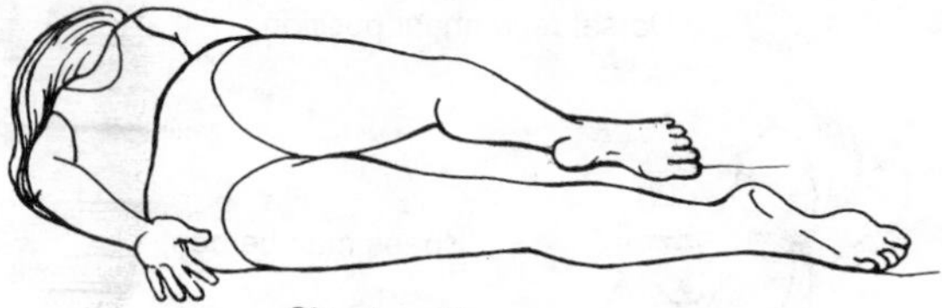

Sims' position

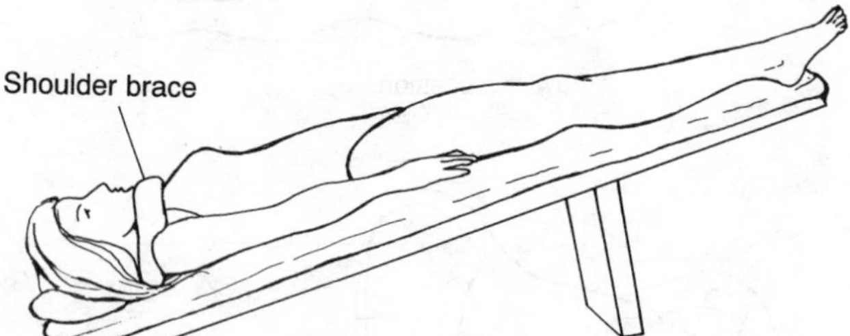

Trendelenburg position

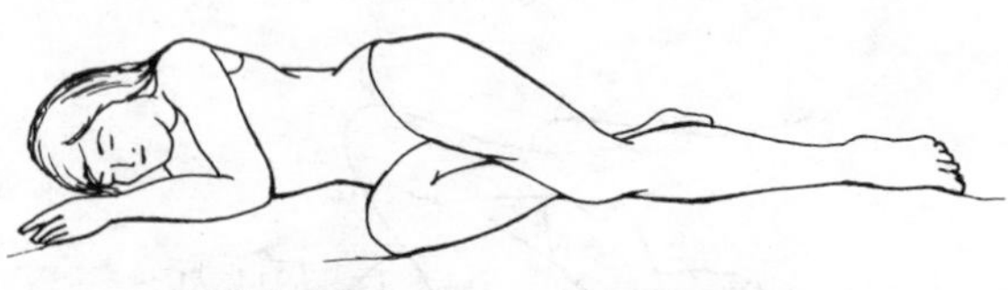

Right lateral recumbent position

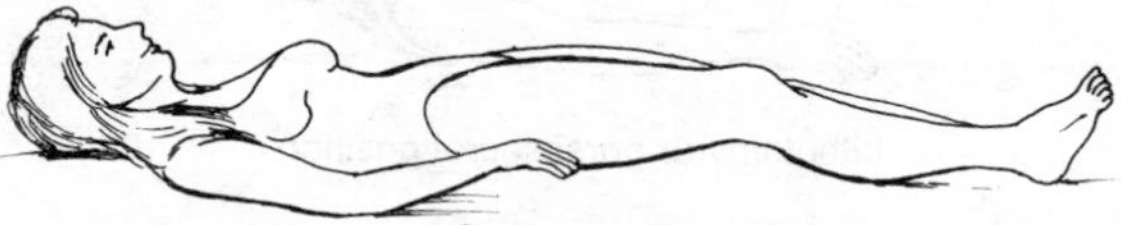

Supine position

Figure 1–32. (continued)

4. Explain treatment or procedures to the patient (even if patient is unconscious).
5. Assess TPR, BP, and LOC every 15 minutes until stable.
6. Monitor I&O (IV fluids, urinary output, and all drains and tubes).
7. Assess surgical site for abnormal drainage or bleeding.
8. Encourage the patient to cough, deep breathe, and turn in bed.
9. Assess pain and provide analgesics as ordered.
10. Document assessment, I&O, behavior, complications, medications given, and patient response.

> _Example_: T—98°F axillary. Apical pulse—98, strong and regular. RR—18, unlabored with regular rate. B/P—118/84 in R arm. Lungs clear. Breath sounds audible in all lung fields. CFT immediate. No bowel sounds heard. No drainage visible on abdominal dressing. Back dry. Responds to verbal stimuli by briefly opening eyes. Moves arms and legs spontaneously. IV of D5NS delivering at 90 mL/hr. No redness or swelling at IV site in L forearm. 250 mL clear light yellow urine in Foley catheter bag.

PREOPERATIVE CARE

1. Remove water pitcher and food from room in accordance with NPO orders. Give the patient instructions and rationale for NPO.
2. Perform or inspect ordered skin prep.
3. Remove nail polish (including toenail polish) and makeup.
4. Place written results of all ordered lab work on chart. If results are not in the chart, contact the lab to obtain results.
5. Complete standard preop list, according to hospital protocol.
6. Prior to administration of preop medications:
   - Ascertain that the patient's surgery-related questions have been answered.

- Teach deep breathing and coughing exercises, and explain the rationale for these actions.
- Make sure that the operative permit has been signed.
- Instruct the patient to void. If he or she is unable to do so, chart the time of the last void. If palpation of bladder, fluid intake (including IV), or time of last void indicates that the bladder may be full, notify the surgeon.
- Assess vital signs. Notify the surgeon if the patient is febrile or if other vital signs vary markedly from the baseline.
- Question the patient regarding the time of last PO intake. Notify the surgeon if intake violates the NPO order.

7. After administering preop meds:
   - Place side rails in the "up" position.
   - Place call bell within the patient's reach.
   - Instruct the patient to stay in bed and to call for assistance if needed.
8. Assess vital signs 15 minutes following the administration of meds.
9. Check to be certain that the preop checklist has been completed.
10. Place addressograph (patient's charge plate) on the chart if hospital policy indicates to do so.

TRACHEOSTOMY SUCTIONING

1. Wash hands.
2. Explain procedure to the patient.
3. Gather equipment.
4. Position the patient in a semi-Fowler's or Fowler's position.
5. Place a towel across the patient's chest.
6. Open sterile irrigation solution.
7. Open suction catheter package.
8. Don sterile gloves. (Only the dominant-hand glove remains sterile throughout the procedure.)
9. Unfold sterile cup.
10. With nondominant hand, pour the sterile irrigation solution into the sterile cup. (The nondominant hand is now contaminated.)

11. With dominant hand, remove the sterile catheter from its wrapper, keeping it coiled.
12. Grasp nonsterile suction tubing in your nondominant hand.
13. Connect suction control port of the suction catheter to the suction tubing, making sure to keep the sterile catheter in your dominant hand.
14. Check equipment by suctioning sterile water or saline through the suction catheter.
15. Some authorities advocate hyperoxygenating the patient for 1 to 2 minutes prior to suctioning.
16. Have assistant disconnect oxygen or ventilator attachment from the trach tube and attach a manual resuscitation bag (MRB) with oxygen connected; deliver three to five ventilations.
17. With finger **off** the opening of the suction port, gently insert the suction catheter into the trach tube using a downward motion.
18. Continue insertion to estimated end of the trach tube.

    NOTE: Many nurses insert the suction catheter until coughing is stimulated or resistance is met; this practice, however, is controversial.

19. Place your thumb over the suction port and encourage the patient to cough while you quickly withdraw the catheter in a circular motion, rotating the catheter between your thumb and finger.

    NOTE: To prevent hypoxemia, never suction longer than 12 seconds at a time; for an infant, not over 5 seconds.

20. Have assistant deliver three to five ventilations with the MRB using oxygen at 100%.
21. Listen to breath sounds and repeat procedure if necessary.
22. Reconnect trach collar or ventilator attachment to the trach tube (if applicable).

    NOTE: Always return oxygen flow to prescribed rate after suctioning procedure is completed.

23. Document amount, color, and consistency of secretions suctioned, character of respirations, breath

sounds after suctioning, patient response, and replacement of oxygen source following the procedure.

> *Example*: Lg amt. thick, green secretions suctioned from trach. RR: 16 and unlabored following suctioning. T collar with O_2 @ 2 L/min replaced to trach. Lungs clear to auscultation following suctioning. Lips and nail beds pink. SaO_2 97%.

VITAL SIGNS

WHEN TO ASSESS

- On admission
- When change in health status occurs
- As ordered
- When chest pains or any abnormal sensations occur
- Before and after administration of preoperative medications
- After surgery or invasive diagnostic procedures
- Before and after administration of blood or medications that could affect the cardiovascular or respiratory system
- Before and after any nursing intervention that may affect the cardiovascular or respiratory system

TEMPERATURE ASSESSMENT

1. Determine whether the patient has consumed any hot or cold food or fluid or has smoked within the last 30 minutes.
2. Wash hands.
3. Don gloves.
4. Electronic temperature devices are appropriate for all temperature assessments. Follow the manufacturer's instructions for use of equipment.
5. Position the patient appropriately:
   - Axillary: Expose axilla.
   - Rectal: Lateral or prone position.
6. Slide the cover over the temperature probe until it snaps into place.

7. Insert the covered thermometer probe:
   - Oral:
     - Place probe at the base of the tongue to the right or left of the frenulum.
     - Have patient close lips around the probe.
   - Axillary:
     - Use patting motion to dry axilla with a towel.
     - Place probe in axilla and hold patient's arm across the chest or to the side to secure the probe.
   - Rectal: Don gloves and lubricate probe; separate buttocks and ask the patient to take a deep breath; insert the probe past the outer rectal sphincter (adult: 1.5 inches; young child: about 0.5 inch).
   - Tympanic:
     - Some devices must be turned on and used only after the "ready" signal appears or a "beep" sounds.
     - Insert probe snugly into the external canal of the ear toward the tympanic membrane (straighten the ear canal of the adult by pulling the pinna of the ear up and back and of the child under age 3 years by pulling the pinna down and back).
8. Listen for the sound indicating that the temperature measurement is complete.
9. Remove the thermometer and determine the reading. (A reading is provided in 2 to 60 seconds depending on the device used.)
10. Discard the probe cover.
11. Replace the temperature unit in its holder to recharge the battery.
12. Document the temperature and the route by which it was assessed.

Norms

- *Oral*: 37°C
  98.6°F
- *Axillary*: About 1°F or 0.5°C lower than oral
- *Rectal*: About 1°F or 0.5°C higher than oral

PULSE ASSESSMENT

1. Wash hands.
2. Place two to three fingertips lightly over a pulse point.
   Never use the thumb because it has a pulse.

   FOR DOPPLER PULSE ASSESSMENT

   - Place a small amount of gel over a pulse point or directly onto the transducer tip.
   - Turn the volume control until static is audible.
   - Slide the transducer tip over the pulse area until "shooshing" is heard.
3. If the pulse is regular, count for 30 seconds and multiply by 2. If it is irregular, count for 1 minute.
4. Assess the pulse rhythm and volume.
5. Document the pulse rate, rhythm, and volume.

> Example: Radial pulse full & bounding. Rate 90 with regular rhythm.

Pulse Rate: Normal adult pulse rate is between 60 and 100 beats per minute. Fewer than 60 beats per minute is known as *bradycardia*. More than 100 beats per minute is known as *tachycardia*.

Pulse Rhythm: Pulse rhythm is normally regular. Irregular rhythm is known as an *arrhythmia*.

Pulse Volume:

0 = absent
1 = weak and thready
2 = normal
3 = bounding

NOTE: For more information on pulse evaluation and location of pulse points, see assessment section.

RESPIRATIONS ASSESSMENT

1. Observe the rise and fall of the chest. Ensure that the patient is resting quietly and is unaware that the respiratory rate is being assessed.
2. Count respiratory rate for 30 seconds and multiply

by 2 if respirations are regular; if they are irregular, count for a full minute.
3. Observe rhythm and character of respirations.
4. Document the respiratory rate, depth, rhythm, and character.

> Example: RR: 16/min, normal depth, unlabored, regular rhythm.

Norms

- *Adult*: 14–20 breaths/min
- *Pediatric*: See Pediatric Fast Facts, Section 3.

Respiratory Assessment Vocabulary

RATE
- *Eupnea*: Quiet, rhythmic, and effortless
- *Tachypnea*: Rapid, quick, and shallow
- *Bradypnea*: Abnormally slow
- *Apnea*: Cessation

VOLUME
- *Hyperventilation*: Prolonged and deep
- *Hypoventilation*: Shallow
- *Hyperpnea*: Deep or rapid
- *Forced*: Voluntary hyperpnea

RHYTHM
- *Biot's*: Alternating periods of apnea and hyperpnea
- *Cheyne-Stokes*: Very deep to very shallow breathing with periods of apnea
- *Cogwheel*: Interrupted
- *Kussmaul's*: Deep, gasping
- *Periodic*: Uneven rhythm (The term *periodic* is also used to describe normal irregular respirations in the newborn, during which apnea may last up to 15 seconds.)

CHARACTER
- *Abdominal*: Abdomen moves, but chest shows little movement
- *Diaphragmatic*: Same as abdominal
- *Dyspnea*: Labored or difficult
- *Labored*: Dyspneic or difficult (Patient appears to "work" at breathing.)

- *Relaxed*: Normal
- *Sonorous*: Loud, low-pitched sound
- *Stertorous*: Rattling or bubbling sounds
- *Stridulous (stridor)*: High-pitched crowing or barking sound on inspiration

BLOOD PRESSURE ASSESSMENT

1. Make sure the patient has not smoked or ingested caffeine within 30 minutes prior to measurement.
2. Position the patient in a comfortable position with the arm slightly flexed and the palm of the hand facing up with the forearm supported at the level of the heart.
3. Expose the upper arm.
4. Make sure the bladder of the cuff encircles at least $^2/_3$ of the arm and that the width of the cuff covers $^1/_2$ to $^2/_3$ of the upper arm.
5. Apply the center of the cuff bladder directly over the medial aspect of the arm about 1 inch above the antecubital space. (When applied, the cuff must not constrict circulation. Any slack between the cuff and the arm results in an invalid reading.)
6. Palpate the brachial artery with your fingertips, close the valve on the pump (turn it clockwise), and inflate the cuff until you feel the pulsation disappear (note the reading on the gauge; this is the palpated systolic pressure).
7. Insert the tips of the stethoscope into your ears.
8. Palpate the brachial artery with your fingertips and place the stethoscope gently over the artery.
9. Close the valve on the pump.
10. Inflate the cuff to at least 30 mm Hg above the palpated systolic pressure.
11. Slowly release the pressure in the cuff, noting the:
    - Point at which sound is first heard
    - Point at which sound becomes muffled (not always heard)
    - Point at which sound completely ceases

NOTE: There is controversy regarding which of the last two "points" should be recorded as the diastolic read-

ing. The best method of recording validates all sounds that are heard.

Example: 142/96/82 or 142/82, if no muffling of sound is heard

Wait 1 minute before taking further blood pressure measurements in the same arm.

12. Remove the cuff from the patient's arm.
13. Document as in step 11, noting the patient's position during assessment and the extremity in which the pressure was assessed. (Readings can vary markedly with position change and extremity.)

Example: BP—130/76, right arm, supine position.

NORMS

- *Adult*: 120/80.
- *Pediatric*: See Pediatric Fast Facts, Section 3.

Pediatric Adaptation

Electronic equipment such as the Doppler or Dynamap is most accurate for BP assessment in the infant or young child. If no such equipment is available and no sounds are audible through the stethoscope, the palpation method of assessment is used. (It is common to hear sounds down to "0" mm Hg in infants when a standard stethoscope is used.)

Recommended Adult Immunization Schedule, United States, by Age Group and Medical Conditions, 2003–2004 (Approved by the Advisory Committee on Immunization Practices [ACIP], and accepted by the American College of Obstetricians and Gynecologists [ACOG] and the American Academy of Family Physicians [AAFP])

Age Group ▶ / Vaccine ▼	19–49 Years	50–64 Years	65 Years and Older
Tetanus, Diphtheria (Td)*	**1 dose booster every 10 years[1]**		
Influenza	1 dose annually[2]	**1 dose annually[2]**	
Pneumococcal (polysaccharide)	1 dose[3,4]		**1 dose[3,4]**
Hepatitis B*	3 doses (0, 1–2, 4–6 months)[5]		
Hepatitis A	2 doses (0, 6–12 months)[6]		

Legend: ☐ *For all persons in this group* ■ (dark) *Catch-up on childhood vaccinations* ■ (light) *For persons with medical/exposure indications*

Measles, Mumps, Rubella (MMR)*	1 dose if measles, mumps, or rubella vaccination history is unreliable; 2 doses for persons with occupational or other indications[7]		
Varicella*	2 doses (0, 4–8 weeks) for persons who are susceptible[8]		
Meningococcal (polysaccharide)	1 dose[9]		

*Covered by the Vaccine Injury Compensation Program. For information on how to file a claim call 800-338-2382. Please also visit www.hrsa.gov/osp/vicp To file a claim for vaccine injury contact: U.S. Court of Federal Claims, 717 Madison Place, N.W., Washington D.C.20005, 202-219-9657.

This schedule indicates the recommended age groups for routine administration of currently licensed vaccines for persons 19 years of age and older. Licensed combination vaccines may be used whenever any components of the combination are indicated and the vaccine's other components are not contraindicated. Providers should consult the manufacturers' package inserts for detailed recommendations.

Report all clinically significant post-vaccination reactions to the Vaccine Adverse Event Reporting System (VAERS). Reporting forms and instructions on filing a VAERS report are available by calling 800-822-7967 or from the VAERS website at www.vaers.org.

For additional information about the vaccines listed above and contraindications for immunization, visit the National Immunization Program Website at www.cdc.gov/nip/ or call the National Immunization Hotline at 800-232-2522 (English) or 800-232-0233 (Spanish).

(*continued on the following page*)

1. **Tetanus and diphtheria (Td)**—Adults including pregnant women with uncertain histories of a complete primary vaccination series should receive a primary series of Td. A primary series for adults is 3 doses: the first 2 doses given at least 4 weeks apart and the 3rd dose, 6–12 months after the second. Administer 1 dose if the person had received the primary series and the last vaccination was 10 years ago or longer. Consult *MMWR* 1991; 40 (RR-10): 1–21 for administering Td as prophylaxis in wound management. The ACP Task Force on Adult Immunization supports a second option for Td use in adults: a single Td booster at age 50 years for persons who have completed the full pediatric series, including the teenage/young adult booster.
   Guide for Adult Immunization. 3rd ed. ACP 1994:20.
2. **Influenza vaccination**—Medical indications: chronic disorders of the cardiovascular or pulmonary system including asthma; chronic metabolic diseases including diabetes mellitus, renal dysfunction, hemoglobinopathies, or immunosuppression (including immunosuppression caused by medications or by human immunodeficiency virus [HIV]), requiring regular medical follow-up or hospitalization during the preceding year; women who will be in the second or third trimester of pregnancy during the influenza season. Occupational indications: health-care workers. Other indications: residents of nursing homes and other long-term care facilities; persons likely to transmit influenza to persons at high risk (in-home care givers to persons with medical indications, household contacts and out-of-home caregivers of children birth to 23 months of age, or children with asthma or other indicator conditions for influenza vaccination, household members and care givers of elderly and adults with high-risk conditions); and anyone who wishes to be vaccinated. For healthy persons aged 5–49 years without high-risk conditions, either the inactivated vaccine or the intranasally administered influenza vaccine (Flumist) may be given.
   MMWR 2003; 52 (RR-8): 1–36; *MMWR* 2003;53 (RR-13): 1–8.
3. **Pneumococcal polysaccharide vaccination**—Medical indications: chronic disorders of the pulmonary system (excluding asthma), cardiovascular diseases, diabetes mellitus, chronic liver diseases including liver disease as a result of alcohol abuse (e.g., cirrhosis), chronic renal failure or nephrotic syndrome, functional or anatomic asplenia (e.g., sickle cell disease or splenectomy), immunosuppressive conditions (e.g., congenital immunodeficiency, HIV infection, leukemia, lymphoma, multiple myeloma, Hodgkin disease, generalized malignancy, organ or bone marrow transplantation), chemotherapy with alkylating agents, antimetabolites, or long-term systemic corticosteroids. Geographic/other indications: Alaskan natives and certain American Indian populations. Other indications: residents of nursing homes and other long-term care facilities.
   MMWR 1997; 46 (RR-8): 1–24.

(continued on the following page)

4. **Revaccination with pneumococcal polysaccharide vaccine**—One-time revaccination after 5 years for persons with chronic renal failure or nephrotic syndrome, functional or anatomic asplenia (e.g., sickle cell disease or splenectomy), immunosuppressive conditions (e.g., congenital immunodeficiency, HIV infection, leukemia, lymphoma, multiple myeloma, Hodgkin's disease, generalized malignancy, organ or bone marrow transplantation), chemotherapy with alkylating agents, antimetabolites, or long-term systemic corticosteroids. For persons 65 years and older, one-time revaccination if they were vaccinated 5 or more years previously and were aged less than 65 years at the time of primary vaccination. *MMWR* 1997; 46 (RR-8): 1–24.
5. **Hepatitis B vaccination**—Medical indications: hemodialysis patients, patients who receive clotting-factor concentrates. Occupational indications: health-care workers and public-safety workers who have exposure to blood in the workplace, persons in training in schools of medicine, dentistry, nursing, laboratory technology, and other allied health professions. Behavioral indications: injecting drug users, persons with more than one sex partner in the previous 6 months, persons with a recently acquired sexually transmitted disease (STD), all clients in STD clinics, men who have sex with men. Other indications: household contacts and sex partners of persons with chronic HBV infection, clients and staff of institutions for the developmentally disabled, international travelers who will be in countries with high or intermediate prevalence of chronic HBV infection for more than 6 months, inmates of correctional facilities. *MMWR* 1991; 40 (RR-13): 1–19.
(www.cdc.gov/travel/diseases/hbv.htm)
6. **Hepatitis A vaccination**—For the combined HepA-HepB vaccine use 3 doses at 0, 1, 6 months). Medical indications: persons with clotting-factor disorders or chronic liver disease. Behavioral indications: men who have sex with men, users of injecting and noninjecting illegal drugs. Occupational indications: persons working with HAV-infected primates or with HAV in a research laboratory setting. Other indications: persons traveling to or working in countries that have high or intermediate endemicity of hepatitis A.
MMWR 1999; 48 (RR-12): 1–37. (www.cdc.gov/travel/diseases/hav.htm)
7. **Measles, Mumps, Rubella vaccination (MMR)**—Measles component: adults born before 1957 may be considered immune to measles. Adults born in or after 1957 should receive at least one dose of MMR unless they have a medical contraindication, documentation of at least 1 dose or other acceptable evidence of immunity. A 2nd dose of MMR is recommended for adults who:
   - Were recently exposed to measles or in an outbreak setting
   - Were previously vaccinated with killed measles vaccine
   - Were vaccinated with an unknown vaccine between 1963 and 1967

(*continued on the following page*)

- Are students in post–secondary educational institutions
- Work in health care facilities
- Plan to travel internationally

Mumps component: 1 dose of MMR should be adequate for protection. Rubella component: give 1 dose of MMR to women whose rubella vaccination history is unreliable and counsel women to avoid becoming pregnant for 4 weeks after vaccination. For women of child-bearing age, regardless of birth year, routinely determine rubella immunity and counsel women regarding congenital rubella syndrome. Do not vaccinate pregnant women or those planning to become pregnant in the next 4 weeks. If pregnant and susceptible, vaccinate as early in postpartum period as possible.

MMWR 1998; 47 (RR-8): 1–57; *MMWR* 2001; 50: 1117.

8. **Varicella vaccination**—Recommended for all persons who do not have reliable clinical history of varicella infection, or serological evidence of varicella zoster virus (VZV) infection who may be at high risk for exposure or transmission. This includes health-care workers and family contacts of immunocompromised persons, those who live or work in environments where transmission is likely (e.g., teachers of young children, day care employees, and residents and staff members in institutional settings), persons who live or work in environments where VZV transmission can occur (e.g., college students, inmates and staff members of correctional institutions, and military personnel), adolescents and adults living in households with children, women who are not pregnant but who may become pregnant in the future, international travelers who are not immune to infection. Note: Greater than 95% of U.S. born adults are immune to VZV. Do not vaccinate pregnant women or those planning to become pregnant in the next 4 weeks. If pregnant and susceptible, vaccinate as early in postpartum period as possible.

   MMWR 1996; 45 (RR-11): 1–36; *MMWR* 1999; 48 (RR-6): 1–5.
9. **Meningococcal vaccine (quadrivalent polysaccharide for serogroups A, C, Y, and W-135)**—Consider vaccination for persons with medical indications: adults with terminal complement component deficiencies, with anatomic or functional asplenia. Other indications: travelers to countries in which disease is hyperendemic or epidemic ("meningitis belt" of sub-Saharan Africa, Mecca, Saudi Arabia for Hajj). Revaccination at 3–5 years may be indicated for persons at high risk for infection (e.g., persons residing in areas in which disease is epidemic). Counsel college freshmen, especially those who live in dormitories, regarding meningococcal disease and the vaccine so that they can make an educated decision about receiving the vaccination. *MMWR* 2000; 49 (RR-7): 1–20.

Note: The AAFP recommends that colleges should take the lead in providing education about meningococcal infection and vaccination and offer it to those who are interested. Physicians need not initiate discussion of the meningococcal quadravalent polysaccharide vaccine as part of routine medical care.

Table 1–9. METHOD OF TRANSMISSION OF SOME COMMON COMMUNICABLE DISEASES

Disease	How Agent Leaves the Bodies of the Sick	How Organisms May Be Transmitted	Method of Entry into the Body
Acquired immunodeficiency syndrome (AIDS)	Blood, semen, or other body fluids, including breast milk	Sexual contact Contact with blood or mucous membranes or by way of contaminated syringes Placental transmission	Reproductive tract Contact with blood Placental transmission Breast-feeding
Cholera	Feces	Water or food contaminated with feces	Mouth to intestine
Diphtheria	Sputum and discharges from nose and throat Skin lesions (rare)	Droplet infection from patient coughing	Through mouth or nose to throat

(continued on the following page)

Table 1–9. METHOD OF TRANSMISSION OF SOME COMMON COMMUNICABLE DISEASES (continued)

Disease	How Agent Leaves the Bodies of the Sick	How Organisms May Be Transmitted	Method of Entry into the Body
Gonococcal disease	Lesions Discharges from infected mucous membranes	Sexual activity Hands of infected persons soiled with their own discharges	Reproductive tract or any mucous membrane
Hepatitis A, viral	Feces	Food or water contaminated with feces	Mouth to intestine
Hepatitis B, viral and delta hepatitis	Blood and serum-derived fluids, including semen and vaginal fluids	Contact with blood and body fluids	Exposure to body fluids including during sexual activity Contact with blood

Hepatitis C	Blood and other body fluids	Parenteral drug use Laboratory exposure to blood Health care workers exposed to blood (i.e., dentists and their assistants, and clinical and laboratory staff)	Infected blood Contaminated needles
Hookworm	Feces	Cutaneous contact with soil polluted with feces Eggs in feces hatch in sandy soil	Larvae enter through skin (esp. of feet), migrate through the body, and settle in small intestine
Influenza	As in pneumonia	Respiratory droplets or objects contaminated with discharges	As in pneumonia
Leprosy	Cutaneous or mucosal lesions that contain bacilli Respiratory droplets	Cutaneous contact or nasal discharges of untreated patients	Nose or broken skin

(continued on the following page)

Table 1–9. METHOD OF TRANSMISSION OF SOME COMMON COMMUNICABLE DISEASES (continued)

Disease	How Agent Leaves the Bodies of the Sick	How Organisms May Be Transmitted	Method of Entry into the Body
Measles (rubeola)	As in streptococcal pharyngitis	As in streptococcal pharyngitis	As in streptococcal pharyngitis
Meningitis, meningococcal	Discharges from nose and throat	Respiratory droplets	Mouth and nose
Mumps	Discharges from infected glands and mouth	Respiratory droplets and saliva	Mouth and nose
Ophthalmia neonatorum (gonococcal infection of eyes of newborn)	Vaginal secretions of infected mother	Contact with infected areas of vagina of infected mother during birth	Directly on conjunctiva
Pertussis	Discharges from respiratory tract	Respiratory droplets	Mouth and nose

Pneumonia	Sputum and discharges from nose and throat	Respiratory droplets	Through mouth and nose to lungs
Poliomyelitis	Discharges from nose and throat, and via feces	Respiratory droplets Contaminated water	Through mouth and nose
Rubella	As in streptococcal pharyngitis	As in streptococcal pharyngitis	As in streptococcal pharyngitis
Streptococcal pharyngitis	Discharges from nose and throat	Respiratory droplets	Through mouth and nose
Syphilis	Lesions Blood Transfer through placenta to fetus	Kissing or sexual intercourse Contaminated needles and syringes	Directly into blood and tissues through breaks in skin or membrane Contaminated needles and syringes

(continued on the following page)

Table 1–9. METHOD OF TRANSMISSION OF SOME COMMON COMMUNICABLE DISEASES (continued)

Disease	How Agent Leaves the Bodies of the Sick	How Organisms May Be Transmitted	Method of Entry into the Body
Trachoma	Discharges from infected eyes	Cutaneous contact Hands, towels, handkerchiefs	Directly on conjunctiva
Tuberculosis, bovine		Milk from infected cow	Mouth to intestine
Tuberculosis, human	Sputum Lesions Feces	Droplet infection from person coughing with mouth uncovered Sputum from mouth to fingers, thence to food and other things	Through nose to lungs or intestines From intestines via lymph channels to lymph vessels and to tissues
Typhoid fever	Feces and urine	Food or water contaminated with feces, or urine from patients	Through mouth via infected food or water and thence to intestinal tract

Source: Thomas, CL (ed): Taber's Cyclopedic Medical Dictionary, ed 18. FA Davis, Philadelphia, 1997, pp 422–423, with permission.

Table 1–10. INCUBATION AND ISOLATION PERIODS IN COMMON INFECTIONS

Infection	Incubation Period	Isolation of Patient
AIDS	Unclear; antibodies appear within 1–3 months of infection	Protective isolation if T-cell count is very low; private room necessary only with severe diarrhea, bleeding, copious blood-tinged sputum if patient has poor personal hygiene habits
Bloodstream (bacteremia, fungemia)	Variable; usually 2–5 days	Contact: private room; gloves and masks; gowns as needed for dealing with drainage or body fluids
Brucellosis	Highly variable, usually 5–21 days; may be months	None
Chickenpox	2–3 weeks	1 week after vesicles appear or until vesicles become dry

(continued on the following page)

Table 1–10. NCUBATION AND ISOLATION PERIODS IN COMMON INFECTIONS (continued)

Infection	Incubation Period	Isolation of Patient
Cholera	A few hours to 5 days	Enteric precautions
Common cold	12 hr–5 days	None
Diphtheria	Usually 2–5 days	Until two cultures from nose and throat, taken at least 24 hr apart, are negative; cultures to be taken after cessation of antibiotic therapy
Dysentery, amebic	From a few days to several months, commonly 2–4 weeks	None
Dysentery, bacillary (shigellosis)	12–96 hr	As long as stools remain positive
Encephalitis, mosquitoborne	5–15 days	None

Giardiasis	3–25 days or longer; median 7–10 days	Enteric precautions
Gonorrhea	2–7 days; may be longer	No sexual contact until cured
Hepatitis A	15–50 days	Enteric (gloves with infected material; gowns as needed to protect clothing)
Hepatitis B	45–180 days	Blood and body fluid precautions (gloves and plastic gowns for contact with infective materials; mask if risk of coughing or sneezing exists)
Hepatitis C	14–180 days	As for hepatitis B
Hepatitis D	2–8 weeks	As for hepatitis B
Hepatitis E	15–64 days	Enteric precautions
Influenza	1–3 days	As practical

(continued on the following page)

Table 1–10. INCUBATION AND ISOLATION PERIODS IN COMMON INFECTIONS (continued)

Infection	Incubation Period	Isolation of Patient
Legionella	2–10 days	None
Lyme disease	3–32 days after tick bite	None
Malaria	7–10 days for *Plasmodium falciparum;* 8–14 days for *P. vivax, P. ovale;* 7–30 days for *P. malariae*	Protection from mosquitoes
Measles (rubeola)	8–13 days from exposure to onset of fever; 14 days until rash appears	From diagnosis to 7 days after appearance of rash; strict isolation from children under 3 years
Meningitis, meningococcal	2–10 days	Until 24 hr after start of chemotherapy
Mononucleosis, infectious	4–6 weeks	None; disinfection of articles soiled with nose and throat discharges

Mumps	12–25 days	Until the glands recede
Paratyphoid fevers	3 days–3 months; usually 1–3 weeks; 1–10 days for gastroenteritis	Until 3 stools are negative
Plague	2–8 days	Strict; danger of airborne spread (pneumonic plague)
Pneumonia, pneumococcal	Believed to be 1–3 days	Enteric precautions in hospital. Respiratory isolation may be required.
Poliomyelitis	3–35 days	1 week from onset
Puerperal fever, streptococcal	1–3 days	Transfer from maternity ward
Rabies	Usually 2–8 weeks; rarely as short as 9 days or as long as 7 years	Strict for duration of illness; danger to attendants

(continued on the following page)

Table 1–10. INCUBATION AND ISOLATION PERIODS IN COMMON INFECTIONS (continued)

Infection	Incubation Period	Isolation of Patient
Rubella (German measles)	16–18 days with range of 14–23 days	None; no contact with nonimmune pregnant women
Salmonellosis	6–72 hr, usually 12–36 hr	Until stool cultures are *Salmonella* free on two consecutive specimens collected in 24-hr period
Scabies	2–6 weeks before onset of itching in patients without previous infections; 1–4 days after re-exposed	Patient is excused from school or work until day after treatment
Scarlet fever	1–3 days	7 days; may be ended in 24 hr
Syphilis	10 days–10 weeks; usually 3 weeks	None; but for hospitalized patients, universal precautions for body secretions

Tetanus	4 days–3 weeks	None
Toxic shock syndrome	Unknown but may be as brief as several hours	None
Trachoma	5–12 days	Until lesions disappear, but usually not practical
Tuberculosis	4–12 weeks to demonstrable primary lesion or significant tuberculin reactions	Variable, depending on conversion of sputum to negative after specific therapy and on ability of patient to understand and carry out personal hygiene methods
Tularemia	2–14 days	None

(continued on the following page)

Table 1–10. INCUBATION AND ISOLATION PERIODS IN COMMON INFECTIONS (continued)

Infection	Incubation Period	Isolation of Patient
Typhoid fever	Usually 1–3 weeks	Until 3 cultures of feces and urine are negative. These should be taken not earlier than 1 month after onset.
Typhus fever	7–14 days	None
Whooping cough	Usually 6–20 days	Respiratory isolation for known cases; for suspected cases, removal from contact with infants and young children

Source: Adapted from Venes, D, and Thomas, CL (eds): Taber's Cyclopedic Medical Dictionary, ed 19. FA Davis, Philadelphia, 2001, p1081–1082, with permission.

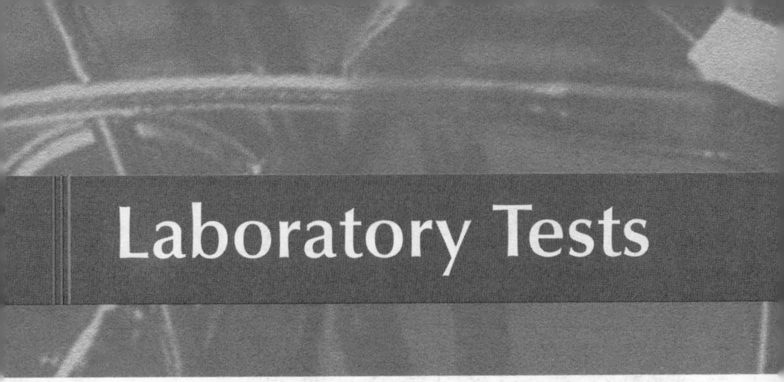

Laboratory Tests

REFERENCE VALUES FOR LABORATORY TESTS (BLOOD OR SERUM) WITH POSSIBLE CAUSES OF INCREASED AND DECREASED VALUES*

It is important to note that, because many tests can be performed by a variety of methods, there can be significant variance in acceptable, or "normal," values. It should also be noted that each lab establishes norms for the population of its geographic area; therefore, when evaluating lab data from individual test(s), norms published by the lab performing the test(s) may generally be considered more accurate than those published here.

Test	*Conventional Units*	*SI Units*	*Causes of Increase*	*Causes of Decrease*
Alanine aminotransferase (ALT or SGPT)	4–36 U/L (varies by method)	0.07–0.6 μkat/L	Liver disorders, muscular dystrophy, muscular trauma, MI, CHF, renal failure, mono, burns, shock, alcohol, numerous meds	Exercise, salicylates

Albumin	3.5–5.0 g/dL or 52–68% of total protein		Dehydration, exercise, meds, prolonged application of tourniquet prior to venipuncture	Malnutrition, chronic diseases, liver disorders, SLE, scleroderma, ascites, burns, nephrotic syndrome, chronic renal failure, Hodgkin's disease, meds
Child	4.0–5.8 g/dL			
Alkaline phosphatase (ALP)	20–90 U/L		Bile duct obstruction, liver disorders, healing fractures, pregnancy, growth in children, hyperparathyroidism, Paget's disease	Hypothyroidism, malnutrition, pernicious anemia, placental insufficiency
Child	60–270 U/L			
Infant	40–300 U/L			
Ammonia	15–70 μg/dL	11–32 μmol/L	Liver disorders, GI bleeding, late CHF, COPD, high-protein diet, erythroblastosis fetalis, meds	Renal failure, hypertension, meds
NB	40–120 μg/dL	64–107 μmol/L		
Amylase	4–25 U/mL	1.36–3.0 μkat/L	Pancreatic disorders, morphine, salivary gland inflammation, burns	Chronic pancreatitis, necrosis of liver, chronic alcoholism, toxic hepatitis, IV D_5W
Child	25–125 U/L	1.88–5.03 μkat/L		
NB	Up to 65 U/L			

(continued on the following page)

REFERENCE VALUES FOR LABORATORY TESTS (BLOOD OR SERUM) WITH POSSIBLE CAUSES OF INCREASED AND DECREASED VALUES* (continued)

Test	*Conventional Units*	*SI Units*	*Causes of Increase*	*Causes of Decrease*
Anti-DNA or Anti-DNP	Neg	<2.0 kU/L	SLE or lupus nephritis	
Antinuclear antibodies (ANA)	Neg at 1 : 10 dilution	Negative	SLE, Sjögren's syndrome, scleroderma, hepatitis, rheumatoid arthritis, cirrhosis, ulcerative colitis, leukemia, infectious mono	
Antistreptolysin O titer (ASO)	≤1 : 160		Recent *Streptococcus pyogenes* infection, rheumatic fever	

Aspartate aminotransferase (AST or SGOT)			Liver or biliary disorder, MI (between 6 hr and 3–4 days), shock, infectious mono, CHF, CVA, infection or inflammation of muscle tissue	Pregnancy, DKA, salicylates
Male	8–46 U/L	0.14–0.78 μkat/L		
Female	7–34 U/L	0.12–0.58 μkat/L		
NB	16–72 U/L	0.27–1.22 μkat/L		
Bicarbonate (HCO_3)			Metabolic alkalosis, compensating respiratory acidosis, meds containing sodium bicarb	Metabolic acidosis, compensating respiratory alkalosis, tissue breakdown, certain types of chemical poisoning
Arterial	22–26 mEq/L	22–26 mmol/L		
Venous	19–25 mEq/L	19–25 mmol/L		
Bilirubin Direct	Up to 0.4 mg/dL	1.7–6.8 μmol/L	Liver disorders, obstructive jaundice	Barbiturates, salicylates, penicillin, caffeine (These can affect all types of bilirubin.)

(continued on the following page)

REFERENCE VALUES FOR LABORATORY TESTS (BLOOD OR SERUM) WITH POSSIBLE CAUSES OF INCREASED AND DECREASED VALUES* (continued)

Test	*Conventional Units*	*SI Units*	*Causes of Increase*	*Causes of Decrease*
Bilirubin (continued)				
Indirect	Up to 0.8 mg/dL	5.0–19.0 μmol/L	Sickle cell anemia, pernicious anemia, hemolytic anemia, septicemia, Rh or ABO incompatibility in newborn, numerous meds	
Total	Up to 1.0 mg/dL	5–20 μmol/L	(See above.)	
NB	1–12 mg/dL	34–102 μmol/L		

Bleeding Time				
Duke	1–3 min		Disorders involved with decreased production or increased destruction of platelets, anti-inflammatory meds	Splenectomy, Hodgkin's disease
Ivy	2–7 min			
Blood gases (ABGs)	See individual gases.		See Table 6–7. *Acid-Base Disorders.*	
Blood urea nitrogen (BUN)	5–25 mg/dL	1.8–7.1 mmol/L	Dehydration, renal disorders (cause usually not renal if serum creatinine normal), tissue necrosis, CHF, shock, MI	Inadequate protein intake, liver disease, water overload, nephrotic syndrome
Child	5–20 mg/dL	2.5–6.4 mmol/L		
Infant	4–18 mg/dL	1.4–6.4 mmol/L		
Calcium (serum)	8.5–10.5 mg/dL	2.25–2.75 mmol/L	Hyperparathyroidism, hyperthyroidism, immobility, tumors, excessive intake	Hypoparathyroidism, hypothyroidism, diarrhea, burns, malabsorption, alcoholism, numerous meds
Child	Slightly higher			

(continued on the following page)

REFERENCE VALUES FOR LABORATORY TESTS (BLOOD OR SERUM) WITH POSSIBLE CAUSES OF INCREASED AND DECREASED VALUES* (continued)

Test	*Conventional Units*	*SI Units*	*Causes of Increase*	*Causes of Decrease*
Carcinoembryonic antigen (CEA)	0–2.5 ng/mL		Cancer, gastric ulcer, smoking	
Chloride	95–107 mEq/L	95–105 mmol/L	Dehydration, acidosis, eclampsia, renal failure, CHF, anemia, hyperventilation	Gastrointestinal loss, diuresis, hypoventilation, burns, fever
Cholesterol				
40–50 yr	140–240 mg/dL	4.37–6.35 mmol/L	Ingested cholesterol, ingested saturated fatty acids, biliary obstruction, hypothyroidism	Malabsorption syndromes, liver disease, hyperthyroidism
Under age 25 yr	125–200 mg/dL			
Infant	70–175 mg/dL	3.27–5.20 mmol/L		

Low density (LDL)			Familial hyperlipoproteinemia, pregnancy, nephrotic syndrome	
Over age 65	Up to 200 mg/dL	2.69–5.12 mmol/L		
To age 40	Up to 180 mg/dL	2.30–4.60 mmol/L		
To age 25	Up to 138 mg/dL	1.87–3.53 mmol/L		
High density (HDL)	32–75 mg/dL (varies with age)	0.82–1.92 mmol/L	Alcohol, chronic hepatitis, hypothyroidism, biliary obstruction	Hyperlipoproteinemia, exogenous estrogens, hyperthyroidism, cirrhosis
CK isoenzyme MB	5% or less		MI, severe angina	
CO_2, venous	23–30 mEq/L	24–30 mmol/L	Metabolic alkalosis, vomiting or gastric suction, steroids, mercurial diuretics	Metabolic acidosis, DKA, diarrhea, renal failure, salicylates, diuretics

(continued on the following page)

REFERENCE VALUES FOR LABORATORY TESTS (BLOOD OR SERUM) WITH POSSIBLE CAUSES OF INCREASED AND DECREASED VALUES* (continued)

Test	*Conventional Units*	*SI Units*	*Causes of Increase*	*Causes of Decrease*
Complete blood count (CBC): See RBC, RBC *indices, hct, hgb,* WBC, WBC *diff, platelets*				
Creatinine	0.6–1.5 mg/dL	53–133 μmol/L	Impaired renal function, massive muscle damage	Muscular dystrophy, pregnancy, eclampsia
Child	0.3–0.7 mg/dL			
NB	0.3–1.0 mg/dL			

Creatine kinase or creatine phosphokinase (CK or CPK)			Exercise, tissue damage or inflammation, MI (>within 4–6 hr, returning to normal within 3–4 days of MI), surgical procedures, pregnancy, muscular dystrophy
Male	55–170 U/L	0.94–2.89 μkat/L	
Female	30–135 U/L	0.51–2.30 μkat/L	
Child	15–50 U/L	0.26–0.85 μkat/L	
NB	30–100 U/L	0.51–1.70 μkat/L	
D-dimer	Negative		DIC and other thrombotic disorders, pulmonary embolism, venous or arterial thrombosis.

(continued on the following page)

REFERENCE VALUES FOR LABORATORY TESTS (BLOOD OR SERUM) WITH POSSIBLE CAUSES OF INCREASED AND DECREASED VALUES* (continued)

Test	Conventional Units	SI Units	Causes of Increase	Causes of Decrease
Erythrocyte count, or red blood cell count				
Male	4.6–6.2 million/mm^3	4.6–6.2 × 10^{12}/L	Polycythemia vera, dehydration, COPD	Anemias, hemodilution
Female	4.2–5.4 million/mm^3	4.2–5.4 × 10^{12}/L		
NB	Up to 7.1 million/mm^3	4.8–7.1 × 10^{12}/L		

Erythrocyte sedimentation rate (ESR or sed rate)				
Westergren Male	Up to 15 mm/h		Inflammation, infection, pregnancy, acute MI, cancer	Polycythemia vera, CHF, sickle cell anemia
Westergren Female	Up to 20 mm/h			
Child	Up to 10 mm/h			
Fibrinogen	200–400 mg/dL		Immune disorders of connective tissue, glomerulonephritis, late pregnancy, oral contraceptives, cancer of breast, stomach, or kidney	DIC, liver disease, cancer of prostate, lung, or pancreas
NB	125–300 mg/dL			
Gamma-glutamyl transpeptidase (GGT)			Liver disease, biliary obstruction, CHF, MI, epilepsy, cancer, mono, diabetes mellitus, alcohol, numerous meds	Late pregnancy, oral contraceptives
Male	6–37 U/L	0.10–0.63 μkat/L		

(continued on the following page)

REFERENCE VALUES FOR LABORATORY TESTS (BLOOD OR SERUM) WITH POSSIBLE CAUSES OF INCREASED AND DECREASED VALUES* (continued)

Test	*Conventional Units*	*SI Units*	*Causes of Increase*	*Causes of Decrease*
Gamma-glutamyl transpeptidase (GGT) (continued)				
Female <45 yr	5–27 U/L	0.08–0.46 μkat/L		
>45 yr	6–37 U/L	0.10–0.63 μkat/L		
Child	3–30 U/L	0.5–0.51 μkat/L		
NB	5 times child's values			

Glucose, whole blood (fasting)	60–100 mg/dL	3.3–5.6 mmol/L	Diabetes mellitus, Cushing's syndrome, MI, trauma, burn, infection, renal failure, numerous meds	Insulin excess, cancer, malnutrition, alcoholism, cirrhosis, adrenal hypofunction
NB 1 day	25–51 mg/dL	1.4–2.8 mmol/L		
Hematocrit (Hct)				
Male	40–54%	0.40–0.54	Polycythemia, dehydration	Anemia, hemodilution, leukemia
Female	36–46%	0.38–0.47		
Child	35–41%	0.35–0.41		
6 mo	30–40%	0.30–0.40		
NB	44–64%	0.44–0.64		
Hemoglobin (Hb or Hgb)				
Male	13.5–18 g/dL	135–180 g/L	Polycythemia, chronic lung disease	Anemia
Female	12–16 g/dL	120–160 g/L		
Child	11–16 g/dL	110–160 g/L		
3 mo	10–11 g/dL	100–110 g/L		
NB	14–24 g/dL	140–240 g/L		
INR	2.0–3.0 INR	2.0–3.0 INR	Refer to Prothrombin time (PT)	Refer to PT

(continued on the following page)

REFERENCE VALUES FOR LABORATORY TESTS (BLOOD OR SERUM) WITH POSSIBLE CAUSES OF INCREASED AND DECREASED VALUES* (continued)

Test	*Conventional Units*	*SI Units*	*Causes of Increase*	*Causes of Decrease*
Iron				
Men	60–170 μg/dL	10.7–30.4 μmol/L	Hemolytic anemia, liver damage, folic acid deficiency, lead poisoning	Iron deficiency anemia, bleeding, rheumatoid arthritis
Women	50–130 μg/dL	9.0–23.3 μmol/L		
Child	40–200 μg/dL	7.2–35.8 μmol/L		
NB	350–500 μg/dL	62.7–89.5 μmol/L		
Total iron-binding capacity (TIBC)	300–360 μg/dL	54–64 μmol/L	Iron deficiency anemia	Anemia of chronic disease, pernicious anemia

Child	100–350 μg/dL	18–63 μmol/L		
Elderly	200–310 μg/dL	35–56 μmol/L		
Lactic or lactate dehydrogenase (LDH)	70–200 U/L	1.21–3.52 μkat/L	Cell damage or destruction, hemolytic anemia, liver disease, pulmonary infarct, shock with necrosis, renal disease, some narcotics	Indicates favorable response to cancer therapy
Child	420–750 U/L			
Infant	500–920 U/L			
Lead	50 μg/dL or less		Lead ingestion or inhalation, heat stroke	
Lipase	14–280 U/L	0–2.72 μkat/L	Pancreatic disorders, renal failure, perforated ulcer, some narcotics, steroids	Hepatitis, late cancer of pancreas
Child	20–136 IU/L			
Infant	9–105 IU/L			
Lipids, total (See also *Cholesterol* and *Triglycerides*.)	400–800 mg/dL		Hyperlipoproteinemia, acute MI, eclampsia, diabetes mellitus, nephrotic syndrome	COPD, abetalipoproteinemia

(continued on the following page)

REFERENCE VALUES FOR LABORATORY TESTS (BLOOD OR SERUM) WITH POSSIBLE CAUSES OF INCREASED AND DECREASED VALUES* (continued)

Test	Conventional Units	SI Units	Causes of Increase	Causes of Decrease
Magnesium (Mg)	1.4–2.4 mEq/L	0.61–1.03 mmol/L	Addison's disease, renal failure, DKA, hypothyroidism, hyperparathyroidism	Hyperaldosteronism, alcoholism, toxemia of pregnancy, nephrotic syndrome, malnutrition
Child	1.2–1.9 mEq/L	0.65–1.07 mmol/L		
Myoglobin				
Male	20–90 ng/mL	20–90 µg/L	Skeletal or cardiac muscle cell injury; increases in 2–6 hr p̄ injury and begins to return to normal in 12–18 hr	
Female	12–75 ng/mL	12–75 µg/L		
Osmolality	285–310 mOsm/Kg	280–300 mmol/kg	Chronic renal disease, diabetes mellitus	Diuretics, Addison's disease

$PaCO_2$	35–45 mm Hg			
NB	27–40 mm Hg			
PaO_2	75–100 mm Hg		Polycythemia vera, splenectomy, fractures, metastatic cancer	Hypoxemia due to impaired lung function, decreased cardiac output
1 day old	60–90 mm Hg			
Partial thrombo-plastin time-activated (PTT)	28–40 sec or within 5 sec of control		Heparin, vit K deficiency, hemophilia, liver disease, DIC, polycythemia, leukemia	Extensive cancer
pH	7.35–7.45		See Table 6–7, *Acid-Base Disorders.*	
1 day old	7.29–7.45			
Phosphorus	2.5–4.5 mg/dL	0.78–1.50 mmol/L	Renal disorders, healing fractures, hypoparathyroidism, numerous meds	Starvation, hyperparathyroidism, continuous D5W IV
Child	4–6 mg/dL	1.45–1.78 mmol/L		
Infant	4.5–6.7 mg/dL	1.45–2.16 mmol/L		

(continued on the following page)

REFERENCE VALUES FOR LABORATORY TESTS (BLOOD OR SERUM) WITH POSSIBLE CAUSES OF INCREASED AND DECREASED VALUES* (continued)

Test	*Conventional Units*	*SI Units*	*Causes of Increase*	*Causes of Decrease*
Platelet count	150,000–450,000 mm^3		Polycythemia vera, splenectomy, fractures, metastatic cancer	ITP, anemias, bone marrow depression, DIC, eclampsia, hepatitis, salicylates
Potassium (K+)	3.5–5.0 mEq/L	3.5–5.0 mmol/L	Renal disorders, acidosis, cell necrosis, DKA, Addison's disease, false > with hemolyzed specimen or vigorous pumping of hand after tourniquet applied	Diuretics, insulin excess, increased corticosteroids, diarrhea, alkalosis, IV therapy without K+ added
Child	3.4–4.7 mEq/L	3.4–4.7 mmol/L		
Infant	4.1–5.3 mEq/L	4.1–5.3 mmol/L		

Protein, total	6–8 g/dL	66–79 g/L	Dehydration, sarcoidosis, macroglobulinemias, numerous meds	Renal disorders, ulcerative colitis, water intoxication, cirrhosis, malnutrition
15 yr	6.5–8.6 g/dL	65–86 g/L		
1 yr	5.0–7.5 g/dL	50–75 g/L		
Prothrombin time (pro time or PT)	11–13 sec or within 2 sec of control		Hemophilia, liver disease, coumadin, numerous meds	Thrombophlebitis, MI, pulmonary embolism, numerous meds
Rapid plasma reagin (RPR)	Negative		Positive may be caused by syphilis, SLE, or other immune complex diseases, or advanced age	
Red blood cell indices				
MCV			Aplastic, hemolytic, or pernicious anemia, liver disease, hypothyroidism, anticonvulsants	Iron deficiency anemia, sickle cell anemia, thalassemia, cancer, rheumatoid arthritis, lead poisoning, radiation
Male	80–94 μm^3			
Female	81–99 μm^3			
NB	96–108 μm^3			
MCH			Aplastic, hemolytic, or pernicious anemia	Hypochromic and microcytic anemias (including iron deficiency)
Male	27–31 pg			
Female	27–31 pg			
NB	32–34 pg			

(continued on the following page)

REFERENCE VALUES FOR LABORATORY TESTS (BLOOD OR SERUM) WITH POSSIBLE CAUSES OF INCREASED AND DECREASED VALUES* (continued)

Test	*Conventional Units*	*SI Units*	*Causes of Increase*	*Causes of Decrease*
Red blood cell indices (continued)			Aplastic, hemolytic, or pernicious anemia	Iron deficiency anemia, thalassemia
MCHC				
Male	32–36%			
Female	32–36%			
NB	32–33%			
Red blood cell count (RBC) (See *Erythrocyte count.*)				

Red blood cell distribution width (RDW)	11.6–14.6 mm	Indicates greater size variability of RBCs; seen with reticulocytosis, iron deficiency, sideroblastic anemia, thalassemia, or after transfusion of normal blood into microcytic or macrocytic cell population (called *anisocytosis*)	
Reticulocyte count	0.5–2.5% of RBCs	Hemolytic anemia, sickle cell anemia	Depressed bone marrow function, defective erythropoietin and/or hgb production
NB	2.5–6.5% of RBCs		
Rheumatoid factor (RF)	<1 : 20 or negative	Rheumatoid arthritis, SLE, scleroderma, dermatomyositis	
SGOT (See *Aspartate aminotransferase.*)			
SGPT (See *Alanine aminotransferase.*)			

(continued on the following page)

REFERENCE VALUES FOR LABORATORY TESTS (BLOOD OR SERUM) WITH POSSIBLE CAUSES OF INCREASED AND DECREASED VALUES* (continued)

Test	*Conventional Units*	*SI Units*	*Causes of Increase*	*Causes of Decrease*
Sickle cell prep and sickledex	Negative		Positive indicates either sickle cell trait or disease.	
Sodium (Na+)	135–145 mEq/L	135–145 mmol/L	Dehydration, CHF, inappropriate IV therapy, nephrotic syndrome, increased corticosteroids	Diuretics and other meds, Addison's disease, renal disorders, burns, DKA, diaphoresis
Infant	134–150 mEq/L	134–150 mmol/L		
Thyroid-stimulating hormone (TSH)	Below 10 mIU/mL	<10m U/L	Hypothyroidism, thyroiditis, autoimmune disease, cirrhosis	Pituitary or hypothalamic dysfunction, hyperthyroidism, aspirin, heparin, corticosteroids
By 3 days old	Below 25 μIU/mL	<25m U/L		

Thyroxine RIA (T_4)	4–12 mg/dL	60–165 nmol/L	Hyperthyroidism, early thyroiditis, pregnancy, estrogen therapy, oral contraceptives, preeclampsia	Hypothyroidism, metastatic cancer, liver or renal disease, cardiovascular disorders, burns, trauma, strenuous exercise, numerous meds
Child	5.5–14.5 μg/dL	60–170 nmol/L		
NB	11–23 μg/dL	140–230 nmol/L		
Triiodothyronine RIA (T_3)	80–200 ng/dL	1.2–3.0 nmol/L	Hyperthyroidism, protein malnutrition, malignancies, liver disease, nephrotic syndrome	Hypothyroidism, thyroiditis, pregnancy, menstruation, oral contraceptives, diuretics
Triglycerides	10–150 mg/dL	0.11–1.68 mmol/L	Hyperlipoproteinemia, acute MI, CVA, hypothyroidism, nephrotic syndrome, pregnancy, numerous meds	Cirrhosis, inadequate dietary protein, hyperthyroidism Fanconi's syndrome, numerous meds
40–60 yr	10–190 mg/dL	0.11–2.21 mmol/L		
Child	10–140 mg/dL	0.11–1.58 mmol/L		
<2 yr	5–40 mg/dL	0.06–0.45 mmol/L		
Troponin T	0–0.1 ng/mL		Cardiac or skeletal muscle injury	

(continued on the following page)

REFERENCE VALUES FOR LABORATORY TESTS (BLOOD OR SERUM) WITH POSSIBLE CAUSES OF INCREASED AND DECREASED VALUES* (continued)

Test	*Conventional Units*	*SI Units*	*Causes of Increase*	*Causes of Decrease*
Troponin I	<1.5 ng/mL		Acute MI and minor myocardial cell damage from a few hours after onset of symptoms up to 5–7 days	
Uric acid			Gout, excessive purine intake, psoriasis, sickle cell anemia, chemotherapy, tissue destruction, eclampsia, alcohol, numerous meds	Fanconi's syndrome, numerous meds
Male	4.0–8.5 mg/dL	0.24–0.51 mmol/L		
Female	2.7–7.3 mg/dL	0.16–0.43 mmol/L		
Child	2.5–5.5 mg/dL	0.15–0.33 mmol/L		

White blood cell count (WBC or leukocytes)	4300–10,800 mm^3	$4.3–10.8 \times 10^9/L$	Infection, inflammation, leukemia, parasitic infestation	Bone marrow depression, tissue damage, viral infection, autoimmune diseases, malignancies, malnutrition, alcoholism, severe infection
1–10 yr	5000–13,000 mm^3	$5.0–13.0 \times 10^9/L$		
6 mo	6000–16,000 mm^3	$6.0–16.0 \times 10^9/L$		
NB	9000–30,000 mm^3	$9.0–30.0 \times 10^9/L$		
White Blood Cell Count Differential				
Neutrophils (polys or segs)	54–75% (lower up to age 2 yr)	0.54–0.75	Bacterial infection, some viral infections, inflammation, tissue necrosis, stress	Bone marrow depression, malnutrition, malignancies, many meds
Bands (stabs)	0–5%	0.03–0.08	Infection, cancer, meds	None
Eosinophils	1–4%	0.01–0.04	Allergy, parasites, sickle cell disease, autoimmune diseases	Disseminated lupus erythromatosus, increased steroid levels, stress, infectious mono

(continued on the following page)

REFERENCE VALUES FOR LABORATORY TESTS (BLOOD OR SERUM) WITH POSSIBLE CAUSES OF INCREASED AND DECREASED VALUES* (continued)

Test	*Conventional Units*	*SI Units*	*Causes of Increase*	*Causes of Decrease*
White Blood Cell Count Differential (continued)				
Basophils	0–1%	0–0.01	Leukemia, chronic hypersensitivity states, polycythemia vera, ulcerative colitis, nephrosis	None
Lymphocytes	25–40% (higher up to age 2 yr)	0.25–0.40	Viral infection, some bacterial infections, ulcerative colitis, chronic illnesses	Immune deficiency disorders, Hodgkin's disease, rheumatic fever, aplastic anemia
Monocytes	2–8%	0.02–0.08	Chronic infections or inflammation, cirrhosis, cancer, hemolytic anemias	None specific

**References for lab tests*: Cavanaugh, BM: Nurses Manual of Laboratory and Diagnostic Tests, ed 4. FA Davis, Philadelphia, 2003; Sacher, RA, and McPherson, RA: Widmann's Clinical Interpretation of Laboratory Tests, ed 11, FA Davis, Philadelphia, 2000.

URINALYSIS (UA)

Urine Test	Norm	Comments
Appearance (clarity)	Clear to slightly hazy	Cloudy urine is most commonly caused by WBCs, RBCs, bacteria, epithelial cells, mucus, or talcum powder.
Bacteria	None–few	Bacteria in urine is usually insignificant (specimen may be contaminated) unless accompanied by excessive number of white blood cells.
Bilirubin	Neg	Bilirubin is found in urine in liver diseases or biliary tract obstruction.
Blood	Neg	Blood may be present because of damage to the genitourinary tract, bleeding disorders, anticoagulant therapy, strenuous exercise, or infection.
Casts	Occ* (hyaline or granular)	Casts are a network of protein, fats, and cells that take the shape of the renal collecting area in which they are formed. They are increased in strenuous exercise, renal disease, CHF, and dehydration.
Color	Pale yellow to amber	*Pale urine*: excess fluid intake, diabetes, nephrotic syndrome, alcohol *Dark yellow*: dehydration, bilirubin, numerous meds *Orange*: bilirubin, meds

(continued on the following page)

URINALYSIS (UA) (continued)

Urine Test	Norm	Comments
		Red: RBCs, hemoglobin, beets, numerous meds *Green: Pseudomonas*, vitamins, numerous meds *Blue*: meds *Brown*: acid hematin, myoglobin, bile pigments, meds *Black or brownish black*: melanin, urobilin, RBCs, iron, and other meds
Crystals	Occ	Crystals form from salts and are increased in concentrated urine or urine allowed to stand for several hours and with certain drug therapy. Certain crystals may indicate liver disease.
Epithelial cells	Few	A few epithelial cells normally slough from the lining of the genitourinary tract. Increased numbers may be seen in tubular necrosis, any damage to kidney, or renal transplant rejection.
Glucose	Neg	Urine glucose is present in uncontrolled diabetes mellitus, gestational diabetes, Cushing's syndrome, severe burns, sepsis, impaired kidney function, and some meds.

Urine Test	*Norm*	*Comments*
Ketones	Neg	Measurable amounts may indicate excessive fat breakdown, inadequate intake or metabolism of carbohydrates, or increased metabolic demand.
Leukocyte esterase	Neg	Dipstick checks are used to test for the presence of white blood cells in urine and to screen for UTI.
Nitrite	Neg	Presence of nitrites may indicate a UTI or contamination of the specimen container. (A first morning urine sample is best to avoid misleading results.)
Odor	Mildly aromatic	A fishy odor is characteristic of bacterial infection, and a fruity odor is characteristic of uncontrolled diabetes mellitus.
pH	4.5–8.0	Acidosis, alkalosis, starvation, diarrhea, dietary intake, and meds can affect pH.
Protein	Neg	Protein is increased with strenuous exercise, renal disease, or systemic disorders.
Red blood cells	0–3/HPF†	The presence of red blood cells may be due to strenuous exercise, damage to glomerular membrane or genitourinary tract, appendicitis, fever, malignant hypertension, or infection.

(continued on the following page)

URINALYSIS (UA) (continued)

Urine Test	*Norm*	*Comments*
Specific gravity (SG)	1.005–1.026	A low SG is seen with overhydration or diabetes insipidus. A high SG is seen with dehydration, uncontrolled diabetes mellitus, and concentrated IV fluids. A persistent SG of 1.010 may indicate damage to renal tubules.
Urobilinogen	0.1–1.0 Ehrlich units/dL	Urobilinogen increases with liver damage, CHF, hemolytic disorders, and alkalosis.
White blood cells	0–4/HPF	Excessive white blood cells can be caused by infection in genitourinary system, glomerulonephritis, or renal calculi.

*The initials "occ" on a UA report stand for "occasional."
†On a UA report, "HPF" stands for "high-powered field" and denotes results detected by microscopic examination.

CEREBROSPINAL FLUID

NOTES: (1) Because the patient is placed in a "head-flexed" position to facilitate the lumbar puncture, the nurse or assistant must continually assess patency of the patient's airway during the procedure. Use of a pulse oximeter assists in monitoring patient status during the lumbar puncture. (2) Several collection tubes are usually partially filled with spinal fluid. It is important to number these tubes to indicate the order in which they were collected as specific tubes are used for specific tests.

Test	*Conventional Units*	*SI Units*	*Comments*
Cell count			
Lymphocytes	Up to $5/mm^3$		Cell count of 10–200 (adult) consisting mostly of lymphocytes indicates viral meningitis.
Child	Up to $20/mm^3$		Cell count of 200–500 consisting mostly of lymphocytes or granulocytes indicates TB meningitis, choriomeningitis, herpes, or syphilitic meningitis.
Granulocytes	None		Cell count over 500 consisting mostly of granulocytes indicates bacterial meningitis. Presence of immature cells (blasts) may indicate CNS leukemia or carcinomatous meningitis.

(continued on the following page)

CEREBROSPINAL FLUID (continued)

Test	*Conventional Units*	*SI Units*	*Comments*
Cell count (continued)			
RBCs	None		Bleeding from a traumatic spinal tap yields high RBC and WBC counts. (Decrease in number of red cells between the first and last fluid collected indicates a traumatic puncture.)
Protein			Inflammation of meninges (meningitis) results in increased permeability of blood-brain barrier and subsequent rise of protein.
Adult	15–45 mg/dL	0.15–0.45 g/L	
Child	14–45 mg/dL	0.14–0.45 g/L	
Infant	30–100 mg/dL	0.30–1.0 g/L	
Glucose			Organisms consume and therefore reduce glucose. Viral meningitis causes less or no change in glucose. Decrease may also result from CNS leukemia, cancer involving meninges, or subarachnoid hemorrhage.
Adult	40–80 mg/dL or less than 50%–80% of blood glucose level 30–60 min earlier	2.22–4.44 mmol/L	

Glucose (continued)			
Child	35–75 mg/dL	1.94–4.16 mmol/L	
Infant	20–40 mg/dL	1.11–2.22 mmol/L	
Lactic acid	10–20 mg/dL	1.1–2.2 mmol/L	Results above 35 mg/dL usually indicate bacterial or fungal meningitis.
Normal flora	None		The presence of organisms indicates contaminated specimen or infection.

NOTES

NOTES

NOTES

NOTES

NOTES

NOTES

NOTES

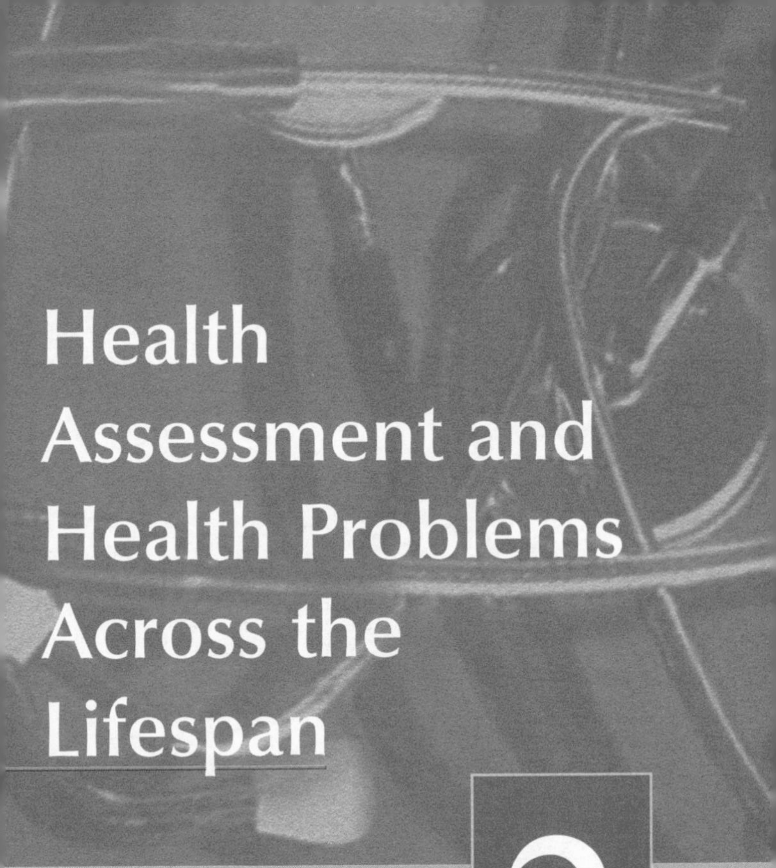

Health Assessment and Health Problems Across the Lifespan

Section 2

HISTORY OF PRESENT ILLNESS (HPI)

The HPI provides information about the patient's chief complaint (CC). A thorough HPI includes:

1. *Statement of general health before illness*: "How had you been feeling before this problem started?"
2. *Date of onset*: "When did this start?"
3. *Characteristics at onset*: "What was it like when this started?"
4. *Severity of symptoms*: "How would you rate the pain on a scale of 1 to 10, with 10 being the worst?"
5. *Course since onset*: "How often does the attack or pain occur?" (Once only, daily, intermittently, continuously) and "Have the symptoms changed since the first attack?"
6. *Associated signs and symptoms*: "Have you noticed any other changes in your health or the way you feel?"
7. *Aggravating or relieving factors*: "Is there anything that seems to make you feel better or worse? Do you feel better or worse at certain times of the day?"
8. *Effect on activities*: "Has this stopped you from going to work or kept you awake?"
9. *Treatments tried and results*: "Have you taken any medications or tried any treatments?" *If so,* "What happened when you took the medication or after the treatment?"

In addition, it is helpful to ask:

- *"What do you think caused this problem?"* The patient may actually know the cause but hesitate to reveal it for numerous reasons; for example, he or she may have feelings of guilt regarding the cause of illness.
- *"Is anyone else in the household sick?"* The answer to this question may give clues to infectious illnesses or reveal information related to stressors that may have contributed to the patient's condition.

If the patient is a child, it is especially important to ask about the following, all of which are usually negatively affected by illness:

1. *Play*
2. *Sleep*
3. *Food and fluid intake*

REVIEW OF SYSTEMS (HEALTH HISTORY)*

Name: ______________________________
Age: ______ DOB: ________ Sex: _____ Race: _____
Admission date: ________ Time: _____ From: ______
Source of information: ________ Reliability (1–4): _____
Family member/Significant other: ____________

ACTIVITY/REST

Occupation: ________ Usual activities/Hobbies: _______
Leisure time activities: ______________________
Complaints of boredom: _____________________
Limitations imposed by condition: _______________
Sleep: Hours: ________ Naps: ________ Aids: _______
Insomnia: ____________ Related to: ____________
Rested upon awakening: ___________________

*Adapted from Doenges, ME, Moorhouse, MF, and Geissler-Murr, AC: Nursing Care Plans, Guidelines for Individualizing Patient Care, ed 6. FA Davis, Philadelphia, 2002, pp. 12–17, with permission.

CIRCULATION

History of: Hypertension: ________ Heart trouble: ____
Rheumatic fever: ___ Ankle/leg edema: ____
Phlebitis: ________ Slow Healing: ________
Claudication: ___________ Other: ________
Extremities: Numbness: __________ Tingling: ________
Cough/hemoptysis: ______________________________
Change in frequency/amount of urine: ______________

EGO INTEGRITY

Report of stress factors: _________________________
Ways of handling stress: _________________________
Financial concerns: _____________________________
Relationship status: _____________________________
Cultural factors: ________________________________
Religion: _______________ Practicing: ___________
Lifestyle: ______________ Recent changes: ________
Feelings of Helplessness: _______ Hopelessness: ______
Powerlessness: _________________________________

ELIMINATION

Usual bowel pattern: ____________ Laxative use: ______
Character of stool: _____________ Last BM: ________
History of bleeding: _____________ Hemorrhoids: ______
Constipation: __________________ Diarrhea: ________
Usual voiding pattern: ____ Incontinence: ____ When: ____
Urgency: _____ Frequency: ______ Retention: ______
Character of urine: ______________________________
Pain/burning/difficulty voiding: ___________________
History of kidney/bladder disease: _________________

FOOD/FLUID

Usual diet (type): _________ No. meals daily: ________
Last meal/intake: _________ Dietary pattern: ________
Loss of appetite: _________ Nausea/vomiting: ________
Heartburn/indigestion: ___ Related to: ___ Relieved by: ___
Allergy/Food intolerance: _________________________
Mastication/swallowing problems: __________________
Dentures: Upper: ______ Lower: _________________

HYGIENE

Activities of daily living: Independent: ______
Dependence (specify): Mobility: ____ Feeding: ____
Hygiene: ____ Dressing: ____
Toileting: ____ Other: ____
Equipment/prosthetic devices required: ______
Assistance provided by: ______
Preferred time of bath: ______ AM ______ PM

NEUROSENSORY

Fainting spells/dizziness: ______
Headaches: Location: ______ Frequency: ____
Tingling/Numbness/Weakness (location): ______
Stroke (residual effects): ______
Seizures: ______ Aura: ____ How controlled: ____
Eyes: Vision loss: R: ______ L: ______
Glaucoma: ______ Cataract: ______
Ears: Hearing loss: R: ______ L: ______
Nose: Epistaxis: ______ Sense of smell: ____

PAIN/COMFORT

Location: ____ Intensity (1–10): ____ Frequency: ____
Quality: ____ Duration: ____ Radiation: ____
Precipitating factors: ______
How relieved: ______

RESPIRATION

Dyspnea (related to): ______
Cough/sputum: ______
History of: Bronchitis: ______ Asthma: ______
Tuberculosis: ______ Emphysema: ____
Recurrent pneumonia: ____ Other: ____
Exposure to noxious fumes: ______
Smoker: ____ Packs/day: ____ Number of years: ____
Use of respiratory aids: ______ Oxygen: ______

SAFETY

Allergies/Sensitivity: ______ Reaction: ______

Previous alteration of immune system: ____ Cause: ____
History of sexually transmitted disease (date/type): ____
Blood transfusion: ____ When: ____
Reaction (described): ____
History of accidental injuries: ____
Fractures/dislocations: ____
Arthritis/unstable joints: ____
Back problems: ____
Changes in moles: ____ Enlarged nodes: ____
Impaired: Vision: ____ Hearing: ____
Prosthesis: ____ Ambulatory devices: ____
Expressions of ideation of violence (self/others): ____

SEXUALITY

Female

Age at menarche: ____ Length of cycle: ____ Duration ____
Last menstrual period: ____ Menopause: ____
Vaginal discharge: ____ Bleeding between periods: ____
Practices breast self-exam: ____ Last PAP smear: ____
Method of birth control: ____

Male

Penile discharge: ____ Prostate disorder: ____
Vasectomy: ____ Use of condoms: ____
Practices self-exam: Breast: ____ Testicles: ____
Last proctoscopic exam: ____ Last prostate exam: ____

SOCIAL INTERACTION

Marital status: ____ Years in relationship: ____
Living with: ____
Concerns/Stresses: ____
Extended family: ____
Other support persons(s): ____
Role within family structure: ____
Report of problems related to illness/condition: ____
Coping behaviors: ____
Do others depend on you for assistance? ____
How are they managing? ____
Frequency of social contacts (other than work): ____

TEACHING/LEARNING

Dominant language (specify): ______
Education level: ______
Learning disabilities (specify): ______
Cognitive limitations (specify): ______
Health beliefs/practices: ______
Special health care practices: ______
Familial risk factors (indicate relationship):
Diabetes: ______ Tuberculosis: ______
Heart disease: ______ Strokes: ______
High BP: ______ Epilepsy: ______
Kidney disease: ______ Cancer: ______
Mental illness: ______ Other (specify): ______
Prescribed medications (circle last dose):

Drug	Dose	Times	Takes regularly	Purpose
____	____	____	____	____
____	____	____	____	____
____	____	____	____	____

Nonprescription drugs: OTC: ______
Street drugs: ______ Smokeless tobacco: ______
Use of alcohol (amount/frequency): ______
Admitting diagnosis (physician): ______
Reason for hospitalization (patient): ______
History of current complaint: ______
Patient expectations of this hospitalization: ______
Previous illness and/or hospitalizations/surgeries: ______
______
Evidence of failure to improve: ______
Last complete physical exam: ______ By: ______

DISCHARGE PLAN CONSIDERATIONS

Date data obtained: ______

1. Anticipated date of discharge: ______
2. Resources available: Persons: ______
   Financial: ______
3. Do you anticipate changes in your living situation after discharge? ______
4. If Yes: Areas may require alteration/assistance:
   Food preparation: ______ Tuberculosis: ______
   Transportation: ______ Ambulation: ______
   Medication/IV therapy: ______ Treatments: ______

Wound care: ______________ Supplies: ____________
Self-care assistance (specify): ______________________
Physical layout of home (specify): ___________________
Homemaker assistance (specify): _____________________
Living facility other than home (specify): ____________

GENOGRAM

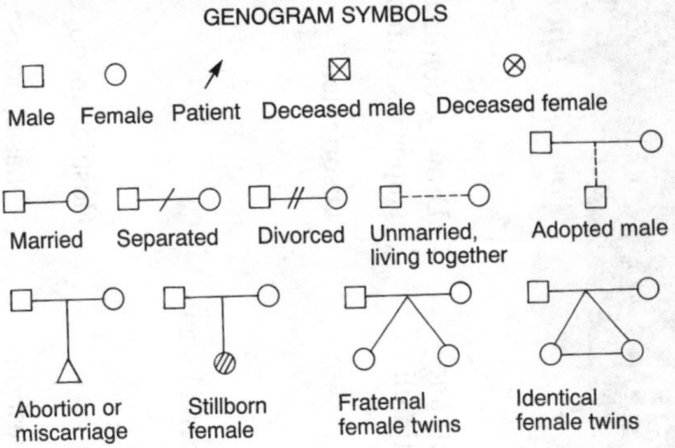

Figure 2–1. Genogram symbols.

- The genogram (see example) should include a minimum of the patient's grandparents, parents, aunts, uncles, and siblings (and children and grandchildren, if applicable).
- The age of each family member or age at the time of death is noted inside each individual's symbol.
- Date of genogram construction is noted.
- Abbreviations should be defined.

Example: Genogram of 3-year-old male with asthma.

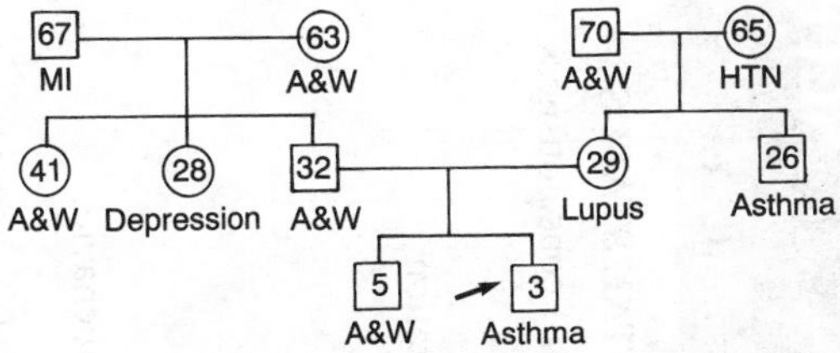

MI = myocardial infarction

HTN = hypertension

A&W = alive and well

PHYSICAL ASSESSMENT ACROSS THE LIFESPAN (CEPHALOCAUDAL APPROACH)

Assessment Area	*Normal Finding or Minor Variation**	*Possible Abnormalities*
MENTAL STATUS		
Level of consciousness	Conscious, awake, alert; aware of self and environment; responds to external stimuli	Drowsy, confused, lethargic, delirious, stuporous, comatose
Orientation	Oriented × 3: 1. Person (self, others) 2. Place 3. Time Appropriate for age in all areas of mental status exam	Disoriented
Mood/behavior	Attentive, cooperative, pleasant	Hostile, uncooperative, restless
Speech (dysphonia)	Articulate, fluent, readily answers questions	Aphasic, hoarse, stutters, hesitates, repeats, slow/fast, slurred, or monotonous speech

Grooming/apparel	Neat, clean; clothes appropriate to occasion, season, and sex	Body odor, one-sided neglect, nail biting, fastidious
Concentration/attention span	Attentive, demonstrates continuity of ideas	Inattentive, unable to follow commands
Memory	Responds appropriately to questions: 1. *Immediate*: "Why are you here?" 2. *Recent*: "What did you eat for breakfast?" 3. *Remote*: "Where were you born?"	Inappropriate responses to questions
Cognitive skills	Responds appropriately: 1. Explain "When the cat's away, the mice will play." 2. How are an apple and orange similar? 3. How are a bush and a tree dissimilar? 4. How many dimes in $1? 5. Read this paragraph, please.	Concrete explanations of symbolic phrases, inappropriate responses to questions ***(Young children are normally concrete thinkers.)***

(continued on the following page)

*A "minor variation," in this context, is one that usually does not require treatment.
Key: Text appearing in blue type refers to pediatric variations. Text appearing in gray type refers to geriatric variations.

PHYSICAL ASSESSMENT ACROSS THE LIFESPAN (CEPHALOCAUDAL APPROACH) (continued)

Assessment Area	*Normal Finding or Minor Variation**	*Possible Abnormalities*
MENTAL STATUS (continued)		
General knowledge/ intellectual level	Responds appropriately: 1. Where does the sun rise? 2. Who is the president? 3. Name three big U.S. cities.	Inappropriate responses to questions
SKIN		
Color	Appropriate for race and genetic norm	Jaundice, cyanosis, pallor, redness, pigment changes (vitiligo), increased vascularity
Moisture	Appropriate to temperature, environment, activity Drier skin, especially over bony prominences and extremities.	Excessively dry/oily, moist, clammy, hot, cold

Temperature	Evenly warm over body (bilateral coolness of hands and feet may be normal)	Unilateral coolness of body parts, excessive warmth or coolness of skin
Texture	Smooth, even Increased wrinkling, thinner	Rough, dry, scaly
Mobility	Moves easily over underlying structures	Skin immovable
Turgor	After skin fold is pinched and released (dorsal surface of hand or inner forearm), skin returns to original place almost immediately Loss of elasticity results in tenting when turgor is assessed	Skin fold remains "tented" (Note number of seconds)

(continued on the following page)

*A "minor variation," in this context, is one that usually does not require treatment.
Key: Text appearing in blue type refers to pediatric variations. Text appearing in gray type refers to geriatric variations.

PHYSICAL ASSESSMENT ACROSS THE LIFESPAN (CEPHALOCAUDAL APPROACH) (continued)

Assessment Area	*Normal Finding or Minor Variation**	*Possible Abnormalities*
SKIN (continued)		
Edema	No edema (Particularly assess dependent areas.) Document as "0" or "none."	Edema present: "Nonpitting": firm, tight, cool skin "Pitting": depression remains Scale: 1+ Trace; disappears rapidly 2+ Moderate; disappears in 10–15 sec 3+ Deep; disappears in 1–2 min 4+ Very deep; remains after 5 min
Lesions	No lesions Cherry angiomas, seborrheic keratosis, sebaceous hyperplasia, cutaneous tags, cutaneous horns, senile lentigines	Describe according to: size, elevation, color, distribution, grouping, sensation. Measure with ruler to detect changes. See Table 2–1 for description of skin lesions.

*A "minor variation," in this context, is one that usually does not require treatment.

Key: Text appearing in blue type refers to pediatric variations. Text appearing in gray type refers to geriatric variations.

Table 2–1.	TYPES OF SKIN LESIONS	
Lesion	**Size in cm**	**Description**
PRIMARY LESIONS		
Macule	<1	Flat, circumscribed, varied in color
Papule	<1	Elevated, firm, solid
Nodule	1 < 2	Elevated, firm, solid
Tumor	>2	Elevated, firm, solid
Wheal	Varied	Transient, irregular, edematous
Vesicle	<1	Elevated, serous fluid filled
Bulla	>1	Elevated, serous fluid filled
Pustule	Varied	Elevated, purulent fluid filled
SECONDARY LESIONS		
Erosion	Varied	Moist epidermal, depression; follows rupture of vesicle, bulla
Excoriation	Varied	Crusted epidermal abrasion
Fissure	Varied	Red, linear dermal break
Ulcer	Varied	Red dermal depression, exudate
Scale	Varied	Flaky, irregular, white to silver
Petechia	<0.5	Flat, red to purple
Purpura	>0.5	Flat, red to purple
Ecchymosis	Varied	Dark red to dark blue; painful

Source: Hogstel, MO, and Curry, LC: Practical Guide to Health Assessment through the Life Span, ed. 3. FA Davis, Philadelphia, 2001, p. 97, with permission.

PHYSICAL ASSESSMENT ACROSS THE LIFESPAN (CEPHALOCAUDAL APPROACH) (continued)

Assessment Area	*Normal Finding or Minor Variation**	*Possible Abnormalities*
HAIR (BODY AND CEPHALIC)		
Texture	Great variation normal Texture coarsens	Extreme changes noted: fine, silky, brittle, coarse, dry
Quantity	Great variation normal Thinning hair	Sparse, dense
Distribution	Well distributed; appropriate for age, sex, body area Symmetric balding common in men	Alopecia, excessive hair growth (especially face or chest hair on females)
Hygiene	Clean, well kept	Lice, nits, dandruff, dirty, strong body odor, unkempt appearance

NAILS		
Color (nail beds)	Pink, CFT < 3 sec May take on yellowish color	Cyanosis, pallor
Consistency	Smooth, flexible Become more brittle	Brittle, pitting, transverse ridges
Contour	Convex	Concave ("spoon nails"), splitting, clubbing
Thickness	Single thickness Nails thicken	Increased thickness (usually indicates fungal infection)
HEAD		
Size/contour	Normocephalic	Hydrocephalic, microcephalic, asymmetric
Scalp	Smooth, nontender	Scaling, masses, tenderness

(continued on the following page)

*A "minor variation," in this context, is one that usually does not require treatment.

Key: Text appearing in blue type refers to pediatric variations. Text appearing in gray type refers to geriatric variations.

PHYSICAL ASSESSMENT ACROSS THE LIFESPAN (CEPHALOCAUDAL APPROACH) (continued)

Assessment Area	*Normal Finding or Minor Variation**	*Possible Abnormalities*
HEAD (continued)		
Head circumference (measured at largest point above eyebrow and behind occiput)	Between 5th and 95th percentile on standardized growth chart. Exceeds chest circumference by 1–2 cm until 18 mo.	Below 5th or above 95th percentile.
Anterior fontanel	3–4 cm in length and 2–3 cm in width until 9–12 mo of age. Soft, flat; bulges while crying. Closes between 9 and 18 mo.	Unusually large fontanel *may indicate hydrocephaly* (*faulty circulation or absorption of CSF*). Unusually small fontanel *may indicate craniosynostosis* (*premature closure of sutures*). Sunken or bulges while at rest. Early or delayed closure.

Posterior fontanel	0.5–1 cm across. May be closed at birth or by 3 mo of age.	Delayed closure *may indicate hydrocephaly*.
FACE		
	Symmetric, with relaxed facial expressions	Asymmetric, weak; involuntary movements; tense or expressionless facies
Cranial nerve (CN) VII: facial, motor	Able to smile, puff cheeks, frown, raise eyebrows, with symmetry noted	Unable to purposely and symmetrically use facial muscles
CN V: trigeminal: motor	Bilateral contractions of temporal and masseter muscles when teeth are clenched	Weak or asymmetric contraction of muscles
CN V: trigeminal: sensory	Able to distinguish touch on both sides of face	Unable to distinguish type and location of touch
Sinuses	Frontal and maxillary sinuses nontender	Tenderness
NOSE (See Fig. 2–2.)		
External	Symmetric alignment, patent nares	Asymmetric, nonpatent nares

(continued on the following page)

*A "minor variation," in this context, is one that usually does not require treatment.
Key: Text appearing in blue type refers to pediatric variations. Text appearing in gray type refers to geriatric variations.

PHYSICAL ASSESSMENT ACROSS THE LIFESPAN (CEPHALOCAUDAL APPROACH) (continued)

Assessment Area	*Normal Finding or Minor Variation**	*Possible Abnormalities*
NOSE (See Fig. 2–2.) (continued)		
CN I: olfactory	With eyes closed, identifies common odors bilaterally (e.g., tobacco, coffee, spices)	Unable to detect and identify odors
Septum	Straight, intact	Deviation, perforation
Mucosa	Moist, pink	Red (infection or irritation); pale (allergies or anemia); crusting; lesions; swelling
Mucus	No obvious mucus drainage	Yellow or green (may indicate bacterial infection), large amount clear (viral infection or allergy)

*A "minor variation," in this context, is one that usually does not require treatment.

Key: Text appearing in blue type refers to pediatric variations. Text appearing in gray type refers to geriatric variations.

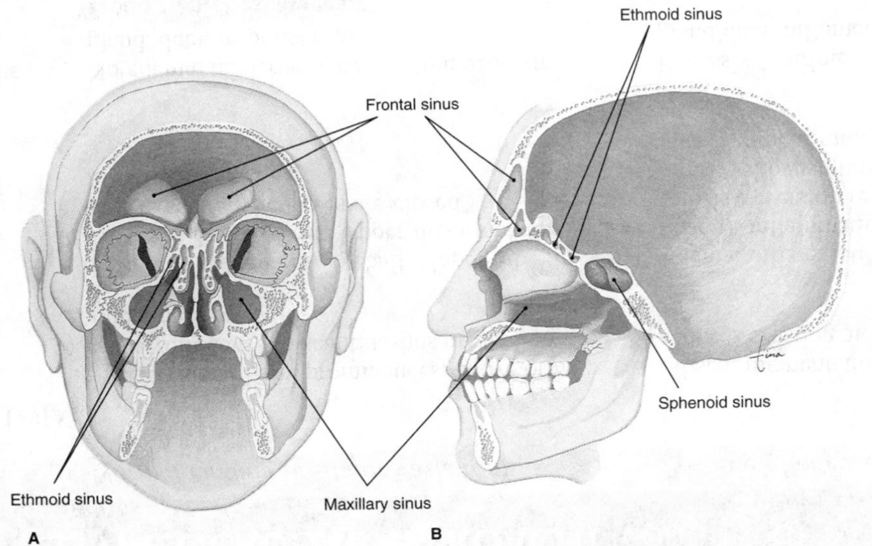

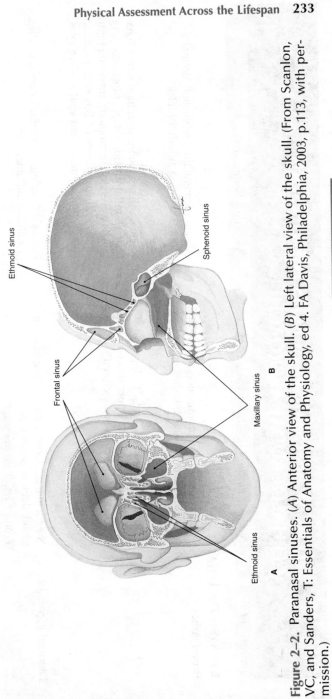

Figure 2–2. Paranasal sinuses. (*A*) Anterior view of the skull. (*B*) Left lateral view of the skull. (From Scanlon, VC, and Sanders, T: Essentials of Anatomy and Physiology, ed 4. FA Davis, Philadelphia, 2003, p.113, with permission.)

PHYSICAL ASSESSMENT ACROSS THE LIFESPAN (CEPHALOCAUDAL APPROACH) (continued)

Assessment Area	Normal Finding or Minor Variation*	Possible Abnormalities
EYES (See Fig. 1–9[A].)		
Brows/lashes	Arched along bony prominences, above orbits; vary from dense to scant; lashes present on upper and lower lids	Absent pigmentation, seborrheic dermatitis, redness/crusting at lash follicles
Lids	Lids are flush against eyeball. Upper lid covers 2–3 mm of iris. Upper lid completely covers sclera when eyes are closed	Edema, inflammation, stye, hard tumor (chalazion), inflammation (blepharitis), drooping (ptosis), eversion (ectropion), inversion (entropion), yellowish tumor on lids near inner canthus (xanthelasma), sclera visible when eyes are closed
Lacrimal apparatus	No edema, tenderness, or swelling of lacrimal gland, duct, or puncta Production of excess tears	Excessive tearing or dryness of eyes, swollen gland/duct, inflamed puncta

Eyeball (globe)	Symmetric (equal amounts of medial and lateral sclera, and symmetric corneal light reflection)	Eyes do not focus in same direction (strabismus), protrusion (exophthalmos), recession (enophthalmos)
Conjunctiva	Inner lid (palpebral) conjunctiva is pink, moist. Eyeball (bulbar) is clear, smooth, shiny, moist.	Pale, red, dull, wrinkled, dry
Sclera	Color varies somewhat according to race (white to light brown), but sclera is clear.	Marked vascularity, jaundice
Iris	Symmetric, clearly defined markings	Absence or dulling of color
Cornea	Opaque, smoothly rounded, Arcus senilis (thin, grayish white circle at edge of cornea)	In young persons, corneal arcus may suggest abnormal lipid metabolism
Lens	Clear	Clouding (cataract)

(continued on the following page)

*A "minor variation," in this context, is one that usually does not require treatment.
Key: Text appearing in blue type refers to pediatric variations. Text appearing in gray type refers to geriatric variations.

PHYSICAL ASSESSMENT ACROSS THE LIFESPAN (CEPHALOCAUDAL APPROACH) (continued)

Assessment Area	Normal Finding or Minor Variation*	Possible Abnormalities
EYES (See Fig. 1–9[A].) (continued)		
CN V: trigeminal	*Corneal reflex*: Blinking occurs when sclera is lightly touched with a wisp of cotton. (Contact lenses should be removed.)	Absence of corneal reflex
Pupils	Equal size (3–6 mm in average room light); round (See Fig. 2–3.)	Significant inequality, constriction (miosis), dilation (mydriasis) to light
CN III: oculomotor	*Light reflex*: Pupil constricts as light is shone directly into it (direct pupillary response); at the same time, the opposite pupil constricts (consensual response).	Absent or sluggish reaction to light
	Accommodation: Patient focuses eye on examiner's finger; eyes converge and pupils constrict as finger is moved toward nose.	Lack of accommodation

*A "minor variation," in this context, is one that usually does not require treatment.
Key: Text appearing in blue type refers to pediatric variations. Text appearing in gray type refers to geriatric variations.

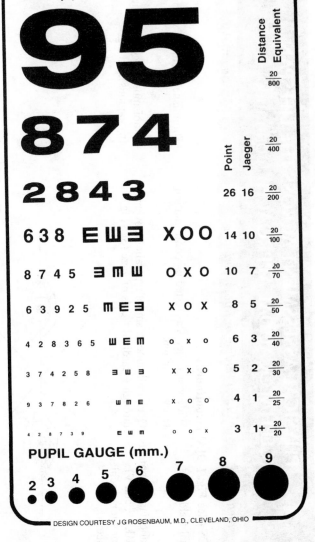

Figure 2–3. Pocket vision screener (actual size).

PHYSICAL ASSESSMENT ACROSS THE LIFESPAN (CEPHALOCAUDAL APPROACH) (continued)

Assessment Area	Normal Finding or Minor Variation*	Possible Abnormalities
EYES (See Fig. 1–9[A].) (continued)		
Visual fields	Wide visual fields as tested by confrontation test with examiner	Diminished fields of vision (glaucoma)
Extraocular movements, CN III, IV, and VI: oculomotor, trochlear, abducens	Ocular alignment; smooth, parallel movement through 6 cardinal fields of gaze (See Fig. 2–4.)	Strabismus; jerky, involuntary movements (nystagmus); lid lag

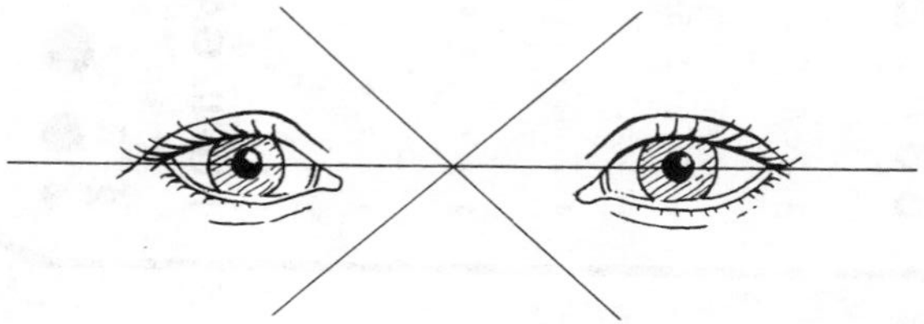

Figure 2–4. Six cardinal fields of gaze.

FUNDUSCOPIC EXAM: INTERNAL EYE (See Fig. 1–9[B].)

Retina (innermost membrane of eye)	Yellowish, pink	Dark color or irregular markings
Optic disk (surrounds convergence point of blood vessels: optic nerve entrance)	Color may be yellowish or pinkish. Rings appear around disk. Medial side may be blurred.	White
Physiologic cup (inside optic disk)	Occupies less than half of optic disk; yellowish white with sharp margins; small vessels visible	White or pink; margins blurred; vessels absent; cup not visible; cup larger than half of disk diameter
Vessels	*Arterioles*: light red and about $^3/_5$ size of veins *Veins*: dark red	Nicking or constriction of vessels, blurred "cottonlike" markings
Macula	Located about 2 disk diameters lateral to disk; no vessels in immediate area	
Fovea	Bright center of macula	

(continued on the following page)

*A "minor variation," in this context, is one that usually does not require treatment.

Key: Text appearing in blue type refers to pediatric variations. Text appearing in gray type refers to geriatric variations.

PHYSICAL ASSESSMENT ACROSS THE LIFESPAN (CEPHALOCAUDAL APPROACH) (continued)

Assessment Area	*Normal Finding or Minor Variation**	*Possible Abnormalities*
VISUAL ACUITY		
CN II: optic (**See Fig. 2–3.**)	"20/20" as tested by the Snellen Eye Chart (The larger the denominator, the worse the vision.)	Squinting; tearing; diminished acuity: nearsighted (myopia), farsighted (hyperopia), loss of accommodation (presbyopia), double vision (diplopia)
	Infant follows objects with eyes or smiles in response to parent's smile. Young child reaches for objects of interest. Child who does not know alphabet but can follow directions can make appropriate responses to Blackbird or Snellen E Eye Chart. Acuity is normally less than 20/20 until age 5 yr.	Does not follow objects or smile.

EARS		
Auricle	Smooth, clear skin; top of pinna in line with inner canthus of eye; no tenderness when manipulated	Unusually small, low-set ears; solid lesions (tophi); tenderness upon movement
Canal	Clear ear canal without redness; small, moderate amount of wax (cerumen); no pain or foul odor	Canal red or white coated (otitis externa), blood or serous fluid present, occluded by wax or foreign body, swelling, pain, foul odor
Tympanic membrane (TM) **(See Fig. 2–5.)** (For 3 yr old and under, hold auricle down and back, for others, hold auricle up and back to inspect TM)	Pearly gray and intact; landmarks visible: umbo, malleus, intact anterior cone of light Tympanic membrane red when child is crying.	Red (infection), dull (fluid), perforations, white markings (old scars), landmarks not visible (bulging membrane), landmarks pronounced (retracted membrane), prominent blood vessels over malleus (may indicate the early stage of an infection: otitis media), interrupted cone of light (serous otitis media) Redness, bulging, and immobility are the 3 characteristics of acute otitis media.

(continued on the following page)

*A "minor variation," in this context, is one that usually does not require treatment.
Key: Text appearing in blue type refers to pediatric variations. Text appearing in gray type refers to geriatric variations.

PHYSICAL ASSESSMENT ACROSS THE LIFESPAN (CEPHALOCAUDAL APPROACH) (continued)

Assessment Area	*Normal Finding or Minor Variation**	*Possible Abnormalities*

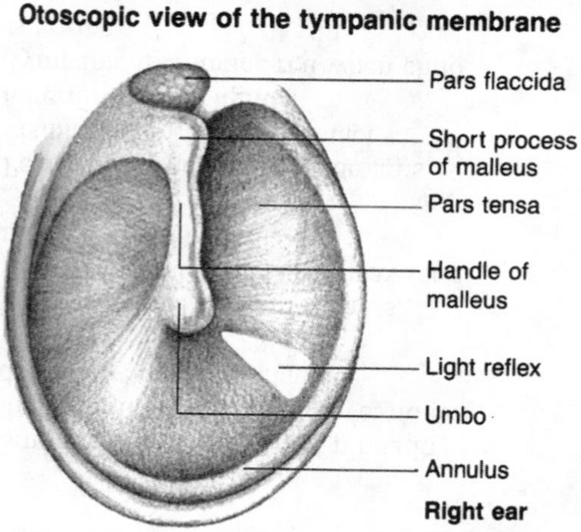

Figure 2–5. Tympanic membrane of the right ear. (From Morton, PG: Health Assessment in Nursing, ed 2. FA Davis, Philadelphia, 1993, p. 233, with permission.)

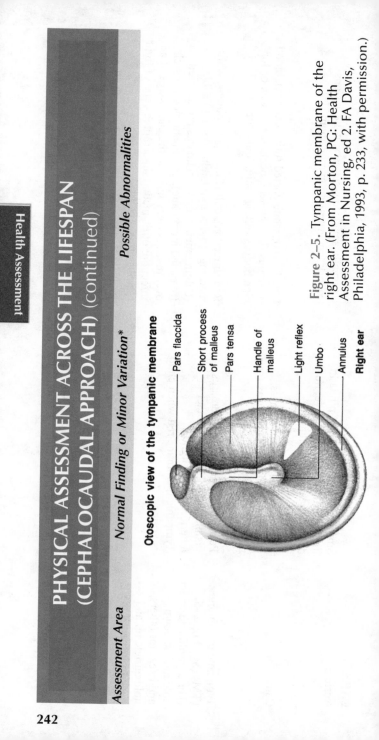

CN VIII: acoustic (auditory acuity)	Hears whispered or spoken voice from about 2 ft away (Have client repeat what was said.)	Diminished hearing. To distinguish between conductive and sensorineural loss, use a tuning fork to perform:
	Infant startles to loud or unexpected noise.	No response to noise.
	Child 6 mo or older turns head toward noise (localization of sound).	Does not turn toward noise
	Older child follows simple directions.	
	Weber test: test for lateralization (Normally, sound heard in midline and equally in both ears.)	
	Rinne test: compares air and bone conduction (Normally, sound heard longer through air than through bone: AC > BC.)	
MOUTH		
Lips	Symmetric, moist, intact, pink	Excessively dry, cyanosis, pallor, lesions (herpes simplex), chancre, irritation of outer corners (angular cheilosis), cleft lip

(continued on the following page)

*A "minor variation," in this context, is one that usually does not require treatment.
Key: Text appearing in blue type refers to pediatric variations. Text appearing in gray type refers to geriatric variations.

PHYSICAL ASSESSMENT ACROSS THE LIFESPAN (CEPHALOCAUDAL APPROACH) (continued)

Assessment Area	*Normal Finding or Minor Variation**	*Possible Abnormalities*
MOUTH (continued)		
Buccal mucosa	Pink, smooth, moist (Patchy brown pigmentation is normal in African-Americans.) Oral hyperpigmentation and leukoedema (grayish white benign lesion of buccal mucosa) increase with age.	Bright cherry red mucosa (associated with carbon monoxide poisoning), lesions, ulcers, white patches (thrush), inflamed parotid ducts
Gums	Pink, moist	Inflammation, swelling, bleeding, retraction from teeth, discoloration
Teeth	White, tight fitting	Discolored, loose, or missing teeth; cavities (caries); cracks; chips
Hard palate	Intact, pink, smooth, moist	Cleft palate, lesions
Soft palate/pharynx	Pink, moist, uvula at midline	Redness, inflammation, exudate, enlarged tonsils

	Pharyngeal tonsils are normally large in toddler. (Mouth of child usually inspected at end of the exam.) Cleft uvula	
CN IX and X: glossopharyngeal and vagus	Symmetric movement of soft palate and uvula as patient says "Ah," swallows without difficulty, gag reflex intact	Absent gag reflex, asymmetry of uvula, difficulty swallowing
Tongue	Pink, rough (dorsal surface), moist, fits easily into mouth	Inflamed, smooth, lesions, ulcerations, white areas, enlarged tongue, twitching (fasciculation)
CN XII: hypoglossal	Tongue protrudes with symmetry	Lateral deviation of protruded tongue
CN VII and IX: facial sensory, glossopharyngeal sensory	Distinguishes tastes of familiar substances	Diminished ability to distinguish tastes
Floor of mouth	Intact frenulum that does not restrict tongue movement	Tight frenulum (restricts tongue movement), white patches, inflamed submaxillary ducts

(continued on the following page)

*A "minor variation," in this context, is one that usually does not require treatment.
Key: Text appearing in blue type refers to pediatric variations. Text appearing in gray type refers to geriatric variations.

PHYSICAL ASSESSMENT ACROSS THE LIFESPAN (CEPHALOCAUDAL APPROACH) (continued)

Assessment Area	*Normal Finding or Minor Variation**	*Possible Abnormalities*
NECK	Supple, and head flexes easily toward chest.	Neck stiff. Shows signs of pain when head flexed onto chest (nuchal rigidity). *May indicate meningitis.*
Trachea	Midline position	Deviation
Carotid arteries/ jugular veins	Lack of audible blood flow with bell of stethoscope; full, regular, equal carotid pulses (palpated bilaterally, one at a time, after auscultation); no distention of jugular veins with head of bed elevated 45 to 60 degrees.	Blowing sound over artery with auscultation; distended, pulsating jugular veins when head of bed elevated >60 degrees (unilateral distention also significant)

CN XI: spinal accessory	Note strength of trapezius muscles while patient shrugs shoulders against examiner's hand. Also, note forceful movement and contraction of opposite sternomastoid muscles as patient turns head to each side against examiner's hand.	Atrophy, fasciculations or weakness of trapezius or sternomastoid muscle, droop of shoulders, downward and lateral displacement of scapula
Lymph nodes (use circular finger motions to examine nodes)	Nonpalpable, or small, nontender, movable (shotty) nodes may be found in normal persons (indicate past infection).	Enlarged, tender, hard, fixed nodes. Tender nodes over 1 cm in size may indicate active infection.
Thyroid gland	Stand behind patient and gently push trachea to one side. Palpate extended side as patient swallows. Repeat on opposite side. There should be no enlargement, masses, or tenderness. (Gland is normally slightly enlarged during pregnancy and puberty. Right lobe may be slightly larger.)	Enlargement (goiter), nodules, tenderness
	Auscultate over gland; lack of audible blood flow with bell of stethoscope.	Blowing sound over gland on auscultation (bruit)
	Thyroid becomes more fibrotic.	

(continued on the following page)

*A "minor variation," in this context, is one that usually does not require treatment.

Key: Text appearing in blue type refers to pediatric variations. Text appearing in gray type refers to geriatric variations.

PHYSICAL ASSESSMENT ACROSS THE LIFESPAN (CEPHALOCAUDAL APPROACH) (continued)

Assessment Area	Normal Finding or Minor Variation*	Possible Abnormalities
THORAX AND LUNGS (ANTERIOR AND POSTERIOR THORAX)		
	Inspection	
	Quiet respirations	Gasping, wheezing, stridor
	Erect posture	Thoracic lateral curve in spine (scoliosis), or "hump back" (kyphosis), may affect breathing
	Slightly convex contour of thorax	Pigeon chest, funnel chest, barrel chest
	AP diameter (in proportion to lateral diameter) 1 : 2	Increased AP diameter seen in barrel chest (more in elderly)
	Infant's thorax is round and develops usual adult shape after age 6 yr.	
	Symmetrical upward and outward movement of thorax with inspiration	Unilateral impairment or lagging of respiratory movement
	Minimal effort used for breathing	Retractions of intercostal space, supraclavicular or sternomastoid contractions, nasal flaring

Rate of respirations between 12 and 20 per minute; smooth, even rhythm	Tachypnea (fast), bradypnea (slow) rate, hypoventilation (shallow), hyperventilation (deep); Cheyne-Stokes, Biot's, apneustic, cluster breathing
Respirations are abdominal until age 6. See *Variations in Respiration with Age* in pediatric section.	Retractions (sinking in of soft tissue of chest) during inspiration.
Palpation Trachea midline	May be displaced laterally because of collapsed lung (atelectasis), air in pleural cavity (pneumothorax), fluid in thoracic cavity (pleural effusion)
Thoracic expansion: Examiner stands behind patient and places thumbs on either side of spine with fingers extending around lower rib cage. During inspiration, examiner's thumbs move upward, outward, and equidistant from midspinal line.	Unilateral lag in chest expansion, no expansion

(continued on the following page)

*A "minor variation," in this context, is one that usually does not require treatment.
Key: Text appearing in blue type refers to pediatric variations. Text appearing in gray type refers to geriatric variations.

PHYSICAL ASSESSMENT ACROSS THE LIFESPAN (CEPHALOCAUDAL APPROACH) (continued)

Assessment Area	*Normal Finding or Minor Variation**	*Possible Abnormalities*
THORAX AND LUNGS (ANTERIOR AND POSTERIOR THORAX) (continued)		
	Thorax nontender, no masses palpated	Tenderness of intercostal spaces (may indicate inflamed pleura), tenderness of ribs (may indicate fracture or arthritis)
	Tactile fremitus: As patient voices "99," mild purrlike vibrations are palpated symmetrically over thorax down to diaphragm. (Fremitus is normally slightly increased on right side.)	Decreased fremitus (pleural effusion, pneumothorax, emphysema, very thick chest wall) Increased fremitus (pneumonia, secretions, tumor)
	Percussion	
	Resonance (loud intensity, low pitch, long duration)	Dullness is heard when fluid or solid tissue replaces air (lobar pneumonia, pleural effusion, hemothorax, emphysema, fibrous tissue, tumor).

	Hyperresonance is heard over hyperinflated lungs (emphysema, asthma, pneumothorax).
Measurement of diaphragmatic excursion: Note distance between levels of dullness on full inhalation and exhalation (assessed on posterior thorax only, normally 5–6 cm).	High level of dullness may suggest pleural effusion or a paralyzed diaphragm.
Auscultation Instruct patient to hold head in midline and to breathe deeply, quietly, and with mouth open.	Sounds may be decreased in obstructive lung disease, muscular weakness, pleural effusion, pneumothorax, emphysema.
Normal Sounds: *Over lung fields*: "Vesicular": inspiration > expiration. *Over main bronchi*: "bronchovesicular": inspiration = expiration. *Over trachea*: "bronchial": inspiration < expiration.	*Adventitious sounds:* rales (crackles), wheezes, coarse sounds (rhonchi)

(continued on the following page)

*A "minor variation," in this context, is one that usually does not require treatment.

Key: Text appearing in blue type refers to pediatric variations. Text appearing in gray type refers to geriatric variations.

PHYSICAL ASSESSMENT ACROSS THE LIFESPAN (CEPHALOCAUDAL APPROACH) (continued)

Assessment Area	*Normal Finding or Minor Variation**	*Possible Abnormalities*
THORAX AND LUNGS (ANTERIOR AND POSTERIOR THORAX) (continued)		
	Vocal fremitus or resonance: As patient voices "99," muffled sounds are auscultated down to level of diaphragm.	Decreased fremitus may suggest pleural effusion, pneumothorax, emphysema, very thick chest wall. Increased fremitus (bronchophony) may suggest pneumonia, secretions, tumor.
HEART AND PULSES		
	Inspection Apical impulse seen in 4th, 5th, or 6th intercostal space, at or medial to the midclavicular line. (May be more easily seen with patient turned slightly on left side.)	Left ventricular enlargement may displace the apical impulse laterally. Impulse may be undetectable in obesity, muscular chest wall, or increased AP diameter.

No lifts/heaves of sternum or ribs	Right-sided heart failure may cause sternum or ribs to lift with each heart beat
Palpation	
Apical impulse usually occupies only 1 interspace.	Apical impulse diameter increased in left ventricular enlargement
No lifts/heaves or thrills ("vibrations")	Thrills may suggest aortic or pulmonic stenosis.
Percussion	
When apical impulse is nonpalpable, percussion may assist examiner in locating left cardiac border. When percussing from lung resonance toward cardiac border, dullness should be elicited at or medial to the midclavicular line.	An enlarged heart may displace the cardiac border laterally.

(continued on the following page)

*A "minor variation," in this context, is one that usually does not require treatment.
Key: Text appearing in blue type refers to pediatric variations. Text appearing in gray type refers to geriatric variations.

PHYSICAL ASSESSMENT ACROSS THE LIFESPAN (CEPHALOCAUDAL APPROACH) (continued)

Assessment Area	*Normal Finding or Minor Variation**	*Possible Abnormalities*
HEART AND PULSES (continued)		
	Ausculation Identify the 4 major auscultatory areas: *Aortic*: 2nd RICS (right intercostal space) near sternum *Pulmonic*: 2nd LICS near sternum *Tricuspid*: 5th LICS near sternum *Mitral*: 5th LICS just medial to midclavicular line (*See Fig. 2–6.*)	

*A "minor variation," in this context, is one that usually does not require treatment.
Key: Text appearing in blue type refers to pediatric variations. Text appearing in gray type refers to geriatric variations.

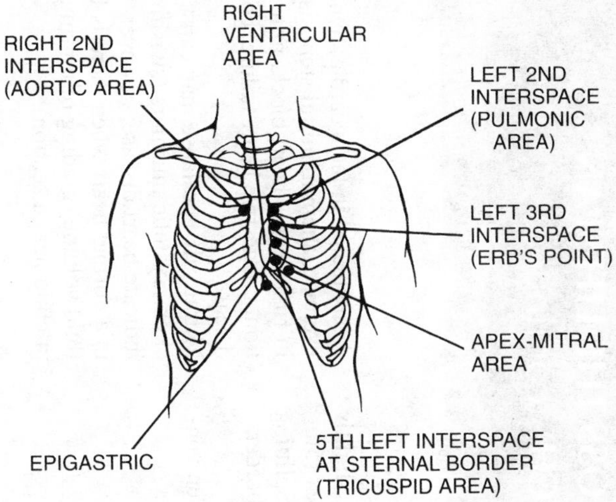

Figure 2–6. Cardiac auscultation sites. (From Hogstel, MO, and Curry, LC: Practical Guide to Health Assessment through the Life Span, ed. 3. FA Davis, Philadelphia, 2001, p. 217, with permission.)

PHYSICAL ASSESSMENT ACROSS THE LIFESPAN (CEPHALOCAUDAL APPROACH) (continued)

Assessment Area	Normal Finding or Minor Variation*	Possible Abnormalities
HEART AND PULSES (continued)	***Listen Carefully To***	
	First heart sound (S_1): Duller, lower pitched, slightly longer duration than S_2, and louder at the apex (5th LICS just medial to the midclavicular line). Splitting may be detected along the lower left sternal border.	Accentuated in tachycardia, hyperthyroidism, exercise, anemia, mitral stenosis; diminished in first-degree heart block, mitral regurgitation, congestive heart failure, coronary heart disease
	Systole: Quiet interval between S_1 and S_2 when ventricles contract and empty	Mitral valve prolapse may cause a systolic click. Systolic murmurs (swishing sound) may indicate heart disease; however, many occur in a normal heart when there is fever or large fluid volume (grading of murmurs described in child health section).

Second heart sound (S_2): Snappier, higher pitched, shorter duration, and louder at the base (upper left chest area). Splitting may be detected bilaterally in the 2nd or 3rd intercostal spaces and is accentuated by inspiration and usually disappears on expiration. S_2 in aortic area is usually louder than in pulmonic area.	Increase in normal splitting that continues throughout respiratory cycle may suggest pulmonic stenosis, right bundle branch block, or mitral regurgitation S_2 loud in pulmonary hypertension
Diastole: Quiet interval between S_2 and S_1 when ventricles relax and fill. Most conditioned athletes have an audible S_3, and many have an S_4. An S_3 may normally be heard in children, young adults to the age of 35–40, and during the last trimester of pregnancy.	An opening snap (very early in diastole) usually suggests a stenotic mitral valve. An S_3 in persons over 40 is almost always pathologic, indicating early ventricular resistance to filling. An S_4 results from increased resistance to ventricular filling after atrial contraction. Diastolic murmurs always indicate heart disease.
Apical heart rate: regular rhythm (may vary with change in respiratory rate)	Irregular heart rate

(continued on the following page)

*A "minor variation," in this context, is one that usually does not require treatment.
Key: Text appearing in blue type refers to pediatric variations. Text appearing in gray type refers to geriatric variations.

PHYSICAL ASSESSMENT ACROSS THE LIFESPAN (CEPHALOCAUDAL APPROACH) (continued)

Assessment Area	*Normal Finding or Minor Variation**	*Possible Abnormalities*
HEART AND PULSES (continued)		
PULSES (See Fig 2–7.)	"Splitting" of sounds (4 distinct sounds)	
	PMI visible in thin child	
	Grade 1 or 2 innocent (no pathology) murmur in up to 30% of children	Grade 3 or greater murmur.
	See *Cardiac Murmurs* in *pediatric section.*	Diastolic murmur
	Innocent murmur is always systolic, usually heard in pulmonic area, and may disappear with position change.	Thrill (vibratory sensation accompanying murmur and palpable in upper left chest)
	Full (volume), regular rhythm; symmetry noted.	Bounding or weak, thready pulse; pulses absent in acute arterial occlusion and arteriosclerosis obliterans
	Pulse is somewhat irregular and varies markedly with respiratory rate.	

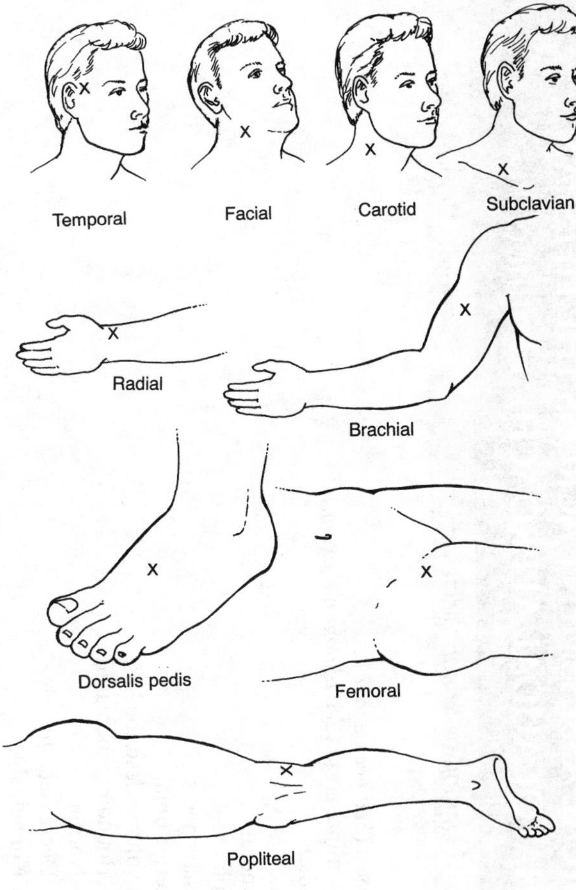

Figure 2–7. Pulse sites.

PHYSICAL ASSESSMENT ACROSS THE LIFESPAN (CEPHALOCAUDAL APPROACH) (continued)

Assessment Area	*Normal Finding or Minor Variation**	*Possible Abnormalities*
HEART AND PULSES (continued)	Carotid (*See neck exam.*) Abdominal aorta (*See abdominal exam.*) Radial Brachial Femoral Popliteal Dorsalis pedis Posterior tibial Pulse volume described as: 3+ Bounding, increased 2+ Normal 1+ Decreased, thready 0 Nonpalpable	

	Dorsalis pedis and posterior tibial pulses may be more difficult to find	
BREASTS AND AXILLAE		
Female breasts	Symmetric (Common for dominant side to be slightly larger.)	
	Skin: intact, no edema, color consistent with rest of body, smooth, convex contour	Redness, inflammation
	Consistency: varies widely (Firm, transverse inframammary ridge along lower breast edge should not be mistaken as abnormal mass.) Inframammary ridge thickens	Any lump or mass that is larger or that significantly differs from other breast tissue should be described according to location, size, shape, mobility, consistency, and tenderness. (Tenderness may be due to premenstrual fullness, inflammation, fibrocystic condition, or sometimes carcinoma.) *Signs of breast cancer:* peau d'orange skin (edema/thickened skin with enlarged pores), retractions, dimpling. Hard, irregular, fixed, noncircumscribed masses

(continued on the following page)

*A "minor variation," in this context, is one that usually does not require treatment.
Key: Text appearing in blue type refers to pediatric variations. Text appearing in gray type refers to geriatric variations.

PHYSICAL ASSESSMENT ACROSS THE LIFESPAN (CEPHALOCAUDAL APPROACH) (continued)

Assessment Area	*Normal Finding or Minor Variation**	*Possible Abnormalities*
BREASTS AND AXILLAE (continued)		
Areola	Small elevations around the nipple (Montgomery's glands) are normal.	Rashes or ulcerations may suggest cancer of mammary ducts (Paget's disease).
Nipple	Usually elastic, everted Nipples become smaller and flatter	Recent changes in size or shape (retraction, flattening, broadening, thickening, loss of elasticity) or the directions in which the nipples point suggest cancer.
	Intact skin, no discharge Occasional hair around nipple	Rashes, ulcerations, or discharge may suggest Paget's disease. Describe any discharge according to color, odor, consistency, quantity, and exact location. A nonmilky discharge may suggest breast disease and should be further evaluated.

Male breasts	Flat or muscular appearance without masses	Gynecomastia: a firm disk-shaped glandular enlargement on one or both sides resulting from imbalance in estrogen/androgen ratio, sometimes drug-related (spironolactone, cimetidine, digitalis preparations, estrogens, phenothiazines, methyldopa, reserpine, marijuana, or tricyclic antidepressants) A hard, irregular, eccentric, or ulcerating nodule suggests breast cancer, not gynecomastia.
Axillae	Smooth, intact skin	Rash (may be caused by deodorant). Velvety, smooth deeply pigmented skin should be further evaluated.
	Small, soft, movable, nontender lymph nodes may be palpated.	Enlarged, tender, hard nodes may be due to hand or arm infection but may also be a sign of breast cancer.

(continued on the following page)

*A "minor variation," in this context, is one that usually does not require treatment.
Key: Text appearing in blue type refers to pediatric variations. Text appearing in gray type refers to geriatric variations.

PHYSICAL ASSESSMENT ACROSS THE LIFESPAN (CEPHALOCAUDAL APPROACH) (continued)

Assessment Area	*Normal Finding or Minor Variation**	*Possible Abnormalities*
ABDOMEN **Note:** Inspect first, as always, but auscultate prior to percussing or palpating		
	Inspection	
Umbilicus	Usually positioned at midline and slightly below center of abdomen, may be normally everted or inverted	A recent change in contour or location may suggest an abnormality such as a hernia or tumor. (Having the patient cough will cause a hernia to bulge farther out. Check for reducibility. Report if hernia cannot be gently reduced or "pushed back" when patient relaxes.)

		Bluish discoloration of periumbilical skin (Cullen's sign) may indicate intraperitoneal hemorrhage, which may be caused by a ruptured ectopic pregnancy or acute pancreatitis.
	Soft (reducible) bulge of umbilicus (hernia) until 4 yr old	Hernia persists after 4 yr of age or is nonreducible. (Hernia cannot be pushed back into abdominal cavity when child is at rest.) **NOTE: Nonreducible hernia may indicate strangulation of tissue and is an emergency situation.**
Contour	Symmetric, slightly rounded or convex, no visible masses or organs Young child has "potbelly"	Enlarged organs or masses cause asymmetry. A distended abdomen may be caused by: fat, flatus, feces, fetus, fluid, or fibroids. Ascites (serous fluid in peritoneal cavity) causes bulging flanks.

(continued on the following page)

*A "minor variation," in this context, is one that usually does not require treatment.
Key: Text appearing in blue type refers to pediatric variations. Text appearing in gray type refers to geriatric variations.

PHYSICAL ASSESSMENT ACROSS THE LIFESPAN (CEPHALOCAUDAL APPROACH) (continued)

Assessment Area	*Normal Finding or Minor Variation**	*Possible Abnormalities*
ABDOMEN *(continued)*		
Skin	Old, silver striae (stretch marks) and a few small visible veins are normal. Describe location and characteristics of scars.	Ascites may cause skin to be tense and to glisten. Bluish discoloration may indicate trauma or intra-abdominal bleeding. Turner's sign is ecchymosis of one or both flanks.
Pulsations	Aortic pulse is a normal finding.	Increased pulsation may be seen with an abdominal aortic aneurysm or in patients with thin-walled, hollow-shaped (scaphoid) abdomens.
Peristalsis	May be visible in very thin patients.	Visible waves may suggest intestinal obstruction.

	Ausculation	
Bowel sounds	Vary in frequency, pitch, and loudness but usually consist of clicks and gurgles from 5–35 per min	*Increased* sounds with gastroenteritis, early intestinal obstruction *Decreased*, then absent sounds, with paralytic ileus, peritonitis Loud, prolonged gurgles (borborygmi) or unusually loud, rushing, high-pitched tinkling sounds, associated with cramping, may indicate intestinal obstruction.
	Listen to the upper abdomen, over the aorta, and to the renal, iliac, and femoral arteries. No vascular sounds should be heard.	An abdominal aortic bruit (swishing noise) associated with decreased pulses in the legs may indicate a dissecting aneurysm.
	Percussion	
	Tympany in all 4 quadrants. The gastric air bubble produces a loud, tympanic sound in upper left quadrant at rib cage. Normal fluid, feces, or distended bladder produces dullness.	Dullness in both flanks (body part between ribs and iliac crest) may indicate ascites. Positive fluid wave and/or shifting dullness indicate ascites.

(continued on the following page)

*A "minor variation," in this context, is one that usually does not require treatment.

Key: Text appearing in blue type refers to pediatric variations. Text appearing in gray type refers to geriatric variations.

PHYSICAL ASSESSMENT ACROSS THE LIFESPAN (CEPHALOCAUDAL APPROACH) (continued)

Assessment Area	Normal Finding or Minor Variation*	Possible Abnormalities
ABDOMEN ***(continued)***		
	Liver dullness percussed at the right midclavicular line (6–12 cm from top to bottom of liver).	Increased liver measurement may suggest hepatomegaly.
	Liver size decreases after age 50	
	Splenic dullness percussed posterior to the left midaxillary line (usually about 4–6 cm).	A large area of dullness may suggest splenomegaly.
	Palpation	
	Lightly palpate to identify skin temperature, areas of tenderness, masses, or muscular resistance.	"Guarding" (increased resistance) may indicate inflammation.
	Deeply palpate to identify masses. The abdominal aortic pulse is also palpated in the upper abdomen, slightly to left of midline.	Describe any mass according to location, size, shape, consistency, tenderness, and mobility.

Adult aorta is not more than 2.5 cm wide.	Increased width of abdominal aorta with expansile pulsation may suggest an aneurysm. Pain in this area may suggest rupture of the aorta. (*Caution: Do not prolong palpation of an enlarged aorta.*) "Rebound" tenderness (pain induced or increased by quick withdrawal of examiner's palpating hand) suggests peritoneal inflammation, such as occurs with appendicitis.
Palpate liver below right costal margin as patient inhales deeply. Palpable up to 2 cm below RCM.	Increased liver size, tenderness, firmness, or irregularity of shape may suggest an abnormality. Liver palpable more than 2 cm below RCM may indicate CHF.
Palpate for spleen below left costal margin; adult spleen is usually nonpalpable. Palpable up to 2 cm below LCM.	A palpable, tender spleen may indicate abnormality.

(continued on the following page)

*A "minor variation," in this context, is one that usually does not require treatment.
Key: Text appearing in blue type refers to pediatric variations. Text appearing in gray type refers to geriatric variations.

PHYSICAL ASSESSMENT ACROSS THE LIFESPAN (CEPHALOCAUDAL APPROACH) (continued)

Assessment Area	Normal Finding or Minor Variation*	Possible Abnormalities
ABDOMEN ***(continued)***		
		Spleen palpable more than 2 cm below LCM may indicate mononucleosis or sickle cell crisis
	As patient inhales deeply, palpate left and right flank to "capture" the kidneys. (A normal right kidney may be palpable. A normal left kidney is rarely palpable.)	Enlargement of kidney may suggest tumors, cysts, hydronephrosis, polycystic disease. Pain on palpation or first percussion may suggest pyelonephritis (kidney infection).

MUSCULO-SKELETAL	Firm muscles palpable; demonstrates ability to resist passive motion All joints show full range of smooth, coordinated, symmetrical movement without swelling, tenderness, increased heat, redness, crepitus, or deformities. (*See Figure 1–25.*) Loss of one or more inches in height common. Joint and muscle agility vary greatly.	Atrophy, naccidity, weakness, or paralysis may suggest a neurologic abnormality. Spastic movements may suggest neurologic abnormality. Tenderness may suggest arthritis, synovitis, tendinitis, or bursitis. Tenderness at the costovertebral angles may suggest a kidney infection rather than a musculoskeletal problem.
Spine	Posture is erect. Spinal column is in alignment. Shoulders and iliac crests are level. Spine shows cervical concavity, thoracic convexity, lumbar concavity. Lordosis ("swayback") may be noted during pregnancy or with marked obesity.	Kyphosis ("hunchback") often seen in the elderly. Scoliosis (lateral curvature) may be associated with vertebral and rib cage deformity or unequal leg length. Often becomes evident during adolescence.

(continued on the following page)

*A "minor variation," in this context, is one that usually does not require treatment.
Key: Text appearing in blue type refers to pediatric variations. Text appearing in gray type refers to geriatric variations.

PHYSICAL ASSESSMENT ACROSS THE LIFESPAN (CEPHALOCAUDAL APPROACH) (continued)

Assessment Area	*Normal Finding or Minor Variation**	*Possible Abnormalities*
MUSCULO-SKELETAL (continued)	Lateral spinal curve that disappears when child bends forward (postural or functional scoliosis) *Functional scoliosis may be due simply to poor posture or may be related to an underlying defect such as unequal leg length.*	Lateral spine curve that does not correct itself when child bends forward (structural scoliosis)
	Small tuft of hair or dimple at lower end of spine with normal leg movement	Tuft of hair or dimple at lower spine without normal leg movement or abnormal urinary or bowel sphincter control may *indicate underlying neurologic defect.*
Extremities	Equal leg lengths Hips symmetric	Unequal leg lengths

Gluteal folds symmetric	Asymmetric gluteal folds
Knees same height when infant supine with knees and hips flexed at 90 degrees	One knee higher when infant supine with knees and hips flexed at 90 degrees (Galeazzi's sign)
	Limited leg abduction
Hips symmetric	One hip prominent. *Findings listed above may indicate dislocated hip* in young child or scoliosis in older child.
Legs flexed at hips and knees when infant held upright with examiner's hands under infant's axillae	Legs adducted (brought toward midline) and extended (straightened) when infant held upright *may indicate paraplegia.*
Knock-knees (genu valgum) are normal until age 7 yr and may be benign past age 7.	Knock-knees after age 7 should be investigated.
Bowlegs (genu varum) are normal throughout toddler period and may be benign thereafter.	Bowlegs that persist past age 3 should be investigated.
Feet in anatomic alignment	Foot turned outward (talipes or pes valgus)
	Foot turned inward (talipes or pes varus)

(continued on the following page)

*A "minor variation," in this context, is one that usually does not require treatment.
Key: Text appearing in blue type refers to pediatric variations. Text appearing in gray type refers to geriatric variations.

PHYSICAL ASSESSMENT ACROSS THE LIFESPAN (CEPHALOCAUDAL APPROACH) (continued)

Assessment Area	*Normal Finding or Minor Variation**	*Possible Abnormalities*
MUSCULO-SKELETAL (continued)	Arch of foot commonly flat (pes planus) prior to 4 yr of age	Persistent flat arch may be benign or problematic.
	Broad-based gait in toddler	
	Toe walking without heels touching floor (pes equinus) common until several months after walking begins	Prolonged toe walking *may indicate cerebral palsy or tight heel cords.*
	Pigeon toe (toeing in) usually benign	Severe toeing in that does not improve after walking begins
	Negative Homans' sign bilaterally (No pain in calf when foot is quickly dorsiflexed.)	Calf pain with upper foot dorsiflexion may suggest thrombophlebitis.

NEUROLOGIC		
Cranial nerves (See *Head and Neck Assessment.*)	Intact	Abnormalities in cranial nerve assessment may suggest neurologic disorders.
Cerebral functioning (See *Mental Status Assessment.*)	Intact	
Cerebellar functioning	Intact	
	Negative Romberg test: maintains upright position with only minimal swaying when standing with feet together and eyes closed	Loss of balance is termed "positive Romberg test" (indicates sensory ataxia).
	Gait is coordinated and balanced, with erect posture, swinging of the arms, and movements of the legs. Tandem walking (heel-to-toe) is intact.	Uncoordinated gait may suggest cerebral palsy, parkinsonism, or drug side effect.
	Coordinated and steady movement while: sliding heel of one foot down opposite shin, rapidly touching thumb to each finger, rapidly touching own nose and then examiner's finger	Inappropriate movements suggest cerebellar disease.

(continued on the following page)

*A "minor variation," in this context, is one that usually does not require treatment.
Key: Text appearing in blue type refers to pediatric variations. Text appearing in gray type refers to geriatric variations.

PHYSICAL ASSESSMENT ACROSS THE LIFESPAN (CEPHALOCAUDAL APPROACH) (continued)

Assessment Area	*Normal Finding or Minor Variation**	*Possible Abnormalities*
NEUROLOGIC (continued)		
Motor system	Intact No involuntary movements *Muscle size, tone, and strength are assessed in musculoskeletal exam.*	Tics, tremors, fasciculations may suggest neurologic involvement.
Sensory system	Intact *Upon symmetric testing of the arms, legs, and trunk, identifies*: *Pain*: "Sharp or dull?" *Temperature*: "Hot or cold?" *Light touch*: "Feel touch?" *Vibration*: "Feel tuning fork vibrating against joint?" *Position sense* (*proprioception*): "Am I moving your toe up or down?"	Inappropriate response indicates neurologic disorder.

Sensory cortex	*Discrimination* (*stereognosis*): "Can you identify the object in your hand?" (e.g., key, paper clip, coin); "What number am I writing on your hand?" (*graphesthesia*) "Can you feel me touch both sides of your body?"	Inabilities suggest a lesion in the sensory cortex.
Reflexes	Symmetric and intact Biceps (inner elbow) Triceps (behind and above elbow) Brachioradialis (lower arm) Patellar (knee) Achilles (ankle) Plantar (sole of foot) ***Reflex Scale*** 0 No response 1+ Diminished 2+ Normal; average 3+ Brisker than normal 4+ Hyperactive; often associated with clonus	Diminished or absent reflexes may suggest upper or lower motor neuron disease; however, this may also be found in normal people. (Reinforcement by isometric contraction such as asking patient to push his or her hands together while knee reflex is checked may increase reflex activity.) A positive Babinski's reflex (toes spread and dorsiflex when sole of foot is stroked) may be seen in pyramidal tract disease or in the unconscious patient.

*A "minor variation," in this context, is one that usually does not require treatment.
Key: Text appearing in blue type refers to pediatric variations. Text appearing in gray type refers to geriatric variations.

Pathologic Conditions

ACQUIRED IMMUNODEFICIENCY SYNDROME (AIDS)

Definition: Immune system disorder occurring in response to exposure to human immunodeficiency virus (HIV) or a similar human retrovirus.

Pathophysiology: Failure of cell-mediated immunity results in serious infections and malignancies that exhaust the body's natural defense mechanisms, resulting in inability to fight infection.

Etiology: Transmitted by exposure to blood and body fluids of HIV-infected persons through sexual contact, sharing of needles, perinatal exposure of infants, and possibly splashing of body fluids into open lesions or mucous membranes.

Manifestations: Fever; diarrhea; malaise; weight loss; lymphadenitis; opportunistic infections and malignancies; positive ELISA/Western blot tests; T4 (CD4) cell count $\leq 200/mm^3$; positive cultures for *Pneumocystis carinii* pneumonia; atypical viral, fungal, and protozoal infections.

Med Tx: Multiple drug therapy regimens may slow progression of illness, but no cure exists. Supplemental nutrition, antibiotics, and chemotherapy as needed.

Nsg Dx: Potential for infection, alteration in nutrition, potential fluid volume deficit R/T diarrhea, altered thought process and resultant potential for injury, numerous psychosocial diagnoses.

Nsg Care: Implement strict infection control practices (universal precautions); monitor for side effects of all medications, I&O, daily weight and nutritional assessment; educate; make support agency referrals for patient and family as needed.

Prognosis: Progressive deterioration with CD4 <100 mm^3 and eventual death.

ANGINA PECTORIS

Definition: Transient chest pain or feeling of constriction about the heart.

Pathophysiology: Deficiency of O_2 to the heart muscle results in pain.

Etiology: CAD; hypertension; CHF; coronary artery spasm usually precipitated by exercise, stress, exposure to cold, or a large meal. Symptoms usually last 1 to 4 minutes.

Manifestations: Pain and/or a feeling of constriction or burning about the heart; typically radiates to the left shoulder and down the left arm, back, or jaw or rarely to the abdomen (mimics MI but does not cause cellular death).

Med Tx: O_2, vasodilators (nitrates), beta-adrenergic blockers, calcium channel blockers, rest, stress reduction programs.

Nsg Dx: Decreased (cardiac) tissue perfusion, pain, activity intolerance, knowledge deficit, anxiety.

Nsg Care: Assess and record details of attacks. Provide for immediate rest and quiet environment during attacks. Monitor effects of medical treatment. Eliminate precipitating factors. Provide education. Instruct the patient to seek immediate medical attention if three doses of nitroglycerin at 5-minute intervals do not provide relief.

Prognosis: Varies. With proper rest and care, recovery is possible, but prognosis may be grave.

ASTHMA (REACTIVE AIRWAY DISEASE)

Definition: An obstructive disease of the airways caused by increased responsiveness of the tracheobronchial tree to various stimuli such as allergens, infection, exercise, cold air, or stress.

Pathophysiology: Airway stimuli result in spasms and edema of the bronchi and bronchioles. There is increased production and viscosity of mucus, and air is trapped distal to the resultant obstruction. There is impaired gas exchange in the alveoli.

Etiology: There is familial predisposition to asthma. Stimuli that may precipitate exacerbations (attacks) include any substance to which the person is allergic, viruses, smoke, dust, cold air, or exercise.

Manifestations: Wheezing, dyspnea, uncontrollable cough, nasal flaring, musical rales, and anxiety.

Med Tx: Prevention of attacks through identification and avoidance of provoking stimuli and with administration of corticosteroids, salmeterol, and cromolyn sodium. Treatment of attacks with bronchodilators (such as albuterol or aminophylline), epinephrine, corticosteroids, expectorants, and antibiotics (if infection is present).

Nsg Dx: Ineffective airway clearance, impaired gas exchange, activity intolerance, anxiety.

Nsg Care: Monitor ongoing respiratory status. Monitor for side effects of medications. Encourage fluids. Plan care to allow for periods of uninterrupted rest. Educate regarding avoidance of and treatments of attacks. Support.

Prognosis: About half will outgrow exacerbations. If asthma persists into the teen years, it will likely continue into adulthood. Persistent asthma may lead to the development of chronic obstructive lung disease.

BRONCHIOLITIS

Definition: Inflammation of the mucous membranes of the bronchioles.

Pathophysiology: Swelling of the small airways leads to hyperinflation (distal to the obstruction) and emphysema. Resultant pneumonitis and patchy areas of atelectasis may be present.

Etiology: Bronchiolitis is usually preceded by an upper respiratory viral infection in children. Respiratory syncytial virus (RSV) is responsible for the majority of cases (believed to be spread by hand to nose or eye transmission). Other causative organisms are adenoviruses and parainfluenza viruses.

Manifestations: Nasal flaring, tachypnea, cough, wheezing, anorexia, and fever. Chest may appear barrel shaped, and suprasternal and subcostal retractions may be present. (Mimics asthma. Usually seen in children under age 2.)

Med Tx: Ribavirin, bronchodilators, corticosteroids, high humidity (croup tent when hospitalized), supplemental O_2 to maintain SaO_2 at 95% or above, and increased fluid intake ($1^1/_2$ times maintenance; see *Pediatric Maintenance Fluid Calculation.*)

Nsg Dx: Ineffective breathing pattern, ineffective airway clearance, impaired gas exchange, potential fluid volume deficit, anxiety.

Nsg Care: Frequently monitor respiratory status. Provide $1^1/_2$ times maintenance fluids. Allow liberal parent visitation to decrease child's anxiety and oxygen needs. Adhere to strict handwashing regimen to avoid transmission of organism. Support. **Warning:** Pregnant personnel should be aware that RSV may be teratogenic.

Prognosis: Most children recover normal lung function after several weeks. Lung problems may persist for years following severe bronchiolitis. A few, especially those who have smoking mothers, have an increased incidence of asthma.

CEREBROVASCULAR ACCIDENT (CVA)

Definition: Occurrence of ischemic or hemorrhagic lesions within the intracranial vasculature (often called a *stroke* or *apoplexy*).

Pathophysiology: Obstruction of the supply of oxygen and nutrients to the brain, which results in varying degrees of cellular injury and neurologic dysfunction.

Etiology: Thrombus, embolism, or bleeding into an intracranial vessel. Predisposing or causative factors include atherosclerosis, hypertension, and AV malformation.

Manifestations: S&S of ICP; headache, altered LOC; pupillary changes; seizures; sensorimotor dysfunctions; alterations in speech, cognition, or cranial nerve functions.

Med Tx: Airway maintenance, ICP management, IV hemodilution, anticoagulation and thrombolytic therapy, vasodilators, diuretics, dexamethasone, anticonvulsants, possible surgery, early institution of rehabilitation therapy.

Nsg Dx: Alteration in tissue perfusion (cerebral), impaired physical mobility, impaired swallowing, impaired verbal communication, alteration in thought processes, numerous psychosocial diagnoses.

Nsg Care: Maintain airway. Monitor VS and neurologic status frequently. Evaluate effects of medical regimen. Monitor I&O and nutritional status. Turn every 1 to 2 hours. Coordinate and support rehabilitative regimens. Provide emotional support and patient and family education.

Prognosis: Varies from full recovery to persistent vegetative state or death depending on type, location, and severity of the event as well as complicating factors.

CHRONIC OBSTRUCTIVE PULMONARY DISEASE (COPD)

Definition: A group of chronic disorders characterized by airflow obstruction that is generally progressive but may be partially reversible; sometimes accompanied by airway hyperreactivity. Diseases included are emphysema, chronic bronchitis, and bronchiectasis. (AKA *chronic obstructive lung disease–[COLD]).*

Pathophysiology: Varies with specific disease. There may be inflammation, mucociliary clearance impairment, and bronchial wall destruction.

Etiology: Varies according to specific disease. History of cigarette smoking or smoke exposure, air pollution or toxic exposure, repeated infection. Risk factors are male sex, nonwhite race, low socioeconomic status, and hyperresponsive airways.

Manifestations: Dyspnea, cough, wheezing, barrel-shaped chest, prolonged expiratory phase of respirations, use of accessory muscles in forced expiration, breath sounds difficult to auscultate, skin color may be deep pink (due to high RBC count stimulated by hypoxia).

Med Tx: Smoking cessation, inhaled ipratropium bromide, pneumococcal vaccine, yearly flu vaccine, chest physiotherapy, supplemental O_2 and antibiotics as needed; acute exacerbations may be treated similarly to asthma.

Nsg Dx: Impaired gas exchange, ineffective airway clearance, activity intolerance, altered nutrition, less than body requirements, risk for infection.

Nsg Care: Small, frequent meals high in calories and protein, fluid intake of at least 3 L per day for adults, encourage avoidance of smoke, monitor for infection and signs of acute air hunger.

Prognosis: Condition, by definition, is chronic and is usually progressive; improvement is possible for some patients with appropriate therapy.

CONGESTIVE HEART FAILURE (CHF)

Definition: Failure of the cardiac muscle to maintain sufficient cardiac output and tissue perfusion.

Pathophysiology: The left ventricle (LV) loses its ability to eject blood into the systemic circulation, resulting in a large volume of blood remaining in the LV after systole. Backup of blood may progress to the left atrium, then to the pulmonary system (left-sided heart failure), then to the right ventricle and atrium, and finally to the systemic circulation (right-sided heart failure).

Etiology: Congenital defects, hypertension, cardiac valvular or peripheral vascular disease, damage to cardiac tissue, rheumatic fever, fluid overload, severe anemia, obstructive lung disease, endocrine disorders, sepsis, or electrolyte imbalances.

Manifestations: Dependent upon the degree of left versus right heart failure and compensatory capability. **Left-sided heart failure** may include: tachycardia, dysrhythmias, tachypnea, orthopnea, anxiety, cyanosis, decreased BP and peripheral pulses, crackles, wheezes, S_3/S_4 gallop, apical murmurs, elevated pulmonary capillary wedge pressure, and decreased cardiac output/index. **Right-sided heart failure** may include: dependent edema, JVD, bounding pulses, oliguria, dysrhythmias, liver/spleen enlargement, increased CVP, and altered liver function tests.

Med Tx: Bed rest if severe, fluid and sodium restriction, O_2, diuretics, inotropics, antihypertensives, vasodilators, antiarrhythmics, fluid restriction, bed rest, intra-aortic balloon pump, possible surgical intervention, and correction of underlying cause.

Nsg Dx: Decreased cardiac output, impaired gas exchange, fluid volume excess or potential deficit R/T diuretic use, activity intolerance, knowledge deficit, anxiety, potential for infection, potential impaired skin integrity related to edema and poor tissue perfusion.

Nsg Care: Monitor VS, peripheral pulses, heart/lung sounds, and I&O. Elevate HOB, assist with ADL, and promote calm environment. Calculate safety of digitalis dose. Monitor response to medications and therapy. Count pulse for a full minute prior to administration of digitalis—decisions to withhold digitalis are based on knowledge of age-appropriate pulse rates. Turn every 1–2 hours. Educate and provide emotional support.

Prognosis: Varies greatly with etiology, severity, compliance, and complicating factors. Many people live productive lives for decades following diagnosis. CHF in children usually resolves after correction of the underlying cause.

CYSTIC FIBROSIS (CF)

Definition: An inherited disease of the exocrine glands.

Pathophysiology: Increased viscosity of mucous gland secretions. Elevated sweat electrolytes and salivary enzymes and abnormalities of the autonomic nervous system result in frequent and severe respiratory infections, progressive lung dysfunction, loss of sodium chloride, and decreased absorption of nutrients.

Etiology: Disease is an inherited autosomal recessive

disorder. Both parents must be carriers. About 1 in 20 whites carry the gene.

Manifestations: Meconium ileus in up to 15% of newborns, failure to thrive, dyspnea, cough, frequent respiratory infection, excessive sodium loss in sweat, bulky, foul-smelling stools containing undigested food, abdominal distention, thin extremities, and rectal prolapse.

Med Tx: Daily percussion and postural drainage of lungs (chest physiotherapy, or CPT), physical exercise, pancreatic enzymes administered with food, multivitamins, increased salt intake, calorie intake increased to 150% of RDA, and aggressive antibiotic therapy during respiratory infections.

Nsg Dx: Ineffective airway clearance; potential for infection; altered nutrition, less than body requirements; knowledge deficit; fear; diversional activity deficit; sleep pattern disturbance.

Nsg Care: Adhere to strict handwashing regimen. Assure compatibility of IV antibiotics. Encourage frequent fluid intake. Offer at least 6 feedings per day. Coordinate activities so that meds and CPT do not interfere with appetite or sleep and rest. Provide teaching and emotional support.

Prognosis: Median survival is 20 to 27 years. Males generally survive longer than females.

DEHYDRATION

Definition: A condition that occurs when output of body fluids exceeds fluid intake.

Pathophysiology: In early dehydration, fluid loss is from both intracellular and extracellular compartments. In chronic dehydration, fluid loss is predominantly cellular. Fluid loss may result in shock, acidosis or alkalosis, kidney and brain damage in children; death occurs much more quickly than in the adult patient.

Etiology: Usual causes are diarrhea, vomiting, extensive burns, or diabetic ketoacidosis.

Manifestations: Poor skin turgor or "tenting" when skin over sternum is lifted by examiner, dry mouth, lack of tears in child over 3 months old, sunken anterior fontanel if fontanel has not closed, weight loss, decreased urine output, and urine specific gravity over 1.023. Decreased blood pressure is not an early, but a late, sign of shock in children because their blood vessels adapt quickly to intravascular fluid loss.

Med Tx: Oral rehydration fluids (ORS) if patient can ingest and retain fluids. IV fluids and electrolytes if patient cannot ingest or retain fluids. For children IV fluids for the first 8 hours include maintenance amount (see *Pediatric Maintenance Fluid Calculation*) plus $^1/_2$ the estimated fluid deficit (using 1 kg of weight loss to represent 1000 mL of fluid loss) administered in the first 8 hours and the remaining $^1/_2$ of estimated deficit added to maintenance fluid administered in the next 24 to 48 hours. Excessive ongoing losses determined by strict I&O must also be factored in calculation. Goal is to achieve 0.5 to 1 mL/h urinary output for each kilogram of body weight and to diagnose and treat underlying cause of dehydration.

Nsg Dx: Fluid volume deficit, altered tissue perfusion.

Nsg Care: Maintain strict I&O. For babies, subtract weight of dry diaper from weight of wet diaper using 1 g of weight to represent 1 mL of output. (Count both urine and liquid stools as fluid output.) Continue to assess for degree of dehydration or overhydration. Calculate appropriateness of ordered IV fluids. ***Warning:*** Avoid IV fluids containing potassium until the patient has voided.

Prognosis: Excellent when fluids and electrolytes are replaced appropriately. ***Warning:*** Children become dehydrated and overhydrated much more quickly than adults.

DIABETES MELLITUS

Definition: A group of syndromes characterized by the inability to metabolize carbohydrates.

Pathophysiology: There is usually inadequate insulin production (by the beta cells of the pancreas) and/or tissue resistance to insulin, which results in the inability of glucose to enter and nourish body cells. Absence of glucose in the cells results in cellular starvation and in fluid and electrolyte imbalances. The body responds to cellular starvation by breaking down fat and protein, which results in muscle wasting and ketone and lactic acid buildup.

Etiology: Cause unknown. Most cases appear to be genetic; others may result from a deficiency of beta cells caused by inflammation, malignancies of the pancreas, or surgery. Onset sometimes follows an apparently unrelated infection. Temporary or permanent gestational diabetes may occur during pregnancy.

Manifestations: Hyperglycemia (elevated blood sugar), glycosuria (sugar in urine), polyuria (excessive urination), polydipsia (excessive thirst), polyphagia (excessive food intake), itching, weight loss, urine SG above 1.020, ketones in urine.

Med Tx: Diet control, exercise, medications, and glucose monitoring.

Nsg Dx: Alteration in elimination, alteration in nutrition, potential fluid volume deficit, potential for infection, knowledge deficit, numerous psychosocial diagnoses.

Nsg Care: Assess frequently for S&S of hyperglycemia, hypoglycemia, dehydration, and acidosis. Provide patient and significant others with extensive education, including specific written information on diet, insulin, exercise, and complications. Provide frequent encouragement and emotional support.

Prognosis: Varies with age of onset, compliance, and complicating factors, but consistent symptom management usually results in an acceptable quality of life for many years.

Table 2–2. COMPARISON OF TYPE 1 INSULIN-DEPENDENT DIABETES MELLITUS AND TYPE 2 NON–INSULIN-DEPENDENT DIABETES MELLITUS

	Type 1	Type 2
Age at onset	Usually under 30	Usually over 40
Symptom onset	Abrupt	Gradual
Body weight	Normal	Obese—80%
HLA association	Positive	Negative
Family history	Common	Nearly universal
Insulin in blood	Little to none	Some usually present
Islet cell antibodies	Present at onset	Absent
Prevalence	0.2%–0.3%	6%
Symptoms	Polyuria, polydipsia, polyphagia, weight loss, ketoacidosis	Polyuria, polydipsia, peripheral neuropathy
Control	Insulin, diet, and exercise	Diet, exercise, and often oral hypoglycemic drugs or insulin
Vascular and neural changes	Eventually develop	Will usually develop
Stability of condition	Fluctuates, may be difficult to control	May be difficult to control in poorly motivated patients

Source: Venes, D, and Thomas, CL (eds): Taber's Cyclopedic Medical Dictionary, ed 19. FA Davis, Philadelphia, 2001, p. 557, with permission.

HYPERTENSION (HTN)

Definition:

For adults:

120–139 systolic or 80–89 diastolic = Prehypertension

140–159 systolic or 90–99 diastolic = Stage 1 HTN

>160 systolic or > 100 diastolic = Stage 2 HTN

For children:

95th percentile or greater adjusted for age, height., and gender.

See *Normal Blood Pressure Readings* chart in pediatric section.

Whichever reading is higher (systolic or diastolic) is used to classify blood pressure.

Pathophysiology and Etiology: Usually unknown (essential, primary, or idiopathic HTN). Excess renin may increase the production of angiotensin II, which raises blood pressure. HTN may be caused by insulin resistance, structural cardiac or vascular defects or disease, pregnancy, obesity, cocaine (most common cause of young adult HTN presentation to ER), sleep apnea, thyroid or parathyroid disease, kidney disease, pheochromocytoma, oral contraceptives, amphetamines, excess alcohol, steroids, erythropoietin, and other pathologies. The term *secondary HTN* is used when cause is known.

Manifestations: Initially, essential HTN is usually asymptomatic except for elevation of blood pressure. Occasionally headache. Late complications of uncontrolled HTN include manifestations of damage to eyes (retinopathy), kidneys, heart, or brain.

Med Tx: Lifestyle changes that include prevention or treatment of obesity and hyperlipidemia by increasing exercise and decreasing dietary calories, fat, and sodium (DASH diet). Smoking cessation and moderation of alcohol consumption. Antihypertensive meds—usually more than one med is needed.

Nsg Dx: Risk for decreased cardiac output (vasoconstriction), risk for sexual dysfunction (atherosclerosis or side effect of meds), pain (headache), knowledge deficit, impaired adjustment.

Nsg Care: Check B/P at every office visit or at least

once per shift when hospitalized. Teach regarding healthy weight, exercise diet, smoking cessation, and alcohol moderation.

Prognosis: Excellent with B/P controlled below <140/90 or <130/80 for those with diabetes or kidney failure. Uncontrolled HTN may result in damage to eyes, kidneys, heart, or brain. These complications are called end-organ damage. Heart failure and death are possible.

HYDROCEPHALUS

Definition: Increased accumulation of cerebrospinal fluid (CSF) within the ventricles of the brain.

Pathophysiology: Hydrocephalus results from obstructed flow of CSF (noncommunicating hydrocephalus) or an imbalance between production and reabsorption of CSF (communicating hydrocephalus). There is increased intracranial pressure, and head size increases abnormally if sutures and fontanels have not closed.

Etiology: *Noncommunicating hydrocephalus* (most common type) may result from development anomalies, tumors, abscesses, or trauma and occurs in about 80% of infants with myelomeningocele. *Communicating hydrocephalus* may result from tumors or infections such as meningitis.

Manifestations: *Infant*: abnormal increase in head circumference, bulging fontanel, enlargement of forehead, "setting sun sign" (sclera is visible above iris of the eye), pupils sluggish and/or unequal, high-pitched cry, irritability, and opisthotonos (head and body arch backward). *Older child*: Headache and nausea on awakening (lessened pain after vomiting), papilledema, strabismus, ataxia, and confusion.

Med Tx: Surgical removal of obstruction if possible or surgical placement of a shunt that drains CSF from the ventricles to the peritoneum or right atrium.

Nsg Dx: Potential for injury related to increased intracranial pressure, potential for infection related to mechanical drainage, knowledge deficit (parents).

Nsg Care: Measure head circumference, daily, of

infants with myelomeningocele or meningitis. Monitor diagnosed infant for signs of increasing intracranial pressure (anorexia, vomiting, irritability, lethargy, seizures, or increased blood pressure). *Postop shunt placement*: Monitor for signs of infection (similar to signs of increased intracranial pressure). Teach parents to monitor for infection and signs of increased intracranial pressure, as shunt infection or malfunction may occur after discharge.

Prognosis: If untreated, outcome is fatal in about half the cases. Seventy percent of surgically treated cases have at least a 5-year survival rate. About one-third of survivors are intellectually and neurologically normal.

IRON DEFICIENCY ANEMIA

Definition: A reduction in the number of circulating red blood cells or the amount of hemoglobin.

Pathophysiology: Iron stores are depleted, serum iron levels fall, and clinical symptoms develop as hemoglobin is inadequate to carry oxygen to body tissues.

Etiology: Inadequate iron intake, malabsorption of iron, chronic blood loss, hemolysis, or pregnancy.

Manifestations: Pallor (paleness), fatigue, vertigo, headache, dyspnea, tachycardia, and amenorrhea.

Med Tx: *Child:* Oral ferrous sulfate or ferrous gluconate, well-balanced diet to include 2 mg/kg of iron each day, vitamin C, intramuscular administration of iron for severe cases, and identification and treatment of excess blood loss. *Adult*: 100 to 200 mg/day in 3 divided doses. Continue treatment 4 to 6 mos after lab values are normal to replace iron stores.

Nsg Dx: Altered nutrition, less than body requirements; activity intolerance; knowledge deficit.

Nsg Care: Administer iron preparation with citrus. Avoid giving iron with alkaline foods or antacids. Give liquid preparation through a straw or behind teeth with dropper. Teach regarding foods high in iron and administration of iron preparations. Monitor response to therapy (adequate response is indicated by reticulocyte count rise, then, after 5 to 10 days of therapy, hemoglobin rise of 0.17 to 0.25 g/dL/day or about 3.4 to 6.25 g/dL/mo).

Prognosis: Excellent with regimen compliance and cessation of excess iron losses that may be caused by bleeding.

LARYNGOTRACHEOBRONCHITIS (CROUP)

Definition: An acute infection and inflammation of the larynx, trachea, and bronchi.

Pathophysiology: Airway mucosa becomes swollen, decreasing airway diameter and greatly increasing the difficulty of respiratory effort.

Etiology: Condition is often preceded by an upper airway viral infection. Common causative organisms are parainfluenza viruses and respiratory syncytial virus.

Manifestations: Harsh, "barking" cough, inspiratory stridor, hoarseness, and tachypnea.

Med Tx: High humidity (steam in bathroom for home treatment, croup tent if hospitalized), oxygen to maintain SaO_2 above 95%, aerosol administration of epinephrine, and IV fluids at $1^1/_2$ times maintenance amount (see *Pediatric Maintenance Fluid Calculation*). Corticosteroids may be ordered.

Nsg Dx: Ineffective airway clearance, potential fluid volume deficit, potential sleep pattern disturbance related to respiratory distress, anxiety.

Nsg Care: Monitor VS and SaO_2 frequently. Assure proper fluid intake (see *Med Tx*). Encourage parent visitation to decrease anxiety and oxygen need. Keep excess humidity wiped from walls of croup tent. Change bedding as needed to keep the child dry and prevent chilling. Elevate head of bed.

Prognosis: Croup can be life-threatening but usually resolves in 3 to 7 days.

Attention: A condition that presents symptoms similar to croup (and is sometimes also called *croup*) is epiglottitis. This condition is caused by a bacteria. Its onset is sudden and it progresses rapidly. The child presents with fever, drooling, muffled voice, retractions, and refusal to lie down. This is a medical emergency, and the nurse should not attempt to examine the throat but should contact the physician immediately and prepare for insertion of an artificial airway (endotracheal tube or tracheostomy).

LEUKEMIA

Definition: Cancer of the blood-forming tissues.

Pathophysiology: Immature leukocytes (white cells) known as *blasts* overproduce and compete with normal white cells, red cells, and platelets as well as other body tissues for space and nutrition. The resultant decrease in normal blood elements results in infections (because of decreased normal white cells), anemia (because of decreased red cells), and bleeding tendencies (because of decreased platelets). Bone marrow and highly vascular organs are heavily infiltrated with the abnormal white cells.

Etiology: Unknown. May be related to genetic abnormality or exposure to environmental factors such as radiation or toxic chemicals. *Acute lymphoid leukemia* (ALL) originates in the lymphatic system. *Acute nonlymphoid leukemia* (ANLL) or *acute myelogenous leukemia* (AML) originates in the bone marrow.

Manifestations: Recurrent or lingering infection, fever, fatigue, pallor, anorexia, bleeding, bruising, petechiae, night sweats, bone and joint pain.

Med Tx: Chemotherapy and possible bone marrow transplantation.

Nsg Dx: Potential for infection, activity intolerance, potential for injury, pain, potential for wide range of psychosocial diagnoses.

Nsg Care: Protect from and monitor for infection. Monitor closely for side effects of chemotherapy. Avoid administration of vesicant chemotherapy in veins that are near joints. Administer antiemetics *before* chemotherapy-induced nausea occurs. Coordinate care to permit periods of uninterrupted rest. Provide emotional support.

Prognosis: Cure rate for childhood ALL is 60% and 50% for ANLL. More deaths are from infection than from leukemia itself.

MENINGITIS

Definition: Inflammation of the membranes covering the spinal cord or brain.

Pathophysiology: Microorganisms invade the meningeal area.

Etiology: Most cases are of hematogenous origin (bloodborne organism is carried to meninges from another body site such as the respiratory or GI tract). *Haemophilus influenzae* (a bacteria) is the most common causative organism. Other bacteria, viruses, and fungi may also cause meningitis.

Manifestations: Anorexia, fever (or decreased temp in the neonate), irritability, tense fontanel, stiff neck (nuchal rigidity), photophobia, seizures, opisthotonos, and positive Kernig's and Brudzinski's signs.

Med Tx: Spinal tap to identify organism, antibiotics if cause is bacterial, isolation, and strict I&O.

Nsg Dx: Pain; potential for injury; hyperthermia (hypothermia may occur in neonate); sleep pattern disturbance.

Nsg Care: Frequently assess vital signs and neurologic status. Strictly monitor I&O. Measure head circumference daily if fontanel has not closed. Keep room quiet and lights dim. Elevate head of bed slightly. Encourage vaccination for *Haemophilus influenzae* in well children as preventive measure.

Prognosis: Prognosis is good with prompt diagnosis and treatment. Residual complications may include hearing problems, seizures, development delays, attention deficit disorder, and mental retardation.

MYOCARDIAL INFARCTION (MI)

Definition: Partial or complete occlusion of one or more of the coronary arteries (a.k.a. *heart attack*).

Pathophysiology: Coronary artery occlusion deprives

the myocardium (muscle tissue of heart) of O_2 and blood. Subsequent death of myocardial tissue occurs.

Etiology: Thrombus (clot) occludes an artery in 90% of cases. CAD, hemorrhage, coronary artery spasm, hypoxia, inflammation from disease, severe exertion or stress in the presence of significant CAD.

Manifestations: Severe and persistent pain (pain does not subside with rest or nitrates). Crushing or squeezing sensation in center of chest behind sternum. Pain may radiate or be localized to the shoulder, neck, arm, back, teeth, jaw, or fourth and fifth fingers of the left hand. N/V, sweating, SOB, pale or ashen color. 15 to 20% of MIs are painless. **ECG:** dysrhythmias; T-wave inversion; ST segment elevation; pathologic, deep Q wave. **Lab:** Elevated troponin, CK-MB, LDH.

NOTE: Validity of lab results is dependent on proper timing of specimen collections. Refer to specific test in Laboratory Tests later in this section.

Med Tx: Medical care should be instituted without delay. Hemodynamic and ECG monitoring, O_2, bed rest, analgesics, nitroglycerin, antiarrhythmics, thrombolytics, tissue plasminogen activator, PTCA, or surgical intervention.

Nsg Dx: Alteration in tissue perfusion (cardiac), pain, potential alteration in cardiac output (decreased), activity intolerance, knowledge deficit, anxiety.

Nsg Care: Promote rest and calm, quiet environment. Assist with ADL. Monitor VS and hemodynamic parameters and response to medical regimen. Provide information including rehabilitation teaching.

Prognosis: Mortality rate is 30 to 40% with over half of the deaths occurring within the first hour after onset of symptoms and prior to arrival at an acute care facility.

PNEUMONIA

Definition: Inflammation of the lungs.

Pathophysiology: Infection and inflammation lead to alveolar edema, promoting spread of the infecting organism. The involved lobe undergoes solidification caused by exudates (referred to as *consolidation* in x-ray reports). Ventilation-perfusion (V/Q) mismatch and right-to-left shunting occur at the site in which alveoli are filled with inflammatory exudates and O_2–CO_2 exchange is impaired.

Etiology: Bacterial or viral infection, chemical irritants, aspiration, stasis of fluids from severely impaired respirations or infrequent turning of immobilized patient. Immunosuppressed patients are at high risk.

Manifestations: Fever, chills, cough, dyspnea, tachypnea, tachycardia, pain in chest, crackles, increased fremitus and egophony, and dullness on percussion of affected lobes.

Med Tx: Antimicrobial agents, O_2, chest physiotherapy, incentive spirometry, hydration, ABG assessment.

Nsg Dx: Impaired gas exchange, ineffective breathing pattern, hyperthermia, fluid volume deficit, pain, anxiety, knowledge deficit.

Nsg Care: Encourage immunization (pneumococcal vaccine) for the aged and those with chronic illnesses. Closely monitor VS, ABG results, and response to medical therapy. Administer analgesics with care and attention to respiratory response. Encourage deep breathing and coughing. Provide education.

Prognosis: Varies greatly and is affected by coexisting and complicating factors. Mortality is high without appropriate antibiotic therapy.

RENAL FAILURE

Definition: Failure of kidneys to perform essential functions.

Pathophysiology: Renal hypoperfusion results in changes in the glomerular-capsular membrane permeability, causing interference with normal glomerular filtration and resulting in inability of the kidneys to perform normal functions, including excretion of toxins, fluids, electrolytes, and hydrogen ions (may be acute or chronic).

Etiology: Decreased cardiac output, renal obstruction, trauma, inflammatory/immunologic factors, chemical or bacterial toxins, tubular necrosis, severe dehydration.

Manifestations: Oliguria (decreased urine production), abnormal UA, signs of dehydration or edema (depending on stage), weight gain, elevated BP, elevated CVP, tachycardia, BUN: Creatine ratio >10 : 1, electrolyte abnormalities, serum K+ grossly elevated, blood pH <7.35, anemia, mental changes, failure to respond to fluid bolus and/or diuretics.

Med Tx: Hemodialysis or peritoneal dialysis, glucose and insulin to drive K+ into cells or Kayexelate enema to remove K+ via the GI tract, antihypertensives, fluid and nutritional restrictions, renal transplant in chronic cases.

Nsg Dx: Fluid volume deficit or excess, altered nutrition, potential for infection, altered thought processes and resultant potential for injury, knowledge deficit, fear.

Nsg Care: Maintain strict compliance with I&O monitoring. Make frequent VS and neuro checks. Assess weight daily. Assist with and monitor response to medical regimen. Educate patient and family. Monitor lab values. Encourage patient to express fears.

Prognosis: Varies greatly with cause, age, promptness of diagnosis, coexisting problems and complications, treatment, and compliance with treatment regimen.

RESPIRATORY DISTRESS SYNDROME (RDS) (HYALINE MEMBRANE DISEASE)

Definition: Severe impairment of respiratory function in premature newborn.

Pathophysiology: Lack of surfactant (a substance that prevents alveolar walls from "sticking together" during expiration) results in atelectasis, impaired perfusion of lungs, and reduced pulmonary compliance.

Etiology: Delivery of infant prior to ability to produce surfactant. Usually occurs in infants weighing less than 5 lb or who are of less than 37 weeks' gestation.

Manifestations: Tachypnea, tachycardia, inspiratory retractions, expiratory grunt, cyanosis, and abnormal ABGs.

Med Tx: Artificial surfactant via ET tube. Theophylline to relax bronchi and pulmonary vessels and to stimulate respiratory center. Supplemental O_2 and assisted ventilation if needed. IV hydration and control of electrolytes.

Nsg Dx: Impaired gas exchange, potential for injury, altered parenting, knowledge deficit (parents).

Nsg Care: Monitor respiratory status. Monitor response to all treatments. Maintain neutral thermal environment. Weigh daily. Monitor I&O. (Urine output = 2 mL/kg/h with sp. gr. of 1.005 to 1.010.). Limit stimuli and handling to reduce O_2 need. Encourage parent-infant bonding.

Prognosis: Mortality during first 24 hours = 50%; after 72 hours' survival, mortality = 10%.

Health Assessment

SICKLE CELL ANEMIA

Definition: A hereditary, chronic form of anemia in which normal hemoglobin is partly or completely replaced by abnormal hemoglobin.

Pathophysiology: Under conditions of dehydration or deoxygenation, red blood cells begin to sickle (assume an odd or irregular shape). These cells carry oxygen poorly and are very fragile, resulting in early cellular destruction. The irregularly shaped cells rupture or become enmeshed with one another, clogging vessels and causing tissue necrosis and pain ("pain crisis" or vaso-occlusive crisis). Major organs such as the spleen, liver, kidneys, and brain may be damaged.

Etiology: The disease is an inherited autosomal recessive disorder; that is, both parents must be carriers. In the United States, about 1 in 12 African-Americans carries the gene (carriers are said to have the "trait").

Manifestations: Hemoglobin S in blood, anorexia, increased susceptibility to infection, small for age, and short trunk and long extremities in older child. "Pain crisis" is manifested by pain (frequently in extremities and abdomen), respiratory distress, and fever.

Med Tx: Goal is to prevent increased sickling and crisis. Daily fluid intake should be at least $1^1/_2$ times normal maintenance amount (see *Pediatric Maintenance Fluid Calculation*). Patient is taught to avoid deoxygenation and resultant crisis by avoiding strenuous exercise, high altitudes, infection, and chilling.

Nsg Dx: Pain, altered tissue perfusion, altered growth and development, potential for infection, constipation related to analgesic use, knowledge deficit, support.

Nsg Care: Force fluids to $1^1/_2$ times normal maintenance (see *Pediatric Maintenance Fluid Calculation*). Monitor need for analgesics. Monitor urine and bowel elimination. Prevent infection. Teach pain crisis prevention. Support.

Prognosis: Mortality rate is about 25% during childhood. Crises are usually less frequent and prognosis is better for adults.

NOTES

NOTES

NOTES

NOTES

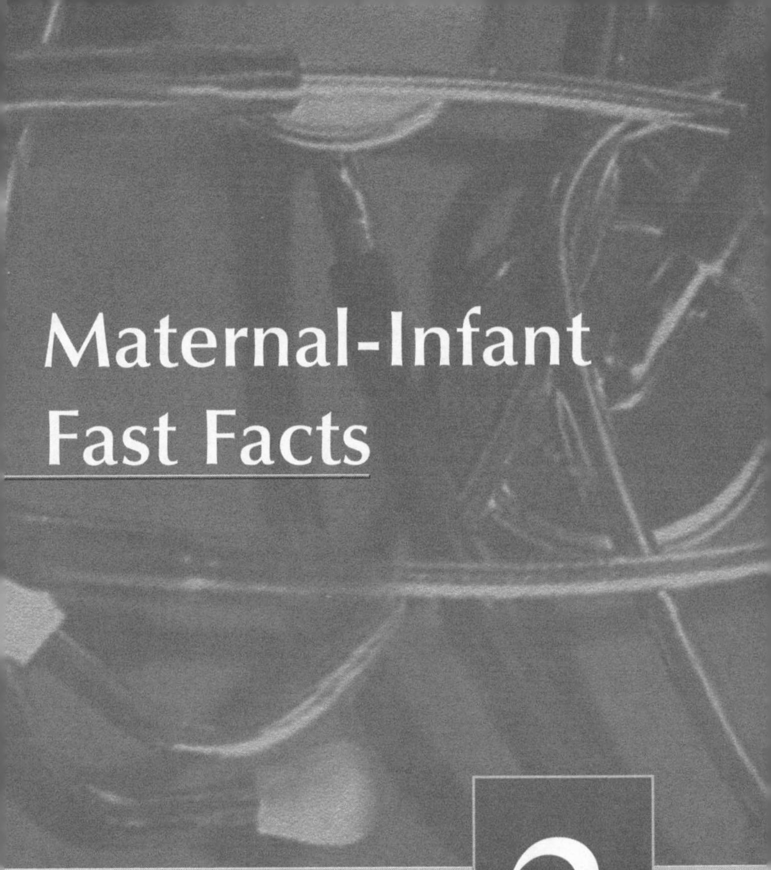

Maternal-Infant Fast Facts

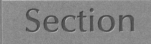

3

Section

SIGNS AND SYMPTOMS OF PREGNANCY

PRESUMPTIVE SIGNS

- *Amenorrhea*: More than 10 days elapsed since the time of expected onset of menstruation
- Fatigue and drowsiness
- Nausea and vomiting
- Urinary frequency increase
- *Breast changes*:
  Feeling of fullness
  Enlargement
  Tenderness
  Enlargement and darkening of areola
  Prominence of veins
  Enlargement of Montgomery's tubercles (small glands around nipple)
- *Vaginal changes*: Bluish color change (Chadwick's sign)
- *Skin changes*:
  Striae (stretch marks)
  Linea nigra (dark pigmented vertical lines on midabdomen)
  Facial melasma (pigment formation on face; also called *chloasma* or *mask of pregnancy*)
- *Quickening*: Mother's perception of fetal movement

PROBABLE SIGNS

- *Uterine changes*:
  Softening of lower uterus, just above cervix (Hegar's sign) and softening of cervix (Goodell's sign)
  False labor (Braxton Hicks' contractions)
- Rebounding of fetus in amniotic fluid (ballottement)
- Palpation of fetal body
- Positive hormonal test for pregnancy

POSITIVE SIGNS

- Fetal heartbeat
- Fetal movements felt by examiner
- Radiograph of fetus
- Sonogram of fetus

Table 3–1. PREGNANCY TABLE FOR ESTIMATING THE EXPECTED DATE OF DELIVERY

Find the date of the last menstrual period in the top line (light-face type) of the pair of lines.
The dark number (bold-face type) in the line below will be expected day of delivery.

Jan.	1	2	3	4	5	6	7	8	9	10	11	12	13	14	15	16	17	18	19	20	21	22	23	24	25	26	27	28	29	30	31	
Oct.	**8**	**9**	**10**	**11**	**12**	**13**	**14**	**15**	**16**	**17**	**18**	**19**	**20**	**21**	**22**	**23**	**24**	**25**	**26**	**27**	**28**	**29**	**30**	**31**	**1**	**2**	**3**	**4**	**5**	**6**	**7**	**Nov.**
Feb.	1	2	3	4	5	6	7	8	9	10	11	12	13	14	15	16	17	18	19	20	21	22	23	24	25	26	27	28				
Nov.	**8**	**9**	**10**	**11**	**12**	**13**	**14**	**15**	**16**	**17**	**18**	**19**	**20**	**21**	**22**	**23**	**24**	**25**	**26**	**27**	**28**	**29**	**30**	**1**	**2**	**3**	**4**	**5**				**Dec.**
Mar.	1	2	3	4	5	6	7	8	9	10	11	12	13	14	15	16	17	18	19	20	21	22	23	24	25	26	27	28	29	30	31	
Dec.	**6**	**7**	**8**	**9**	**10**	**11**	**12**	**13**	**14**	**15**	**16**	**17**	**18**	**19**	**20**	**21**	**22**	**23**	**24**	**25**	**26**	**27**	**28**	**29**	**30**	**31**	**1**	**2**	**3**	**4**	**5**	**Jan.**
April	1	2	3	4	5	6	7	8	9	10	11	12	13	14	15	16	17	18	19	20	21	22	23	24	25	26	27	28	29	30		
Jan.	**6**	**7**	**8**	**9**	**10**	**11**	**12**	**13**	**14**	**15**	**16**	**17**	**18**	**19**	**20**	**21**	**22**	**23**	**24**	**25**	**26**	**27**	**28**	**29**	**30**	**31**	**1**	**2**	**3**	**4**		**Feb.**
May	1	2	3	4	5	6	7	8	9	10	11	12	13	14	15	16	17	18	19	20	21	22	23	24	25	26	27	28	29	30	31	
Feb.	**5**	**6**	**7**	**8**	**9**	**10**	**11**	**12**	**13**	**14**	**15**	**16**	**17**	**18**	**19**	**20**	**21**	**22**	**23**	**24**	**25**	**26**	**27**	**28**	**1**	**2**	**3**	**4**	**5**	**6**	**7**	**Mar.**
June	1	2	3	4	5	6	7	8	9	10	11	12	13	14	15	16	17	18	19	20	21	22	23	24	25	26	27	28	29	30		
Mar.	**8**	**9**	**10**	**11**	**12**	**13**	**14**	**15**	**16**	**17**	**18**	**19**	**20**	**21**	**22**	**23**	**24**	**25**	**26**	**27**	**28**	**29**	**30**	**31**	**1**	**2**	**3**	**4**	**5**	**6**		**April**

July	1	2	3	4	5	6	7	8	9	10	11	12	13	14	15	16	17	18	19	20	21	22	23	24	25	26	27	28	29	30	31	
April	**7**	**8**	**9**	**10**	**11**	**12**	**13**	**14**	**15**	**16**	**17**	**18**	**19**	**20**	**21**	**22**	**23**	**24**	**25**	**26**	**27**	**28**	**29**	**30**	**1**	**2**	**3**	**4**	**5**	**6**	**7**	**May**
Aug.	1	2	3	4	5	6	7	8	9	10	11	12	13	14	15	16	17	18	19	20	21	22	23	24	25	26	27	28	29	30	31	
May	**8**	**9**	**10**	**11**	**12**	**13**	**14**	**15**	**16**	**17**	**18**	**19**	**20**	**21**	**22**	**23**	**24**	**25**	**26**	**27**	**28**	**29**	**30**	**31**	**1**	**2**	**3**	**4**	**5**	**6**	**7**	**June**
Sept.	1	2	3	4	5	6	7	8	9	10	11	12	13	14	15	16	17	18	19	20	21	22	23	24	25	26	27	28	29	30		
June	**8**	**9**	**10**	**11**	**12**	**13**	**14**	**15**	**16**	**17**	**18**	**19**	**20**	**21**	**22**	**23**	**24**	**25**	**26**	**27**	**28**	**29**	**30**	**1**	**2**	**3**	**4**	**5**	**6**	**7**		**July**
Oct.	1	2	3	4	5	6	7	8	9	10	11	12	13	14	15	16	17	18	19	20	21	22	23	24	25	26	27	28	29	30	31	
July	**8**	**9**	**10**	**11**	**12**	**13**	**14**	**15**	**16**	**17**	**18**	**19**	**20**	**21**	**22**	**23**	**24**	**25**	**26**	**27**	**28**	**29**	**30**	**31**	**1**	**2**	**3**	**4**	**5**	**6**	**7**	**Aug.**
Nov.	1	2	3	4	5	6	7	8	9	10	11	12	13	14	15	16	17	18	19	20	21	22	23	24	25	26	27	28	29	30		
Aug.	**8**	**9**	**10**	**11**	**12**	**13**	**14**	**15**	**16**	**17**	**18**	**19**	**20**	**21**	**22**	**23**	**24**	**25**	**26**	**27**	**28**	**29**	**30**	**31**	**1**	**2**	**3**	**4**	**5**	**6**		**Sept.**
Dec.	1	2	3	4	5	6	7	8	9	10	11	12	13	14	15	16	17	18	19	20	21	22	23	24	25	26	27	28	29	30	31	
Sept.	**7**	**8**	**9**	**10**	**11**	**12**	**13**	**14**	**15**	**16**	**17**	**18**	**19**	**20**	**21**	**22**	**23**	**24**	**25**	**26**	**27**	**28**	**29**	**30**	**1**	**2**	**3**	**4**	**5**	**6**	**7**	**Oct.**

Source: Venes, D, and Thomas, CL (eds): Taber's Cyclopedic Medical Dictionary, ed 19. FA Davis, Philadelphia, 2001, p. 1731, with permission.

PURPOSE

Fundal height is measured to assess fetal growth.

METHOD

Measure from the top of the symphysis pubis to the top of the fundus. Height is assessed in centimeters.

NOTE: Some authorities state that the top of the fundus may be palpated near the umbilicus at 22–24 weeks' gestation.

CLASSIC MILESTONES

12 *weeks*: Fundus is just above symphysis pubis.
16 *weeks*: Fundus is midway between symphysis and umbilicus.
20 *weeks*: Fundus is at umbilicus.
20 *to* 36 *weeks*: Height in centimeters equals gestational age in weeks, approximately.

CAUSES OF DEVIATIONS FROM USUAL FUNDAL HEIGHT

Fundal Height Greater than Expected

- Multiple pregnancy
- Miscalculated due date
- Polyhydramnios
- Hydatidiform mole

Fundal Height Less than Expected

- Fetal failure to grow
- Miscalculated due date

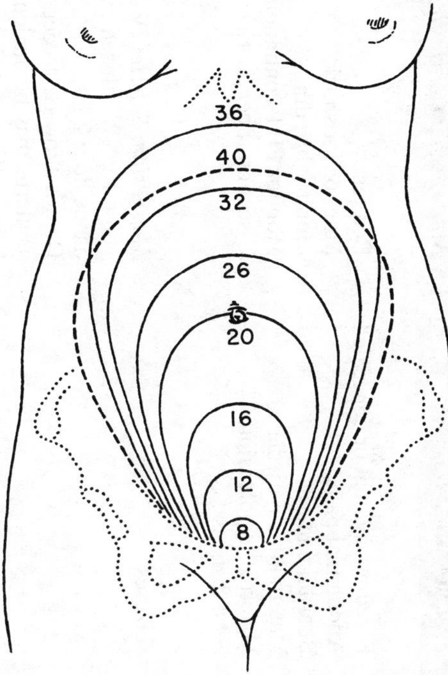

Figure 3–1. Usual fundal height at various gestational stages. (From Scott, JR, et al: Danforth's Obstetrics and Gynecology, ed 6. JB Lippincott, 1990, p 135, with permission.)

COMPLICATIONS OF PREGNANCY

Complication	*Manifestations*	*Management and Nursing Care*
ABRUPTIO PLACENTAE Premature separation of placenta	Bleeding, evident or concealed Abdominal pain Boardlike uterus Maternal tachycardia Maternal hypotension Fetal distress	Bed rest. Monitor for shock. Monitor bleeding. Monitor FHT continuously. C-section if cervix firm and undilated.
ECLAMPSIA Seizures between 20th wk of pregnancy and first postpartal wk; with or following manifestations of pregnancy-induced hypertension.	Seizures	*Magnesium Sulfate*: IV loading dose 4–6 g in 100 mL D_5W infused over 20–30 min; maintenance dose 2 g/h. Do not allow BP to decrease to less than 130/80, as uterus may be inadequately perfused. Frequently assess VS and DTRs. Report abnormal findings. Restrict hourly fluid intake to a total of 125 mL/h; urinary output should be at least 30 mL/h.

GESTATIONAL ONSET DIABETES Impaired ability to metabolize carbohydrate because of inadequate production of or resistance to insulin; with onset or first recognized during pregnancy.	Diagnostic values vary according to criteria used. Screening with 1-hour glucose level following 50-g glucose load. Diagnosis with 3-hour GTT after 100-g load. Polyuria Polydipsia Polyphagia Glycosuria (may also occur with normal blood glucose because of lowered renal threshold)	Dietary management. Exercise. Insulin if needed. Monitor weight Teach and continue to assess glucose monitoring and diet.
PLACENTA PREVIA Implantation of placenta in lower part of uterus; completely or partially covering the internal os	Painless vaginal bleeding	Bed rest. Monitor maternal VS. Monitor FHTs. Never perform vaginal exam if placenta previa is suspected.

(continued on the following page)

COMPLICATIONS OF PREGNANCY (continued)

Complication	Manifestations	Management and Nursing Care
GROUP B STREPTPCOCCAL INFECTION 10–30% of pregnant women are colonized; 70% of infants are colonized but few develop sepsis. CDC recommends screening by rectovaginal swab at 36 wks' gestation	Women are asymptomatic; infected infants may have respiratory problems that mimic RDS.	Women are given antibiotics during labor. Septic infants are treated with antibiotics.
PREGNANCY-INDUCED HYPERTENSION (PIH, PRE-ECLAMPSIA, TOXEMIA) Syndrome of hypertension, edema, and proteinuria; occurs after the 20th wk of pregnancy	Blood pressure of 140/90 or greater, or an increase of 30 mm Hg systolic or 15 mm Hg diastolic at two readings Nondependent edema; not relieved by bed rest Headache	Bed rest. Assess BP. Antihypertensives. Check urine for protein. Increased dietary protein and calories. I&O. Daily weight.

	Proteinuria Weight gain above 2 lb/wk Visual disturbance Epigastric pain	Check DTRs. Magnesium sulfate.
HELLP SYNDROME Related to severe preeclampsia	Hemolysis, elevated liver enzymes, low platelet count	Delivery
PRETERM LABOR (PTL) Labor between 20 and 37 wks' gestation	Contractions (less than 10 min apart) between 20 and 37 wks' gestation Cervical dilation of 2 or more cm or effacement of 75% See *True and False Labor Compared.*	Rule out UTI. Bed rest; left lateral position. Hydrate. Monitor FHTs. Monitor for ruptured membranes. Terbutaline. Magnesium sulfate.

LABOR AND DELIVERY TERMINOLOGY

Attitude: Degree of flexion of the fetus or relationship of fetal parts to each other. (In a "good" attitude, the fetus is in complete flexion or the classic fetal position.)

Dilation: Opening of the cervix from closed (0.0 cm) to completely open (10.0 cm).

Duration: Length of time a contraction lasts (should be less than 70 seconds).

Effacement: Thinning and shortening of the cervix and lower uterine segment. Extent of effacement is expressed as a percentage.

Engagement: Entrance of the fetal head or presenting part into superior pelvic opening.

Frequency of contractions: Time from the beginning of one contraction to the beginning of the next.

Intensity: Strength of a contraction. To assess, the fingers of the examiner are placed on the fundus of the uterus throughout a contraction.

Lie: Comparison of the long axis of the fetus to the long axis of the mother. Lie is described as either "transverse" or "longitudinal."

Position: Landmark of fetal presenting part to the right or left and anterior, posterior, or transverse portion of the mother's pelvis. (See abbreviations such as LOA, ROP, etc.)

Presentation: Portion of the infant that is deepest in the birth canal and is palpable upon vaginal examination.

Show: The blood-tinged mucus that is discharged as the cervix begins to dilate.

Station: The position of the presenting part in relation to the ischial spines; progresses from −5 to 0 to +5 (see Fig. 3–2).

PRELIMINARY EVENTS TO LABOR

- Backache.
- Braxton Hicks' contractions increase.
- Cervix becomes soft and effaced.
- Lightening (settling of fetus into lower uterus or pelvis).

- Membranes may rupture.
- Urinary frequency increases.
- Vaginal secretions increase.
- Passage of mucous plug occurs.
- "Bloody show" occurs.
- Weight loss of 1 to 3 lb.
- Energy surge may occur (termed "nesting").

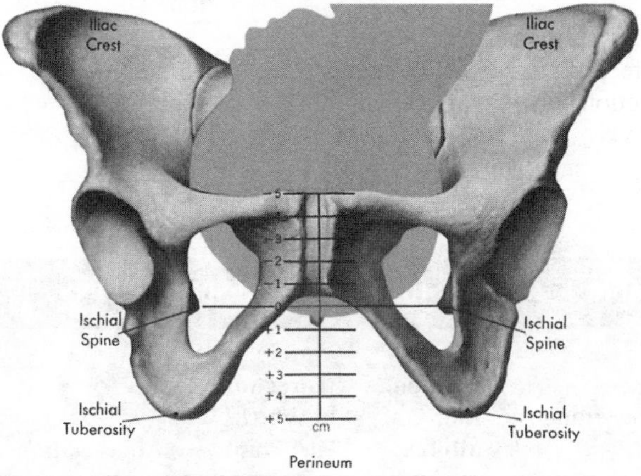

Figure 3–2. Stations of the presenting part. (Reprinted with permission of Ross Laboratories, Columbus, OH 43216.)

TRUE AND FALSE LABOR COMPARED

	True Labor	*False Labor*
Location of contractions	Back and abdomen	Lower abdomen
Frequency of contractions	Regular with decreasing intervals	Irregular with unchanging or increasing intervals
Intensity of contractions	Increases over time Increases with walking Little or no effect from sedation	Remains the same, is unaffected by, or decreases with walking Relieved by sedation
Effect of contractions on cervix	Dilation and effacement	No dilation or effacement

Table 3–2. POSSIBLE FETAL PRESENTATIONS

Presenting Part	Position, R or L of Mother	Variety (Direction in Which Part Points)	Abbreviation
Vertex (occipital)	Left	Anterior	LOA
	Left	Transverse	LOT
	Left	Posterior	LOP
	Right	Anterior	ROA
	Right	Transverse	ROT
	Right	Posterior	ROP
Face (mentum or chin)	Left	Anterior	LMA (example)
Shoulder (scapula)	Left	Anterior	LScA (example)
Breech (sacrum)	Left	Anterior	LSA (example)

Other Possible Abbreviations

Sa: Sacrum
A (when used as the middle letter): Acromion process (shoulder)

Other Cephalic Presentations

Face
Brow
The most efficient presentation for delivery is vertex, which occurs in about 95% of term pregnancies.

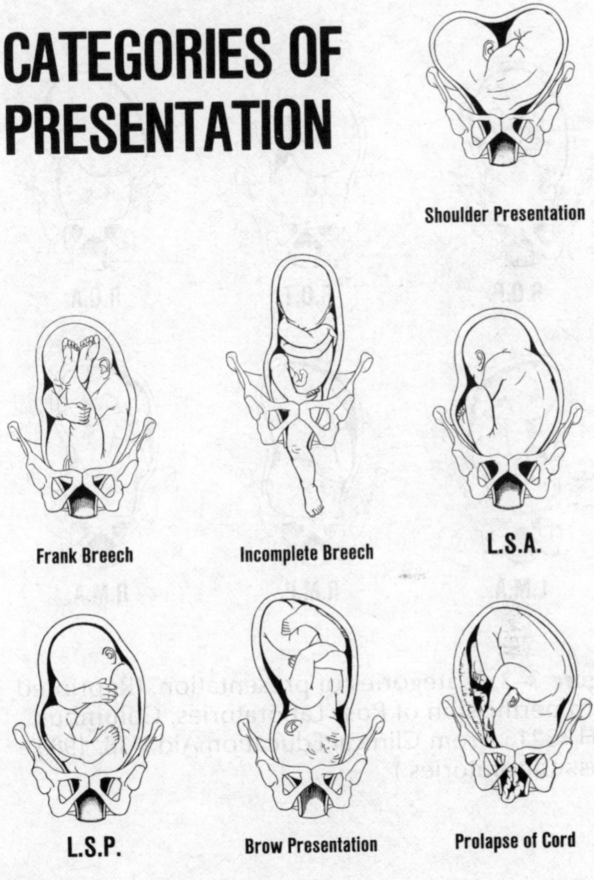

Figure 3–3. (continued)

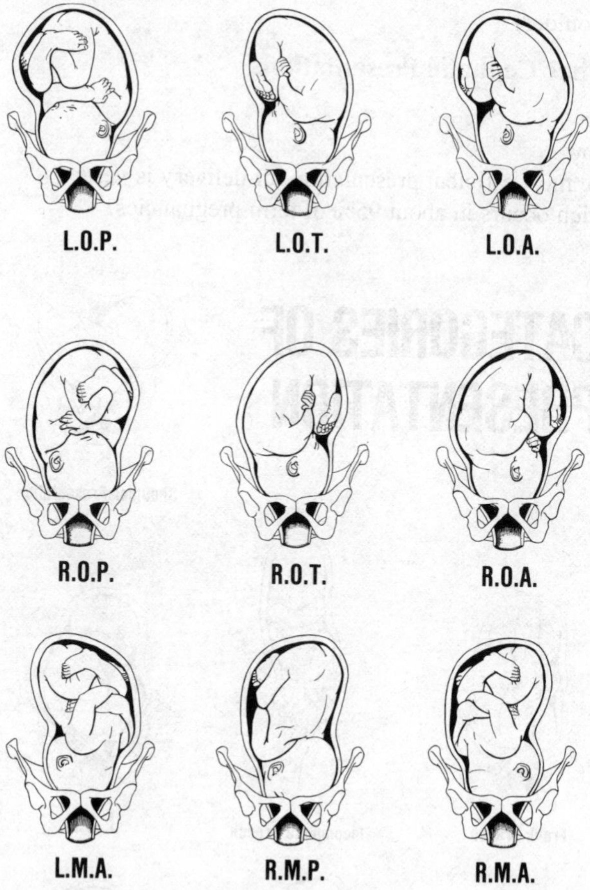

Figure 3–3. Categories of presentation. (Reprinted with permission of Ross Laboratories, Columbus, OH 43216. From Clinical Education Aid # 18, 1980, Ross Laboratories.)

TERMINOLOGY

Baseline fetal heart rate (FHR): Rate of fetal heartbeats between contractions.
Normal FHR: 120 to 160 or greater for short periods.
Tachycardia: Sustained (10 minutes or more) FHR of 160 or greater. *Etiology*: Early fetal hypoxia, immaturity, amnionitis, maternal fever, and/or terbutaline.
Bradycardia: Sustained (for 10 minutes or more) baseline FHR below 120. *Etiology*: Late or profound fetal hypoxia, maternal hypotension, prolonged umbilical cord compression, and/or anesthetics.

METHODS

External Monitoring

Contractions and FHR are monitored and recorded through transducers applied to the mother's abdomen. Quality of tracing is affected by many variables.

Internal Monitoring

FHR is monitored by an electrode attached to the fetal scalp or presenting part, and contractions are measured using a sterile water-filled pressure catheter placed in the uterine cavity alongside the fetus (should not be used if mother tests positive for group B *Streptococcus*).

INTERPRETATION

Variability

The term *variability* refers to cardiac rhythm irregularities. *Beat to beat variability* refers to the difference between successive heartbeats. To the extents described here, variability of cardiac rhythm is considered normal or abnormal:

No variability: 0 to 2 variations per minute (abnormal)
Minimal variability: 3 to 5 variations per minute (abnormal)

Average variability: 6 to 10 variations per minute (normal)

Moderate variability: 11 to 25 variations per minute (normal)

Marked variability: Above 25 variations per minute (abnormal)

NOTE: Decreased or marked variability may be the first sign of fetal distress. Place mother on her left side and hydrate.

Deceleration

The term *deceleration* refers to decreases in the fetal heart rate. Deceleration may be further described as follows:

Early deceleration: Can be detected in the monitor tracing appearance (mirror image of the contraction is seen). *Etiology*: Usually caused by head compression. *Treatment*: None (Fig. 3–4A).

Late deceleration: Can be detected in the monitor tracing appearance (reverse mirror image of the contraction seen late in the contraction). *Etiology*: Usually uteroplacental insufficiency. *Treatment*: Change mother's position from supine to lateral, slow or stop oxytocin, give IV fluids. Give O_2 at 6–10 L/min via face mask if fetal distress suspected. C-section may be needed if not corrected (Fig. 3–4B).

Variable deceleration: Occurs at unpredictable times during contractions. *Etiology*: Usually cord compression. *Treatment*: Change mother's position from supine to lateral or Trendelenburg. Give O_2 at 6–10 L/min via face mask. Perform pelvic exam to assess for descent of fetal presenting part or prolapsed cord. If cord is palpable, lift presenting part above it, place mother in Trendelenburg position and avoid manipulating cord. C-section is usually needed (see Fig. 3-4C).

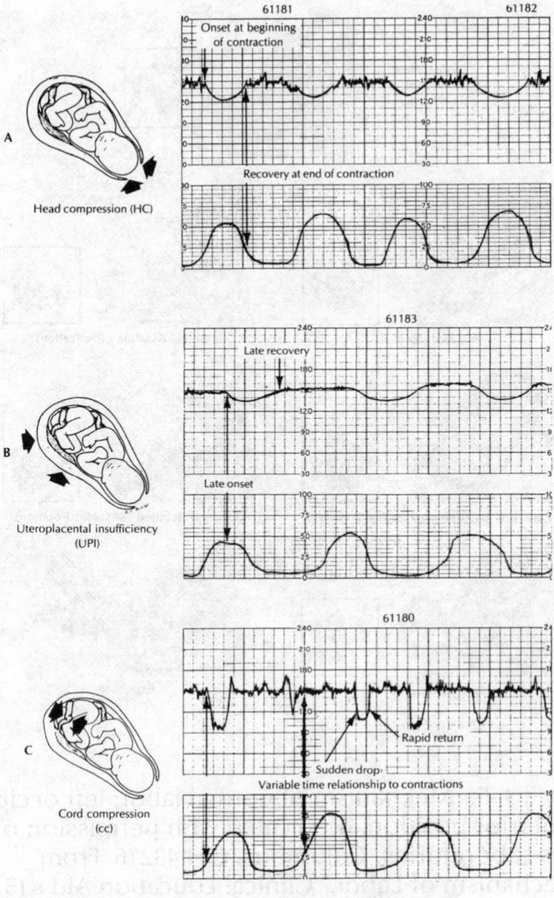

Figure 3–4. Fetal heart rate tracings. (From Tucker, SM: Fetal monitoring and fetal assessment in high-risk pregnancy. In Jansen, MM, and Bobak, MM (eds): Maternity and Gynecologic Care. St. Louis, 1978. CV Mosby, with permission.)

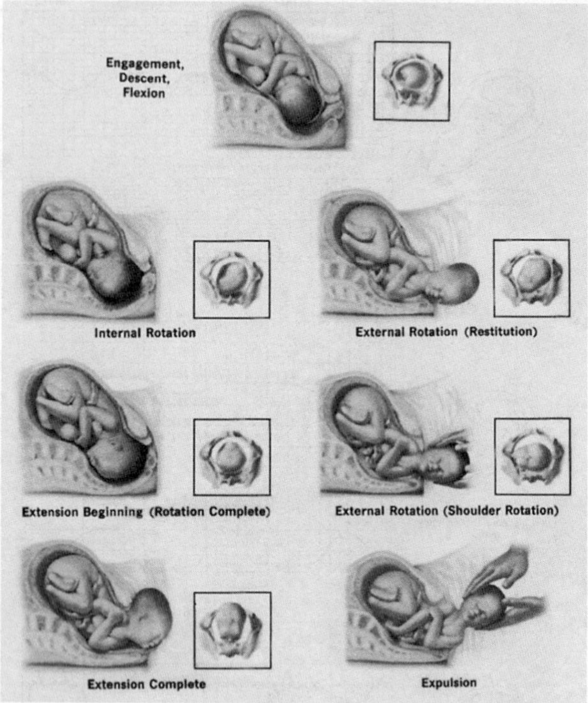

Figure 3–5. Mechanism of normal labor: left occipitoanterior position. (Reprinted with permission of Ross Laboratories, Columbus, OH 43216. From "Mechanism of Labor," Clinical Education Aid #13, 1980, Ross Laboratories.)

Table 3–3. FOUR STAGES OF LABOR: CHARACTERISTICS AND NURSING ACTIONS

A. First Stage: The first stage consists of three phases—latent, active, and transition. This stage of labor begins with the first true labor contraction and ends with complete effacement and dilation to 10 cm.

	First Stage: Latent Phase (Early Labor)	**First Stage: Active Phase**	**First Stage: Transition Phase**
Contractions			
Intensity	Mild	Mild to moderate	Moderate to severe
Frequency	5–10 min apart	2–5 min apart	2–3 min apart
Duration	20–30 seconds	30–50 sec	50–60 sec
Phase duration			
Primipara	10–12 h	2–4 h	1–2 h
Multipara	8–10 h	2–4 h	1–2 h
Cervical dilation	0–3 cm	4–7 cm	8–10 cm

(continued on the following page)

Table 3–3. FOUR STAGES OF LABOR: CHARACTERISTICS AND NURSING ACTIONS (continued)

A. First Stage: The first stage consists of three phases—latent, active, and transition. This stage of labor begins with the first true labor contraction and ends with complete effacement and dilation to 10 cm.

	First Stage: Latent Phase (Early Labor)	First Stage: Active Phase	First Stage: Transition Phase
Nursing actions	BP, P, RR, q 1/h Temp q 4 h ($\overline{q}$ 1–2 hr $\overline{p}$ membrane rupture) Time contractions q 30 min FHT q 15 min or continuous monitor I&O Urine for protein and glucose Encourage diversional activities.	BP, P, RR q 30/min Temp q 4 h or q 2 h if membranes ruptured Contractions q 15 min FHT q 15 min or continuous Position on left side to improve uterine circulation	VS and FHT same as active phase Contractions q 5–10 min Keep environment quiet; patient behavior changes as discomfort increases.
	Teach breathing: *In:* Deep, through mouth at start of contraction. *Out:* Pursed lips. *Then:* Slow, rhythmic chest breathing.	*Breathing:* Encourage same as for latent phase or shallow, light breathing; no more than 16 breaths per minute.	*Breathing:* *In:* 4–8 short breaths. *Out:* One "puff."

B. Second through Fourth Stages

	Second Stage	Third Stage	Fourth Stage
Begins with	Complete dilation	Delivery of infant	Delivery of placenta
Ends with	Delivery of infant	Delivery of placenta	Postpartum stabilization
Duration			
Primiparas	30–90 min	Up to 20 min	Usually 1–2 h after delivery
Multiparas	15–20 min	Up to 20 min	Usually 1–2 h after delivery
Nursing actions	Assess fetal well-being continuously. Encourage pushing. Encourage deep, full breaths (not to hold breath longer than 5 secs when pushing). Commend mother's efforts.	Observe for placental separation. Observe mother for signs of altered LOC or altered respirations (may indicate aneurysm or emboli). Allow maternal-infant interaction as soon as possible.	Administer oxytocin product if ordered (enhances contractions; increased BP is side effect). Maternal VS q 15 min for first hour, then q 30 min if stable (watch for shock).

(continued on the following page)

Table 3–3. FOUR STAGES OF LABOR: CHARACTERISTICS AND NURSING ACTIONS (continued)

B. Second through Fourth Stages (continued)

Second Stage	Third Stage	Fourth Stage
		Assess fundus q 15 min; if soft, massage with side of hand. Assess lochia, checking peri pad and under lower back. Assess bladder for distention (full bladder will prevent contractions and increase bleeding). Assess episiotomy for intactness and possible bleeding.

DELIVERY ROOM CARE OF THE NEONATE

1. Note the exact time of delivery.
2. Suction excess mucus from mouth and nose.
3. Dry the infant and place him or her in a warm environment. (Evaporative heat loss can have profound negative effects on an infant's glucose, bilirubin, and respiratory status.)
4. Assess and record first Apgar at 1 minute past delivery (see Table 3–4).
5. Collect cord blood if indicated (mother Rh negative or desires to store for possible future stem cell use).
6. Count vessels in cord (should have two arteries and one vein).
7. Place ID bands on the infant and mother.
8. Record footprints (if indicated by agency policy).
9. Assess and record second Apgar at 5 minutes past delivery.
10. Follow hospital protocol for prophylactic treatment of eyes (antibiotic ointment or silver nitrate), and record.
11. Allow the mother to see and touch her infant if condition allows.

NOTE: Some agencies require a third Apgar assessment at 10 minutes.

APGAR SCORING

Apgar scoring is performed at 1 and 5 minutes of age (and at 10 minutes in some hospitals). The infant is observed and rated in each of the five categories (called *signs*), and the ratings are then totaled.

A = Appearance (color)
P = Pulse (heart rate)
G = Grimace (reflex)
A = Activity (muscle tone)
R = Respiratory effort

Table 3–4.	APGAR SCORING		
	Apgar Score		
Sign	0	1	2
Heart rate	Absent	Slow (less than 100)	Greater than 100
Respiratory effort	Absent	Slow, irregular	Good; crying
Muscle tone	Limp	Some flexion of extremities	Active motion
Reflex irritability (response to catheter in nostril)	No Response	Grimace	Cough or sneeze
Color	Blue or pale	Body pink; extremities blue	Completely pink

Ranges for scores:
7–10: Good score, no immediate danger
4–6: Condition guarded, moderately depressed
<4: Condition serious, resuscitation needed, severely depressed

NURSERY ADMISSION CARE OF THE NEONATE

1. Weigh the infant.
2. Place him or her in warm environment.
3. Assess vital signs.
4. Measure length and head and chest circumference.
5. Give vitamin K injection (to prevent hemorrhage).
6. Check ID band.
7. Perform complete assessment (see *Physical Assessment of the Newborn*).

PHYSICAL ASSESSMENT OF THE NEWBORN

Assessment	*Normal or Minor Variation*	*Abnormal*
VITAL SIGNS		
Temperature	36.5–37°C or 97.8–98.6°F (axillary)	Sustained temp below or above stated limits
Pulse	120–160 min (apical)	Sustained pulse below or above stated limits
Respirations	30–60 min	Sustained rate below or above stated limits
	Vigorous cry	Weak cry
Blood pressure	55–68 systolic	Marked deviations from stated norm
	24–48 diastolic	
MEASUREMENTS		
Weight	2.5 kg (5.5 lb) to 4.3 kg (9.5 lb)	Deviation from stated norms
Length	46 cm (18 in) to 54.4 cm (21.5 in)	Deviation from stated norms
Head circumference	32 cm (12.5 in) to 37 cm (14.5 in)	Deviation from stated norms
Chest circumference	2–3 cm (0.75–1.00 in), smaller than head circumference	Deviation from norm

(continued on the following page)

PHYSICAL ASSESSMENT OF THE NEWBORN (continued)

Assessment	*Normal or Minor Variation*	*Abnormal*
SKIN	Pink Acrocyanosis (extremities blue) Mongolian spots (dark discolorations in sacral and gluteal areas) Milia (white, pinpoint papules on face) Vernix caseosa (cheesy coating on skin) Telangiectasia (flat, reddish birthmark, "stork bite") Mottling ("splotchy" discolored skin) Lanugo (soft downy hair on body)	Pallor General cyanosis Marked peeling (sign of postmaturity) Meconium on skin Jaundice before 24 h of age

HEAD	Molding (shaping of skull with overlapping of cranial bones) Caput succedaneum (swelling of tissue over presenting portion of head; usually crosses suture line) Fontanels (soft spots): • Anterior is diamond-shaped and about 4 cm at widest point. • Posterior is triangular and 1 cm or less at widest point.	Cephalohematoma (collection of blood between skull and periosteum—usually does not cross suture line) Hydrocephaly (enlargement of head because of excess or poor absorption of CSF) Microcephaly Bulging fontanel Closed fontanel
EARS	Tops of ears in line with inner canthus of eye Preauricular skin tags Preauricular sinus Startle reflex can be elicited by loud, sudden noise.	Low-set ears No response to sound (Amniotic fluid in ear canal may diminish ability to hear for several hours after birth.)
EYES	Lid edema Subconjunctival hemorrhage Red reflex present PERL Able to focus briefly on object or face	Conjunctivitis with purulent discharge Cataracts Absence of red reflex Fixed, constricted, or dilated pupil Unable to focus

(continued on the following page)

PHYSICAL ASSESSMENT OF THE NEWBORN (continued)

Assessment	*Normal or Minor Variation*	*Abnormal*
NOSE	Patent	Choanal atresia (blockage of posterior nares) Flaring
MOUTH	Intact lips and palate Epstein's pearls (small cysts on hard palate)	Cleft lip or palate White coating (thrush) Excessive saliva (esophageal atresia) Large, protruding tongue
NECK	Short	Excessive tissue on back of neck (chromosomal abnormalities) Resistance to flexion (meningitis) Masses
CHEST	A-P: lateral diameter equal Chest circumference 2–3 cm smaller than head or equal for first few days	

	Symmetric expansion Slight retractions Breast engorgement Milk in breasts Extra nipple	Asymmetric chest Marked retractions Fractured clavicle
LUNGS	Abdominal breathing Bilateral bronchial sounds Rhonchi shortly after birth Periodic breathing (periods of apnea up to 15 secs)	Grunting Absence of bilateral breath sounds Marked adventitious sounds with other signs of distress (flaring, grunting, cyanosis, tachypnea)
	Resp rate, 30–60	Sustained rate below or above limits
HEART	PMI at 5th left intercostal space Soft murmur during first few days of life	Displacement of PMI Loud murmur Thrill (palpable vibration caused by murmur)
	Heart rate, 120–160	Sustained rate above or below limits
ABDOMEN	Slightly protuberant Soft Liver 2–3 cm below right costal margin Tip of spleen may be palpable.	Distended or flat Masses Liver more than 3 cm below costal margin

(continued on the following page)

PHYSICAL ASSESSMENT OF THE NEWBORN (continued)

Assessment	*Normal or Minor Variation*	*Abnormal*
	Umbilical cord has three vessels. Umbilical cord gray Umbilical hernia	Umbilical cord has two vessels Dark umbilical cord Nonreducible umbilical hernia
GENITALIA	Testicles descended or in inguinal canal Urethral opening in center of penis	Testes not palpable in scrotum or inguinal canal Hypospadias (urethra on ventral or lower side of penis) Epispadias (urethra on dorsal or upper side of penis) Swollen scrotum Hernia (abdominal contents protrude between muscles) Hydrocele (accumulation of fluid in scrotum)
	Hymenal tag Large labia minora Large clitoris in premature infant Vaginal discharge of mucus or blood	Large clitoris in term infant

EXTREMITIES	Flexed with spontaneous movement Full ROM Equal leg length Symmetric gluteal folds	Flaccid, extended Limited ROM Unequal leg length (dislocated hip) Asymmetric gluteal folds (dislocated hip)
REFLEXES	(See *Neonatal Reflexes*.)	
GESTATIONAL AGE	Forms for gestational age assessment are available from major infant formula companies.	

Table 3–5. WEIGHT CONVERSION TABLE FOR NEONATES (POUNDS AND OUNCES TO GRAMS)

	Pounds														
Ounces	**0**	**1**	**2**	**3**	**4**	**5**	**6**	**7**	**8**	**9**	**10**	**11**	**12**	**13**	**14**
0	0	454	907	1361	1814	2268	2722	3175	3629	4082	4536	4990	5443	5897	6350
1	28	482	936	1389	1843	2296	2750	3204	3657	4111	4565	5018	5472	5925	6379
2	57	510	964	1418	1871	2325	2778	3232	3686	4139	4593	5046	5500	5954	6407
3	85	539	992	1446	1899	2353	2807	3260	3714	4167	4621	5075	5528	5982	6435
4	113	567	1021	1474	1928	2381	2835	3289	3742	4196	4649	5103	5557	6010	6464
5	142	595	1049	1503	1956	2410	2863	3317	3771	4224	4678	5131	5585	6039	6492
6	170	624	1077	1531	1985	2438	2892	3345	3799	4253	4706	5160	5613	6067	6521
7	198	652	1106	1559	2013	2466	2920	3374	3827	4281	4734	5188	5642	6095	6549

8	227	680	1134	1588	2041	2495	2948	3402	3856	4309	4763	5216	5670	6124	6577
9	255	709	1162	1616	2070	2523	2977	3430	3884	4338	4791	5245	5698	6152	6606
10	284	737	1191	1644	2098	2552	3005	3459	3912	4366	4820	5273	5727	6180	6634
11	312	765	1219	1673	2126	2580	3033	3487	3941	4394	4848	5301	5755	6209	6662
12	340	794	1247	1701	2155	2608	3062	3515	3969	4423	4876	5330	5783	6237	6691
13	369	822	1276	1729	2183	2637	3090	3544	3997	4451	4905	5358	5812	6265	6719
14	397	851	1304	1758	2211	2665	3119	3572	4026	4479	4933	5387	5840	6296	6747
15	425	879	1332	1786	2240	2693	3147	3600	4054	4508	4961	5415	5868	6322	6776

NEONATAL REFLEXES

Reflex	*How to Elicit*	*Normal Findings*
Arm recoil	Grasp infant's wrists and pull downward.	Brisk flexion of elbows when released.
Babinski's	Stroke lateral sole upward and across ball of foot.	Hyperextension and spreading of toes.
Crawling	Place infant in prone position.	Makes crawling movements.
Gallant	Place infant in prone position, and firmly stroke back to side of spine in downward motion. Check both sides.	Body curves to side stroked.
Magnet reflex	With infant supine, press against soles of feet to flex legs.	Pushes (extends) legs.
Moro (startle)	Strike flat surface near infant.	Symmetric "embracing" motion.
Palmar grasp	Place finger in infant's palm.	Grasps finger.
Plantar grasp	Press thumbs at base of infant's toes.	Toes curl downward.
Rooting	Stroke cheek or lip.	Turns head toward stimuli.
Stepping	Hold infant upright and allow one foot to touch a flat surface.	Movements are similar to walking.

Reflex	*How to Elicit*	*Normal Findings*
Sucking	Place gloved finger or bottle in infant's mouth.	Infant sucks.
Swallowing	Observe during feeding.	Swallows without gagging coughing, or vomiting.
Tonic neck	Turn infant's head to side while he or she is supine.	Extremities on same side extend, and those on other side flex.
Traction	Pull infant up by lower arms from supine position.	Head lags, then is pulled forward and falls onto chest.

COMPLICATIONS OF THE NEONATE PERIOD

Condition	*Etiology*	*Manifestations*	*Management and Nursing Care*
ABO INCOMPATIBILITY (Both Rh and ABO incompatibility are known as "hemolytic disease of the newborn.")	Fetus and mother have different ABO types. Maternal antibodies destroy infant's RBCs.	Positive Coombs' Jaundice within first 24 h after delivery Poor feeding Dark amber urine	Assess bilirubin levels closely. Administer phototherapy (cover eyes). Increase fluids. Prevent chilling. Exchange transfusion (rarely needed).
INFANT OF DIABETIC MOTHER (IDM)	In response to high maternal glucose, the fetus hypersecretes insulin.	LGA Hypoglycemia Jitteriness Cardiomegaly	Monitor glucose (maintain above 40 mg/dL) Feed early or administer IV glucose. Prevent chilling.

MECONIUM ASPIRATION Aspiration of meconium before or at birth	Stress may cause passage of meconium into amniotic fluid. Infant aspirates meconium while in utero or at birth.	Respiratory distress Tachycardia	Administer respiratory support. Continuously monitor for apnea. Administer antibiotics.
NEONATAL SEPSIS Generalized infection of bloodstream (Term is frequently used to denote any serious infection.)	Contact with infectious agent prior to, at, or after birth (Grp B strep common).	Poor feeding Decreased or increased temp (Temp may be normal.) Apnea Diarrhea Seizures Hypotonia	Obtain blood, urine, and CSF cultures (sepsis workup) to identify organism. Treat with appropriate antibiotic. Maintain temp at 97.8–98.6°F (Ax). Monitor continuously for apnea. IV hydration.
PHYSIOLOGIC JAUNDICE (OR HYPERBILIRUBINEMIA)	Fetal RBCs have shorter life than adult cells. Liver is unable to handle the large amount of bilirubin produced by massive RBC breakdown.	Jaundice after first 24 h of life	Provide early feeding. Prevent chilling. Assess bilirubin level. Provide phototherapy if severe.

(continued on the following page)

COMPLICATIONS OF THE NEONATE PERIOD (continued)

Condition	*Etiology*	*Manifestations*	*Management and Nursing Care*
RESPIRATORY DISTRESS SYNDROME (RDS) OR HYALINE MEMBRANE DISEASE (HMD) Acute lung disease of newborn involving atelectasis	Believed to be due to lack of surfactant in lungs (most common in premature infants).	Nasal flaring Tachypnea Retractions Expiratory grunt	Administer artificial surfactant via ET tube. Provide respiratory support. Monitor for apnea. Prevent chilling. IV hydration. Monitor I&O (urine should = 2 mL/kg/h). Limit stimuli and handling.
RH INCOMPATIBILITY	*Mother*: Rh negative *Infant*: Rh positive Maternal antibodies destroy infant's RBCs.	See *ABO Incompatibility*	See *ABO Incompatibility*

POSTPARTUM ASSESSMENT AND NURSING CONSIDERATIONS

Assessment	*Nursing Considerations*
Vital signs	Temp of 100.4°F during first 24 h after delivery considered normal. Encourage fluids. If temp is above 100.4°F, check the following for possible infection: lacerations, sutures, breasts, lochia (foul odor of lochia may indicate infection), urine. Pulse elevation may be first sign of hemorrhage. Decreased pulse rate (as low as 50) is considered normal during first postpartal week. Decreased BP and/or narrowed pulse pressure are signs of shock. Orthostatic hypotension is common during the early postpartal period. The patient should rise slowly from lying or sitting to prevent “blackouts” or falls. Assess BP every hour if patient has been preeclamptic.
I&O	Accurate I&O for at least 12 h (urinary retention may occur).
Head	Assess for headache resulting from anesthesia or elevated BP. Visual light flashes may indicate preeclampsia
Lungs	Check for adventitious sounds. Prolonged bed rest, labor, vomiting, or anesthesia may predispose to pneumonia (women who have had spinal or epidural anesthesia may have difficulty coughing or clearing the lower airway until anesthesia wears off). Chest pain and dyspnea are common symptoms of pulmonary embolism.

(continued on the following page)

Maternal-Infant

Assessment	*Nursing Considerations*
Breasts	Colostrum appears within first 12 h. Breast milk appears by about 72 h. Breast engorgement occurs on the 3rd or 4th postpartal day and should resolve spontaneously within 36 h. Assess for infection (warm, painful, reddened area). Assess for irritation of nipples. Bra should be worn by all women during the postpartal period.
Abdomen	Assess fundus. Should be firm and at umbilicus immediately after delivery, then fall 1 cm (1 fingerbreadth) each day for next 10 days. If fundus is boggy, assess first for bladder fullness, and have patient void if indicated. If fundus is boggy and bladder is empty, massage top of fundus with fingers held together. (Patient may be taught to massage fundus.) Auscultate to assess peristalsis. Assess daily for BM. (Analgesics and other aspects of labor and delivery make constipation very common.) Increase fiber and fluid intake to prevent constipation. Encourage early ambulation.
Perineum	Assess episiotomy for edema, bleeding, or redness. Assess for hematoma (purplish mass may be seen at introitus of vagina) if patient complains of severe perineal pain or a feeling of fullness in the vagina. Assess for hemorrhoids. Assess lochia. Patients who report or are observed to have heavy bleeding should be placed on pad count.

Assessment	Nursing Considerations
	A continuous flow of bright red lochia or the passage of large and/or frequent clots is abnormal and indicates hemorrhage. Occasional passage of clots in the absence of heavy flow may be normal. Lochia should progress as follows: Lochia rubra: Dark red, 2–3 days Lochia serosa: Paler, brownish pink, 4–10 days Lochia alba: Whitish or yellowish, up to 3 wks **Lochia should be odorless.**
Lower extremities	Assess veins for redness and extreme warmth (signs of phlebitis). Assess for pain while dorsiflexing foot. Pain indicates positive Homans' sign, which is sign of thrombophlebitis. Ambulation and/or early leg exercises help prevent venous stasis and clot formation.
Psyche	Assess mood. Mild "let-down feeling" is usually considered normal. Watch for signs of parent-infant bonding: Parents hold baby so that mutual gazing can occur ("enface" position). Parents talk to baby. Parents stroke baby. Parents make positive statements about baby. Parents give baby cherished name.

NOTES

NOTES

NOTES

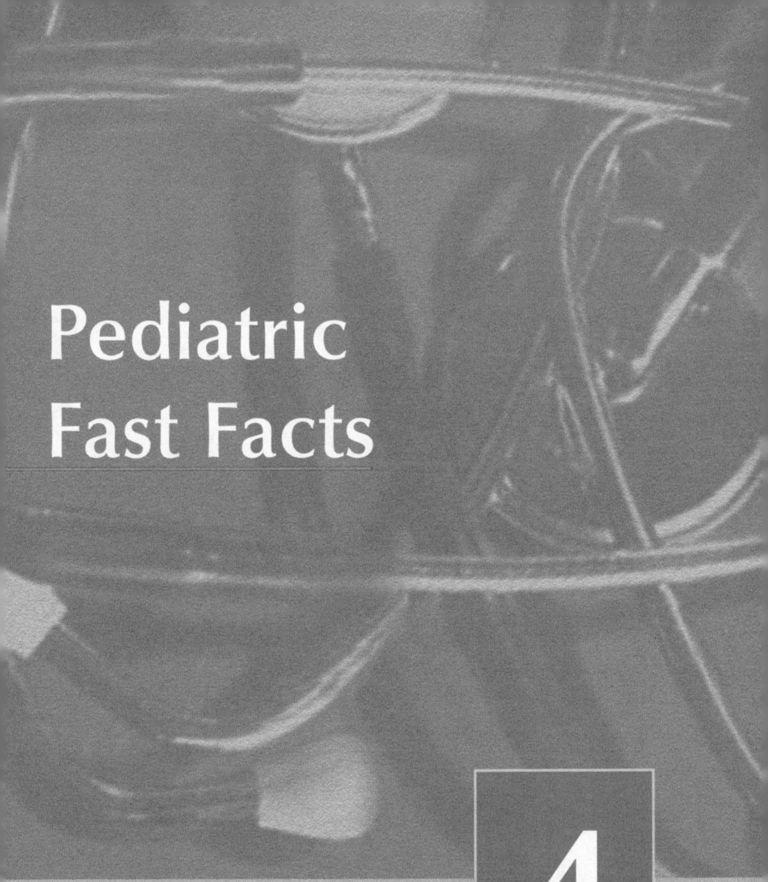

Pediatric Fast Facts

Section 4

COMMUNICATING WITH CHILDREN

1. Avoid "rushing in" on a child. Give the child time to adjust to your presence before touching him or her.
2. Be aware of body language, the child's and your own.
3. Meet the child at his or her eye level.
4. Use simple language appropriate to his or her development level.
5. If the child draws away from you, talk to the parents and appear to ignore him or her for a while.
6. Use a toy or a game to begin an interaction.
7. Call the child by his or her name often.
8. Do not laugh at a child, but do laugh with him or her.
9. Demonstrate any unfamiliar procedure on a doll if possible.
10. Always tell the truth. Do not say a procedure will not hurt if it will hurt.
11. Tell the child it is okay to cry if a procedure will hurt.
12. Unless a child objects to being touched, a gentle pat on the back or shoulder can communicate caring.
13. Make positive rather than negative statements. *Example*: Say "Put your feet on the floor" rather than "Don't put your feet on the table."
14. Avoid moralizing. Such phrases as "You're such a good boy (or girl) for not crying" may imply that he or she is not a "good" child if he or she cries the next time.
15. When correcting negative behavior, do not demean. *Example*: Say "You may not hit Susan. It hurts to be hit" rather than "Don't hit Susan. That's an ugly thing to do."
16. Don't give a choice when there is none. *Example*: Say "It's time to take your medicine" rather than "Will you take your medicine for me?"

If a child has well-developed language skills but is non-communicative, one of the following techniques may enhance communication:

1. Provide supplies, and ask the child to draw a picture about how he or she feels, what the hospital is like, or something his or her family likes to do.
2. Ask the child to tell a story about the picture he or she has drawn.
3. Ask the child "If you could have three wishes, what would they be?"
4. Ask the child "What makes you angrier (or happier) than anything else?"
5. Use the third person to question a suspected problem. Example: "Sometimes people are afraid when they are in the hospital. Do you ever feel that way?"
6. An adolescent may be hesitant to discuss his or her feelings. Ask him or her to explain what things would be like for you if you had just been diagnosed with the same condition that afflicts him or her.

GROWTH AND DEVELOPMENT TERMINOLOGY

Cephalocaudal: Head to toe direction in which development always proceeds; that is, child holds head up before sitting alone.

Critical period (sensitive period): Time period during which child is ready for growth or development. Future growth and development may be jeopardized if opportunity for growth and development is denied during a critical period.

Development: Progress in skill and complexity of functioning; a result of growth, maturation, and learning.

Development milestones: Important skills associated with a particular age range; that is, sitting, crawling, and walking.

Growth: Increase in size.

Maturation: Physical qualitative changes determined by genetics and brought about by aging.

Proximodistal: Center to outer direction in which development always proceeds.

DEVELOPMENTAL ASSESSMENT

The normal range of development timing is wide but in all children follows the directions of:

Cephalocaudal: Head to toe
Proximodistal: Center to periphery

Children who lag markedly behind in major developmental milestones should be evaluated by a child health professional. See *Developmental Milestones* for a partial listing of these milestones.

Common tools used to detect development delays and to monitor children at risk for delays are the Denver Developmental Tests. These are standardized tools for detecting problems in areas identified as *personal-social, fine motor–adaptive, language,* and *gross motor.* A standardized score sheet and an approved kit are needed to conduct tests.

DEVELOPMENTAL THEORIES

ERIKSON'S PSYCHOSOCIAL DEVELOPMENT

Erikson's theory is based on the belief that each stage or conflict is the result of the child's need to adapt to the social environment and that the conflict of each stage must be resolved before the next stage can be successfully achieved.

Approximate Age	*Stage or Conflict*
Birth–1 yr	Trust vs mistrust
1–3 yr	Autonomy vs shame and doubt
4–5 yr	Initiative vs guilt
6–11 yr	Industry vs inferiority
12–18 yr	Identity vs identity confusion

FREUD'S STAGES OF PSYCHOSEXUAL DEVELOPMENT

Freud's theory emphasizes the importance of sex and control over aggressive impulses in the child's development.

Approximate Age	*Stage*
Birth–2 yr	Oral
2–3 yr	Anal
3–6 yr	Phallic
6–12 yr	Latent
12–18 yr	Genital

PIAGET'S COGNITIVE THEORY

Piaget defined stages of intellectual thought development. At the end of each stage, a brief period of equilibrium is said to exist. Disequilibrium resumes when the child becomes dissatisfied with old answers and finds new ways to solve problems.

Approximate Age	*Stage*
Birth–2 yr	*Sensorimotor*: Senses and motor activity
2–7 yr	*Preoperational or preconceptual*: Intellectual development
7–11 yr	*Concrete operations*: Reasoning and organizing thoughts
11 yr through adulthood	*Formal operations*: Abstract thinking and deductive reasoning

AGE-RELATED STAGES USED TO CATEGORIZE CHILDREN

Age	*Stage*	*Age*	*Stage*
Conception–birth	Prenatal	3–6 yr	Preschool
Birth–1 mo	Neonatal	6–12 yr	School age
Birth–1 yr	Infancy	12–18 yr	Adolescent
1–3 yr	Toddler		

DEVELOPMENTAL MILESTONES

Milestones are based on averages. Each child progresses at his or her own rate. Children who vary markedly from averages should be assessed by a child health professional.

Age	*Milestone*
Birth–1st mo	Lies in flexed position
	Demonstrates reflex activities
	Maintains eye contact (Vision is poor.)
	Communicates by crying
	Growth:
	Average weight gain is 3–5 oz weekly during first 6 mo.
2 mo	Lifts head for short periods when prone
	Visually follows moving objects
	Smiles and frowns
	Coos
3 mo	Turns from back to side
	Sits with support
	Focuses on own hands
	Recognizes parent
	Demonstrates pleasure by squealing
4 mo	Turns from back to prone position
	Lifts head and chest 90 degrees and bears weight on forearms
	Holds head erect while in sitting position
	Reaches for objects, usually without success
	Grasps objects with both hands
	Intentionally carries objects to mouth
	Plays with fingers
	Laughs aloud
	Makes consonant sounds
5 mo	Turns from abdomen to back
	Holds object in one hand and reaches for another object with other hand
	Plays with toes
	Puts feet into mouth

(continued on the following page)

Age	*Milestone*
6 mo	Sits alone leaning forward on both hands Reaches for and grasps objects with whole hand Holds bottle Extends arms when he or she wishes to be picked up Briefly looks for dropped objects Begins to fear strangers Enjoys caregiver's briefly placing towel over face to play peekaboo Begins to make wordlike sounds *Growth:* Birth weight has doubled. Average weekly weight gain is 3–5 oz during 6–18 mo. Teething: See Figure 4–11, p. 374.
7 mo	Begins to crawl Bears weight on feet when placed upright on surface Transfers object from one hand to the other
8 mo	Pulls to standing position Sits alone without support Releases object intentionally Begins to use pincer grasp (picks objects up with fingers) Shows marked stranger anxiety Says "dada" without meaning
9 mo	Walks sideways while holding on Crawls well Bangs 2 blocks together Drinks from cup Attempts to feed self Searches for hidden object
10 mo	May begin to walk May begin to climb Neat pincer grasp Demonstrates one-hand dominance Plays pat-a-cake Initiates peekaboo game May say 1–2 words with meaning

Age	*Milestone*
11 mo	Cooperates with dressing activities Attempts to feed self with spoon Can follow simple directions Understands meaning of "no" Shakes head to indicate "no"
12 mo	Walks alone or with one hand held Falls frequently while walking Drinks well from a cup Points with one finger Pulls off socks *Growth*: Birth weight has tripled. Birth length has increased by 50%. Head and chest circumference are equal.
15 mo	Walks without assistance Pulls or pushes toys Throws ball overhanded Builds tower of 2 blocks Scribbles with crayon or pencil
18 mo	Runs clumsily Jumps in place with both feet Builds tower of 3–4 blocks May be able to control anal and urinary sphincters Says about 10 words
2 yr	Runs well with wide stance Climbs stairs by placing both feet on each step Attains bladder and bowel control sometime between 2 and 3 yrs Names some familiar objects Has vocabulary of about 300 words Combines 2–3 words into meaningful phrases *Growth*: Weighs about 4 times birth weight. Average weight gain is 4–6 lb/yr during ages 2–6 yr. Has attained about $^1/_2$ of expected adult height.

(continued on the following page)

Age	*Milestone*
$2^1/_2$ yr	Jumps from chair or step Stands on one foot briefly
3 yr	Rides tricycle Climbs stairs by alternating feet on steps Turns doorknobs Dresses self Speaks in short sentences *Growth*: All 20 deciduous teeth have erupted.
4 yr	Hops on one foot Catches ball Recognizes colors *Growth*: Birth length has doubled.
5 yr	Skips well Jumps rope Balances with eyes closed Sentences contain all parts of speech Has vocabulary of about 2100 words

NOTE: When the child is school age, most motor milestones have been attained and the child fine tunes previously attained skills. Development focus moves largely to cognitive and social skills.

6–12 yr	*Can learn to*: Swim Skate Ride bicycle Ties shoes Uses pencil or crayon well Forms clubs or gangs Demonstrates awareness of rule-governed behavior Has strong sense of "what's fair" Uses complex sentences Reads Counts

Age	*Milestone*
	Growth: Average weight gain is 4–6 lb/yr during ages 6–12 yr.
Adolescent	Major development task is learning to care for self independently while learning to effectively interact with society.

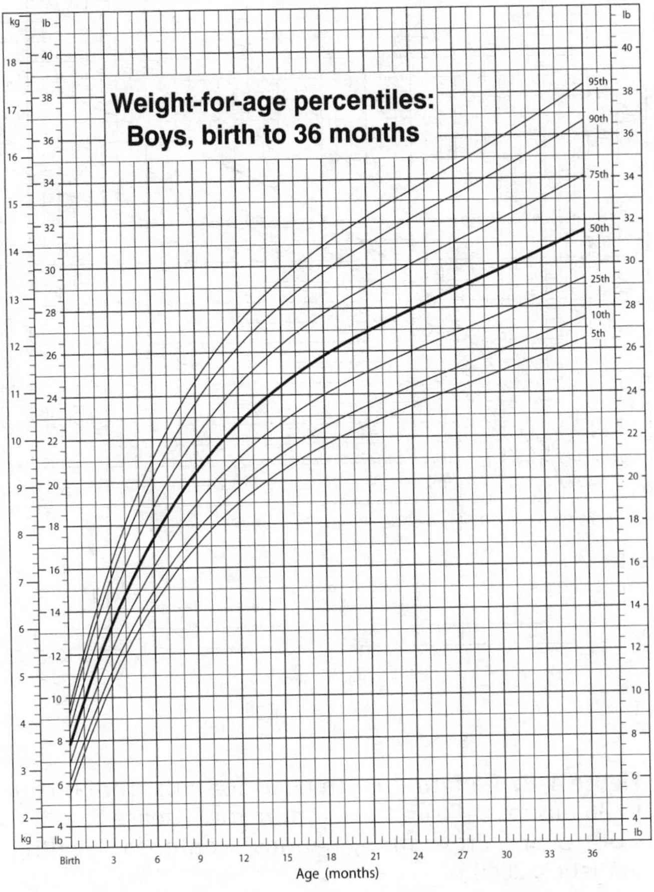

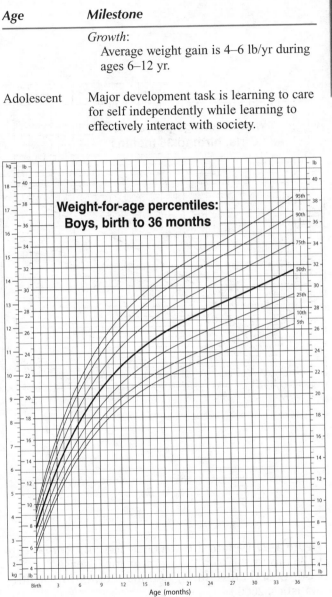

Figure 4–1. Weight growth chart for boys from birth to 36 months. (From the Centers for Disease Control and Prevention, National Center for Health Statistics, 2000.)

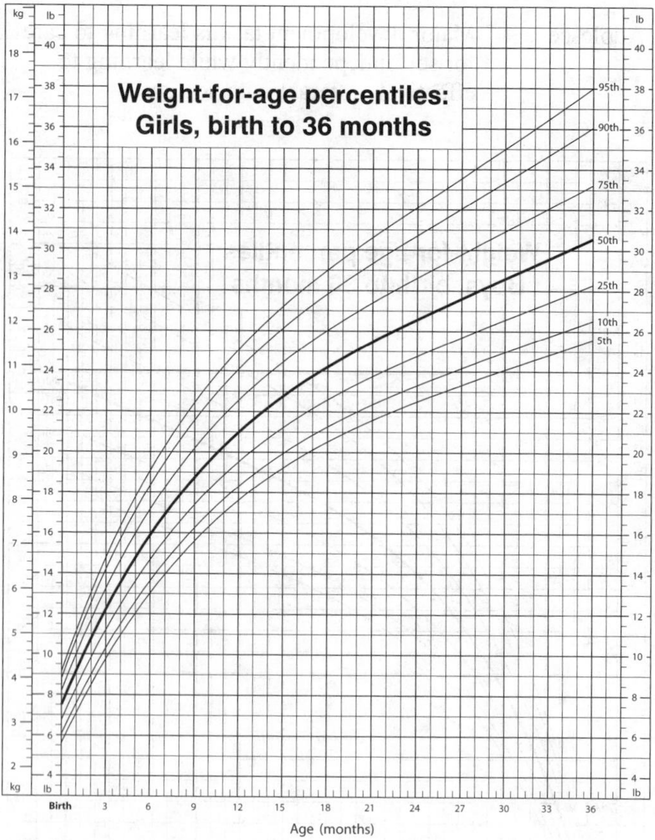

Figure 4–2. Weight growth chart for girls from birth to 36 months. (From the Centers for Disease Control and Prevention, National Center for Health Statistics, 2000.)

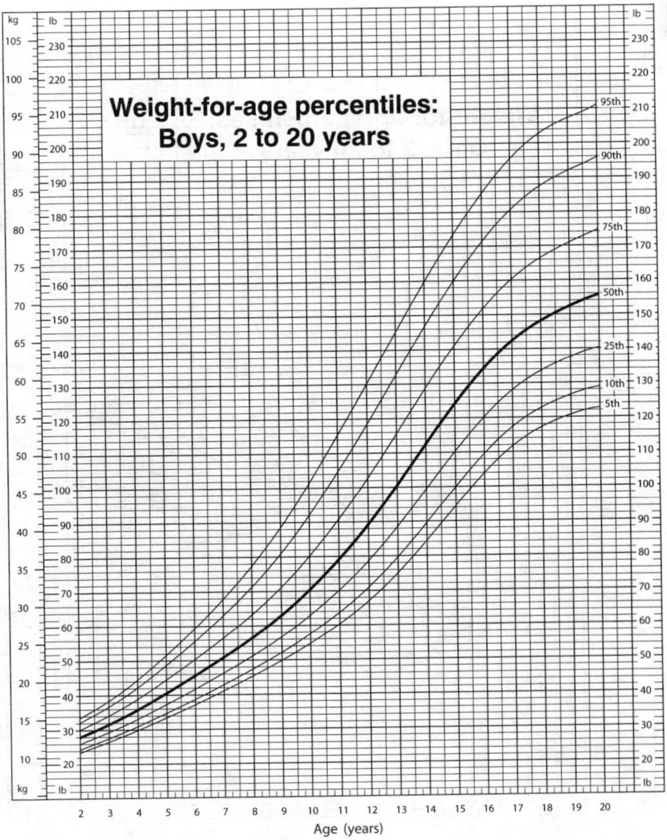

Figure 4–3. Weight growth chart for boys from 2 to 20 years. (From the Centers for Disease Control and Prevention, National Center for Health Statistics, 2000.)

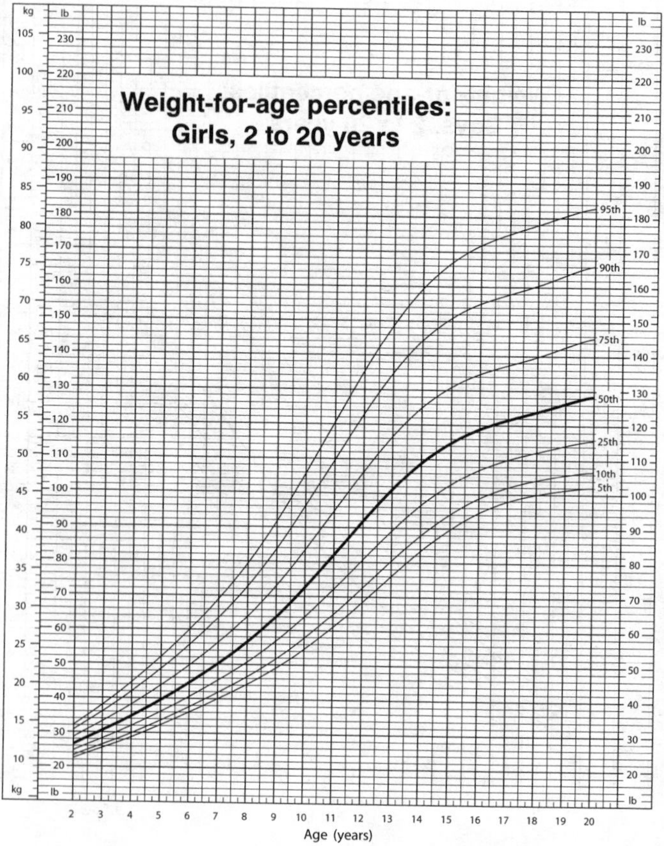

Figure 4–4. Weight growth chart for girls from 2 to 20 years. (From the Centers for Disease Control and Prevention, National Center for Health Statistics, 2000.)

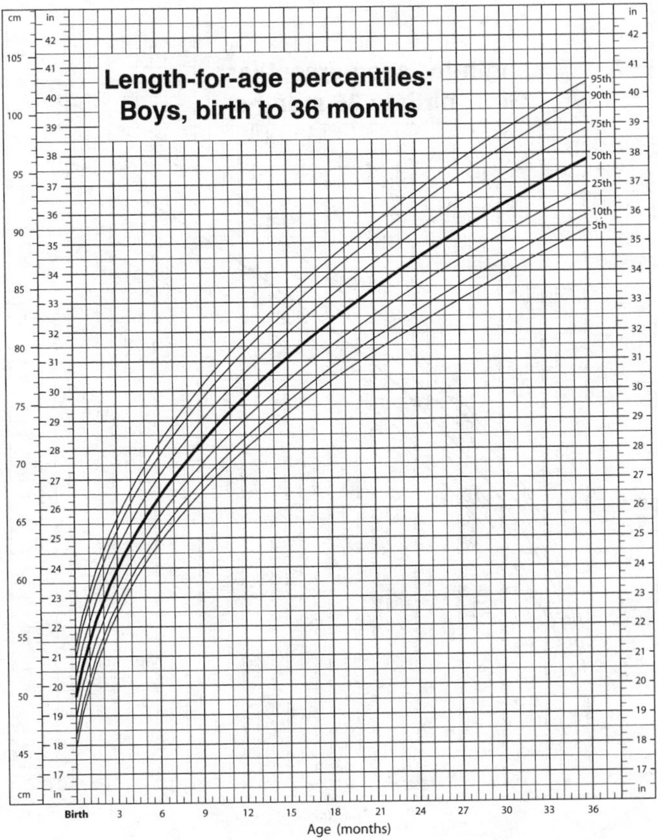

Figure 4–5. Length growth chart for boys from birth to 36 months. (From the Centers for Disease Control and Prevention, National Center for Health Statistics, 2000.)

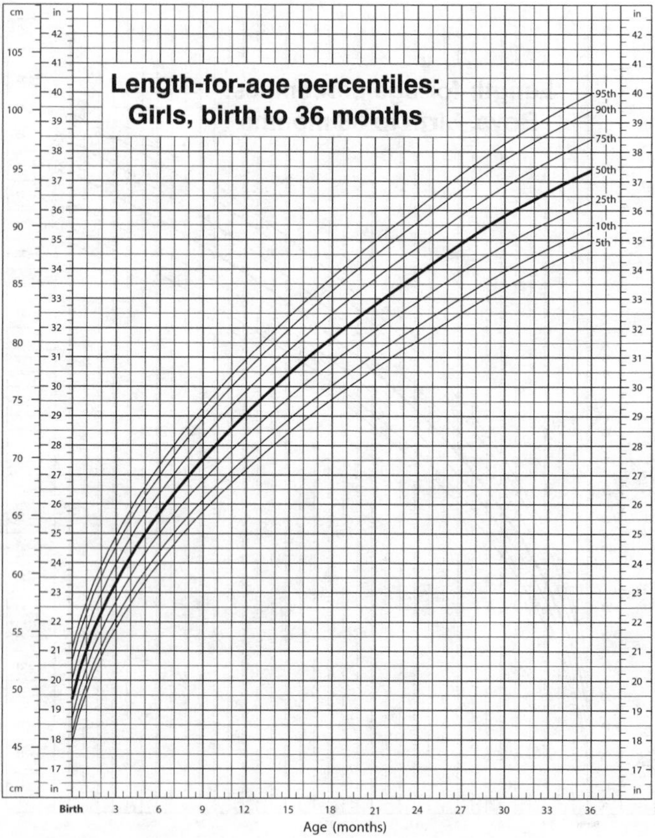

Figure 4–6. Length growth chart for girls from birth to 36 months. (From the Centers for Disease Control and Prevention, National Center for Health Statistics, 2000.)

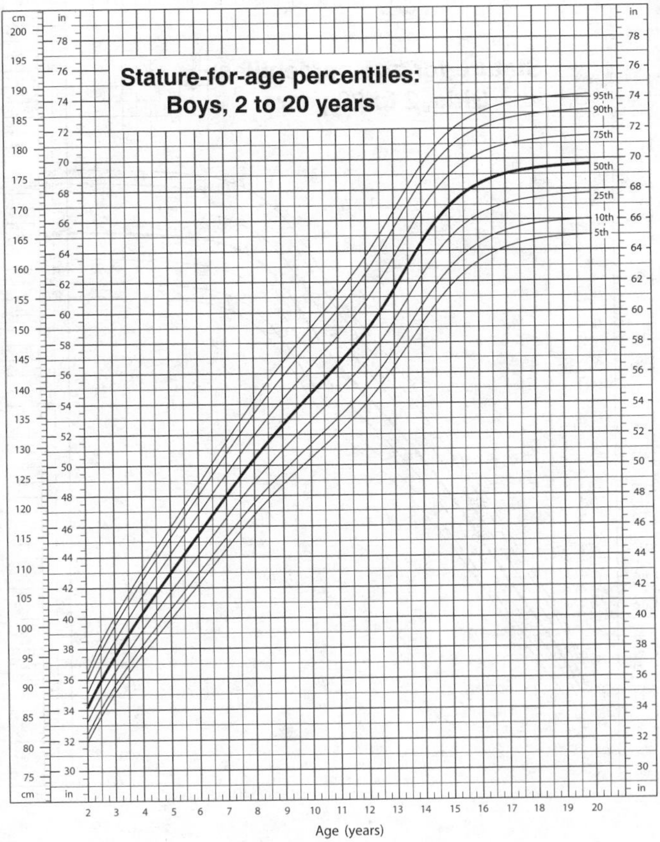

Figure 4–7. Height growth chart for boys from 2 to 20 years. (From the Centers for Disease Control and Prevention, National Center for Health Statistics, 2000.)

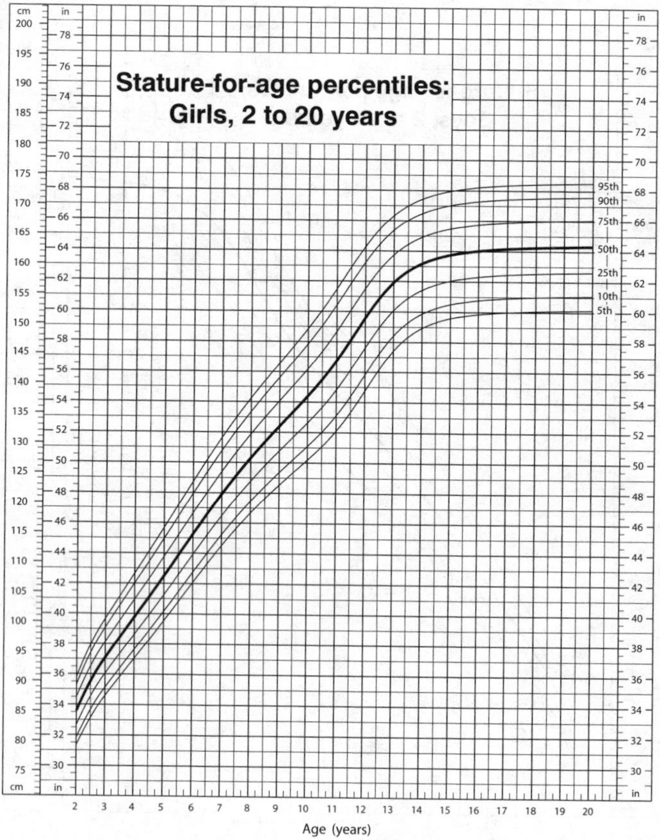

Figure 4–8. Height growth chart for girls from 2 to 20 years. (From the Centers for Disease Control and Prevention, National Center for Health Statistics, 2000.)

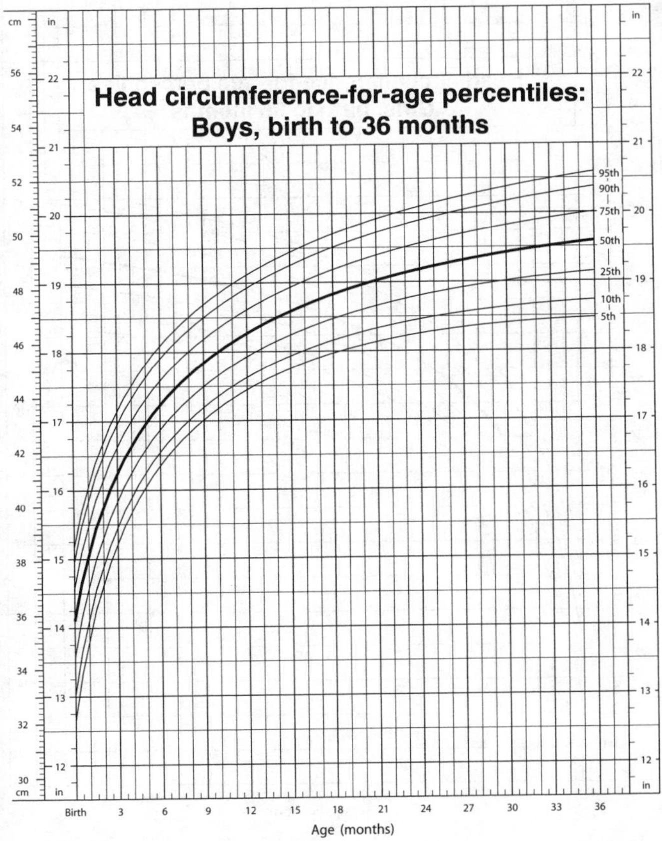

Figure 4–9. Head circumference growth chart for boys from birth to 36 months. (From the Centers for Disease Control and Prevention, National Center for Health Statistics, 2000.)

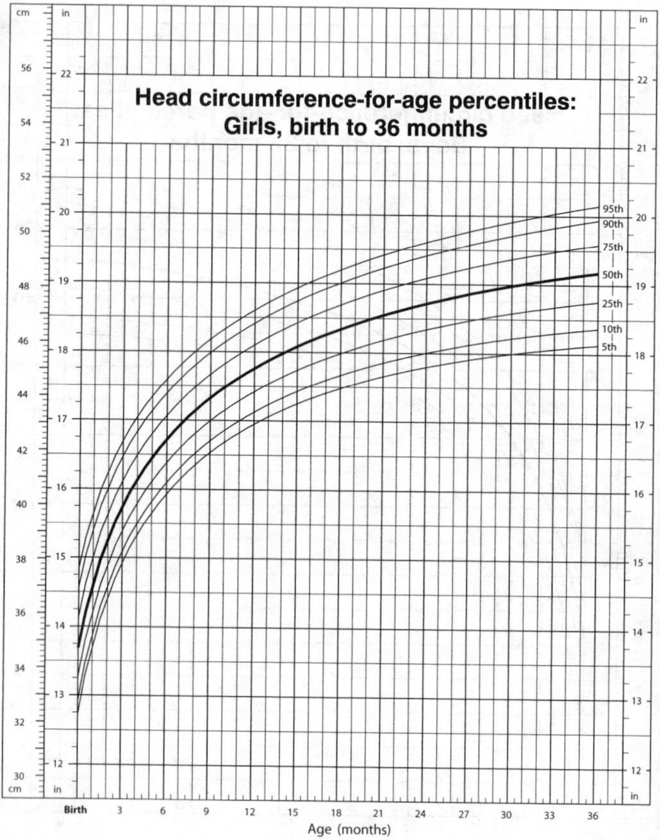

Figure 4–10. Head circumference growth chart for girls from birth to 36 months. (From the Centers for Disease Control and Prevention, National Center for Health Statistics, 2000.)

HOW TO CONDUCT THE ASSESSMENT

Assessment techniques must be geared to the child's developmental level and temperament. The traditional head-to-toe examination is usually not possible. Guidelines to alleviate fear and facilitate the exam in children are listed below.

For specific techniques and possible findings, see *Section 2: Physical Assessment and Health Problems Across the Lifespan.*

1. Approach the child on eye level.
2. If the child turns away from you, sit several feet away from the child and talk to the parent to allow the child time for adjustment. This is usually an ideal time to take the health history. Make all assessments possible *before* touching the child.
3. If the child is in the parent's lap, complete all assessments possible before moving the child to the examination table.
4. Allow the child to touch or play with any safe equipment.
5. Pretend to listen to the parent's or older sibling's heart or look into his or her ears.
6. Explain all procedures in a soft voice.
7. Use play whenever possible. *Example*: "Open your mouth like a big bear."
8. Do not give a choice if there is none. *Example*: Say "I'm going to look in your ears," not "Would you let me look in your ears?"
9. Save invasive procedures (such as looking into ears or mouth) and procedures that require clothing to be removed until the end of the exam.
10. Allow the child or parent to remove the child's clothing when necessary.
11. Weigh the child under the age of 1 year *without* clothing.
12. Praise the child for his or her efforts.

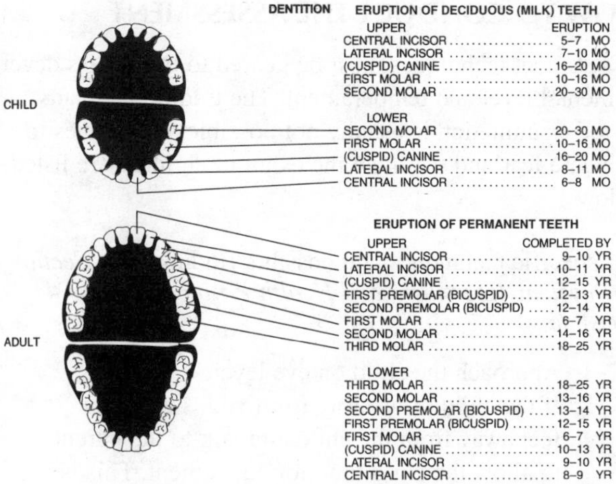

DENTITION
CHILD
ADULT
ERUPTION OF DECIDUOUS (MILK) TEETH
UPPER ERUPTION
CENTRAL INCISOR .... 5–7 MO
LATERAL INCISOR .... 7–10 MO
(CUSPID) CANINE .... 16–20 MO
FIRST MOLAR .... 10–16 MO
SECOND MOLAR .... 20–30 MO
LOWER
SECOND MOLAR .... 20–30 MO
FIRST MOLAR .... 10–16 MO
(CUSPID) CANINE .... 16–20 MO
LATERAL INCISOR .... 8–11 MO
CENTRAL INCISOR .... 6–8 MO
ERUPTION OF PERMANENT TEETH
UPPER COMPLETED BY
CENTRAL INCISOR .... 9–10 YR
LATERAL INCISOR .... 10–11 YR
(CUSPID) CANINE .... 12–15 YR
FIRST PREMOLAR (BICUSPID) .... 12–13 YR
SECOND PREMOLAR (BICUSPID) ..... 12–14 YR
FIRST MOLAR .... 6–7 YR
SECOND MOLAR .... 14–16 YR
THIRD MOLAR .... 18–25 YR
LOWER
THIRD MOLAR .... 18–25 YR
SECOND MOLAR .... 13–16 YR
SECOND PREMOLAR (BICUSPID) ..... 13–14 YR
FIRST PREMOLAR (BICUSPID) .... 12–15 YR
FIRST MOLAR .... 6–7 YR
(CUSPID) CANINE .... 10–13 YR
LATERAL INCISOR .... 9–10 YR
CENTRAL INCISOR .... 8–9 YR

Figure 4–11. Dentition. (From Venes, D, and Thomas, CL [eds]: Taber's Cyclopedic Medical Dictionary, ed. 19. FA Davis, Philadelphia, 2001, p. 557, with permission.)

VITAL SIGNS

AVERAGE HEART RATES FOR INFANTS AND CHILDREN AT REST

Age	*Average Rate*	*Age*	*Average Rate*
Birth	140	2–4 yr	105
1st mo	130	6–10 yr	95
1–6 mo	130	10–14 yr	85
6–12 mo	115	14–18 yr	82
1–2 yr	110		

Source: Adapted from Lowrey, GH: Growth and Development of Children, ed 8. Mosby-Year Book, Chicago, 1986, p 246, with permission.

VARIATIONS IN RESPIRATION WITH AGE

Age	*Rate per Minute*	*Age*	*Rate per Minute*
Premature	40–90	5 yr	20–25
Newborn	30–80	10 yr	17–22
1 yr	20–40	15 yr	15–20
2 yr	20–30	20 yr	15–20
3 yr	20–30		

Source: Adapted from Lowrey, GH: Growth and Development of Children, ed 8. Mosby-Year Book, Chicago, 1986, p 277.

NOTE: A sustained respiratory rate above 60 in the newborn may indicate distress.

BLOOD PRESSURE ASSESSMENT FOR CHILDREN

A child's blood pressure should be assessed with a cuff that covers $^2/_3$ the distance from the shoulder to the elbow. A cuff that is too small will result in a false high reading. A cuff that is too large will result in a false low reading. If a perfect-sized cuff is not available, it is better to use a cuff slightly too large than too small.

Table 4–1. NORMAL BLOOD PRESSURE READINGS FOR GIRLS

	Systolic Blood Pressure Percentile					Diastolic Blood Pressure* Percentile					
Age	5th	10th	50th	90th	95th	Age	5th	10th	50th	90th	95th
1 day	46	50	65	80	84	1 day	38	42	55	68	72
3 days	53	57	72	86	90	3 days	38	42	55	68	71
7 days	60	64	78	93	97	7 days	38	41	54	67	71
1 mo	65	69	84	98	102	1 mo	35	39	52	65	69
2 mo	68	72	87	101	106	2 mo	34	38	51	64	68
3 mo	70	74	89	104	108	3 mo	35	38	51	64	68
4 mo	71	75	90	105	109	4 mo	35	39	52	65	68

5 mo	72	76	91	106	110	5 mo	36	39	52	65	69
6 mo	72	76	91	106	110	6 mo	36	40	53	66	69
7 mo	72	76	91	106	110	7 mo	36	40	53	66	70
8 mo	72	76	91	106	110	8 mo	37	40	53	66	70
9 mo	72	76	91	106	110	9 mo	37	41	54	67	70
10 mo	72	76	91	106	110	10 mo	37	41	54	67	71
11 mo	72	76	91	105	110	11 mo	38	41	54	67	71
1 yr	72	76	91	105	110	1 yr	38	41	54	67	71
2 yr	71	76	90	105	109	2 yr	40	43	56	69	73
3 yr	72	76	91	106	110	3 yr	40	43	56	69	73

(continued on the following page)

Table 4–1. NORMAL BLOOD PRESSURE READINGS FOR GIRLS (continued)

	Systolic Blood Pressure Percentile					Diastolic Blood Pressure* Percentile				
Age	**5th**	**10th**	**50th**	**90th**	**95th**	**Age**	**5th**	**10th**	**50th**	**90th**	**95th**
4 yr	73	78	92	107	111	4 yr	40	43	56	69	73
5 yr	75	79	94	109	113	5 yr	40	43	56	69	73
6 yr	77	81	96	111	115	6 yr	40	44	57	70	74
7 yr	78	83	97	112	116	7 yr	41	45	58	71	75
8 yr	80	84	99	114	118	8 yr	43	46	59	72	76
9 yr	81	86	100	115	119	9 yr	44	48	61	74	77
10 yr	83	87	102	117	121	10 yr	46	49	62	75	79

11 yr	86	90	105	119	123	11 yr	47	51	64	77	81
12 yr	88	92	107	122	126	12 yr	49	53	66	78	82
13 yr	90	94	109	124	128	13 yr	46	50	64	78	82
14 yr	92	96	110	125	129	14 yr	49	53	67	81	85
15 yr	93	97	111	126	130	15 yr	49	53	67	82	86
16 yr	93	97	112	127	131	16 yr	49	53	67	81	85
17 yr	93	98	112	127	131	17 yr	48	52	66	80	84
18 yr	94	98	112	127	131	18 yr	48	52	66	80	84

*K4 was used for children younger than 13 years; K5 was used for children 13 years and older.

Source: Second Task Force on Blood Pressure Control in Children, National Heart, Lung and Blood Institute, Bethesda, Md. Tabular data prepared by Dr. B. Rosner, 1987.

Table 4–2. NORMAL BLOOD PRESSURE READINGS FOR BOYS

	Systolic Blood Pressure Percentile					Diastolic Blood Pressure* Percentile					
Age	5th	10th	50th	90th	95th	Age	5th	10th	50th	90th	95th
1 day	54	58	73	87	92	1 day	38	42	55	68	72
3 days	55	59	74	89	93	3 days	38	42	55	68	71
7 days	57	62	76	91	95	7 days	37	41	54	67	71
1 mo	67	71	86	101	105	1 mo	35	39	52	64	68
2 mo	72	76	91	106	110	2 mo	33	37	50	63	66
3 mo	72	76	91	106	110	3 mo	33	37	50	63	66
4 mo	72	76	91	106	110	4 mo	34	37	50	63	67

5 mo	72	76	91	105	110
6 mo	72	76	90	105	109
7 mo	71	76	90	105	109
8 mo	71	75	90	105	109
9 mo	71	75	90	105	109
10 mo	71	75	90	105	109
11 mo	71	76	90	105	109
1 yr	71	76	90	105	109
2 yr	72	76	91	106	110
3 yr	73	77	92	107	111

5 mo	35	39	52	65	68
6 mo	36	40	53	66	70
7 mo	37	41	54	67	71
8 mo	38	42	55	68	72
9 mo	39	43	55	68	72
10 mo	39	43	56	69	73
11 mo	39	43	56	69	73
1 yr	39	43	56	69	73
2 yr	39	43	56	68	72
3 yr	39	42	55	68	72

(continued on the following page)

Table 4–2. NORMAL BLOOD PRESSURE READINGS FOR BOYS (continued)

	Systolic Blood Pressure Percentile						Diastolic Blood Pressure* Percentile				
Age	**5th**	**10th**	**50th**	**90th**	**95th**	**Age**	**5th**	**10th**	**50th**	**90th**	**95th**
4 yr	74	79	93	108	112	4 yr	39	43	56	69	72
5 yr	76	80	95	109	113	5 yr	40	43	56	69	73
6 yr	77	81	96	111	115	6 yr	41	44	57	70	74
7 yr	78	83	97	112	116	7 yr	42	45	58	71	75
8 yr	80	84	99	114	118	8 yr	43	47	60	73	76
9 yr	82	86	101	115	120	9 yr	44	48	61	74	78
10 yr	84	88	102	117	121	10 yr	45	49	62	75	79

11 yr	86	90	105	119	123	11 yr	47	50	63	76	80
12 yr	88	92	107	121	126	12 yr	48	51	64	77	81
13 yr	90	94	109	124	128	13 yr	45	49	63	77	81
14 yr	93	97	112	126	131	14 yr	46	50	64	78	82
15 yr	95	99	114	129	133	15 yr	47	51	65	79	83
16 yr	98	102	117	131	136	16 yr	49	53	67	81	85
17 yr	100	104	119	134	138	17 yr	51	55	69	83	87
18 yr	102	106	121	136	140	18 yr	52	56	70	84	88

*K4 was used for children younger than 13 years; K5 was used for children 13 years and older.

Source: Second Task Force on Blood Pressure Control in Children, National Heart, Lung and Blood Institute, Bethesda, Md. Tabular data prepared by Dr. B. Rosner, 1987.

ROUTINE PEDIATRIC IMMUNIZATION SCHEDULE

Recommendations regarding immunization schedules are issued by the Centers for Disease Control (CDC) and are subject to change. Actual schedules may vary somewhat from state to state. Always check current recommendations of the CDC and your local board of health. Possible updates to CDC recommendations and links to individual state requirements may be accessed at http://www.cdc.gov/nip.

Contraindications to Immunizations—For details, refer to: http://www.cdc.gov/nip/recs/contraindication.htm

DTaP,DT,	Previous CNS damage, uncontrolled convulsions, progressive neurologic disorder
Td	(defer until stabilized). Pertussis usually not given after age 7.
HepB	Allergy to yeast products, infant weighing <2000 g
Hib	Allergy to diphtheria toxoid or thimerosal (merthiolate), age <6wks
IPV	Pregnancy
MMR	Allergy to egg or neomycin, severe immunosuppression, pregnancy

NOTE: Moderate or severe acute illness, with or without fever, is a contraindication to immunizations. Previous severe reaction to the vaccine or any of its components is a contraindication. The common cold without fever is NOT a contraindication to immunization.

Recommended Childhood and Adolescent Immunization Schedule— United States, 2003 (approved by the Advisory Committee on Immunization Practices (www.cdc.gov/nip/acip<www.edc.gov/nip/acip>), the American Academy of Pediatrics (www.aap.org <www.acp.org>, and the American Academy of Family Physicians (www.aafp.org). <www.aafp.org).>)

range of recommended ages | catch-up-vaccination | preadolescent assessment

Vaccine ▼ Age ►	Birth	1 mo	2 mos	4 mos	6 mos	12 mos	15 mos	18 mos	24 mos	4–6 yrs	11–12 yrs	13–18 yrs
Hepatitis B[1]	Hep B #1	only if mother HBsAg (–)									Hep B series	
			Hep B #2			Hep B #3						
Diphtheria, Tetanus, Pertussis[2]			DTaP	DTaP	DTaP		DTaP			DTaP	Td	
Haemophilus influenzae Type b[3]			Hib	Hib	Hib		Hib					
Inactivated Polio			IPV	IPV			IPV			IPV		
Measles, Mumps, Rubella[4]							MMR #1			MMR #2	MMR #2	
Varicella[5]							Varicella				Varicella	
Pneumococcal[6]			PCV	PCV	PCV		PCV		PCV		PPV	
----- Vaccines below this line are for selected populations -----												
Hepatitis A[7]											Hepatitis A series	
Influenza[8]									Influenza (yearly)			

This schedule indicates the recommended ages for routine administration of currently licensed childhood vaccines, as of December 1, 2002, for children through age 18 years. Any dose not given at the recommended age should be given at any subsequent visit when indicated and feasible. Indicates age groups that warrant special effort to administer those vaccines not previously given. Additional vaccines may be licensed and recommended during the year. Licensed combination vaccines may be used whenever any components of the combination are indicated and the vaccine's other components are not contraindicated. Providers should consult the manufacturers' package inserts for detailed recommendations.

1. **Hepatitis B vaccine (HepB).** All infants should receive the first dose of hepatitis B vaccine soon after birth and before hospital discharge; the first dose may also be given by age 2 months if the infant's mother is HBsAg-negative. Only monovalent HepB can be used for the birth dose. Monovalent or combination vaccine containing HepB may be used to complete the series. Four doses of vaccine may be administered when a birth dose is given. The second dose should be given at least 4 weeks after the first dose, except for combination vaccines which cannot be administered before age 6 weeks. The third dose should be given at least 16 weeks after the first dose and at least 8 weeks after the second dose. The last dose in the vaccination series (third or fourth dose) should not be administered before age 6 months.
   Infants born to HBsAg-positive mothers should receive HepB and 0.5 mL Hepatitis B Immune Globulin (HBIG) within 12 hours of birth at separate sites. The second dose is recommended at age 1–2 months. The last dose in the vaccination series should not be administered before age 6 months. These infants should be tested for HBsAg and anti-HBs at 9–15 months of age.
   Infants born to mothers whose HBsAg status is unknown should receive the first dose of the HepB series within 12 hours of birth. Maternal blood should be drawn as soon as possible to determine the mother's HBsAg status; if the HBsAg test is positive, the infant should receive HBIG as soon as possible (no later than age 1 week). The second dose is recommended at age 1–2 months. The last dose in the vaccination series should not be administered before age 6 months.
2. **Diphtheria and tetanus toxoids and acellular pertussis vaccine (DTaP).** The fourth dose of DTaP may be administered as early as age 12 months, provided 6 months have elapsed since the third dose and the child is unlikely to return at age 15–18 months. **Tetanus and diphtheria toxoids (Td)** is recommended at age 11–12 years if at least 5 years have elapsed since the last dose of tetanus and diphtheria toxoid-containing vaccine. Subsequent routine Td boosters are recommended every 10 years.

(continued on the following page)

3. ***Haemophilus influenzae* type b (Hib) conjugate vaccine.** Three Hib conjugate vaccines are licensed for infant use. If PRP-OMP (PedvaxHIB® or ComVax® [Merck]) is administered at ages 2 and 4 months, a dose at age 6 months is not required. DTaP/Hib combination products should not be used for primary immunization in infants at ages 2, 4 or 6 months, but can be used as boosters following any Hib vaccine.
4. **Measles, mumps, and rubella vaccine (MMR).** The second dose of MMR is recommended routinely at age 4–6 years but may be administered during any visit, provided at least 4 weeks have elapsed since the first dose and that both doses are administered beginning at or after age 12 months. Those who have not previously received the second dose should complete the schedule by the 11–12 year old visit.
5. **Varicella vaccine.** Varicella vaccine is recommended at any visit at or after age 12 months for susceptible children, i.e. those who lack a reliable history of chickenpox. Susceptible persons aged ≥ 13 years should receive two doses, given at least 4 weeks apart.
6. **Pneumococcal vaccine.** The heptavalent **pneumococcal conjugate vaccine (PCV)** is recommended for all children age 2–23 months. It is also recommended for certain children age 24–59 months. **Pneumococcal polysaccharide vaccine (PPV)** is recommended in addition to PCV for certain high-risk groups. See *MMWR* 2000;49(RR-9);1–38.
7. **Hepatitis A vaccine.** Hepatitis A vaccine is recommended for children and adolescents in selected states and regions, and for certain high-risk groups; consult your local public health authority. Children and adolescents in these states, regions, and high risk groups who have not been immunized against hepatitis A can begin the hepatitis A vaccination series during any visit. The two doses in the series should be administered at least 6 months apart. See *MMWR* 1999;48(RR-12);1–37.
8. **Influenza vaccine.** Influenza vaccine is recommended annually for children age ≥6 months with certain risk factors (including but not limited to asthma, cardiac disease, sickle cell disease, HIV, diabetes, and household members of persons in groups at high risk; see *MMWR* 2002;51(RR-3);1–31), and can be administered to all others wishing to obtain immunity. In addition, healthy children age 6–23 months are encouraged to receive influenza vaccine if feasible because children in this age group are at substantially increased risk for influenza-related hospitalizations. Children aged ≤ 12 years should receive vaccine in a dosage appropriate for their age (0.25 mL if age 6–35 months or 0.5 mL if aged ≥3 years). Children aged ≤8 years who are receiving influenza vaccine for the first time should receive two doses separated by at least 4 weeks.

For additional information about vaccines, including precautions and contraindications for immunization and vaccine shortages, please visit the National Immunization Program Website at www.cdc.gov/nip or call the National Immunization Information Hotline at 800-232-2522 (English) or 800-232-0233 (Spanish).

PEDIATRIC CALORIC REQUIREMENTS

Age, Years	*Calories per Kilogram of Body Weight*	*Average Caloric Need**
0–6 mo	108	650
6 mo–1 yr	98	850
1–3 yr	102	1300
4–6 yr	90	1800
7–10 yr	70	2000
FEMALE		
11–14 yr	47	2200
15–18 yr	40	2200
MALE		
11–14 yr	55	2500
15–18 yr	45	3000

*Average caloric needs are based on median weights and heights of children living in the United States.

Source: Adapted from Recommended Daily Allowances, Food and Nutrition Board, National Academy of Sciences, National Research Council, Washington, DC. Revised 1990.

NOTE: The American Academy of Pediatrics recommends that premature infants receive 120 calories per kilogram per day.

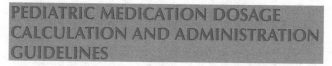

PEDIATRIC MEDICATION DOSAGE CALCULATION AND ADMINISTRATION GUIDELINES

Safe dosages (based on body weight) should always be calculated prior to the administration of medications ordered for children. Dosage information based on the child's weight in kilograms is available for most medications in current medication manuals. If no information is available for a specific medication, the **body surface area** is sometimes used to calculate dosages. The calculation method is as follows:

1. Use a nomogram to calculate body surface area (see Figs. 1–26 and 1–27).

2. Divide the surface area in meters by 1.7.
3. Multiply the quotient from step 2 by the adult dose.

Tips for Administrating Medications

1. Never ask a child if he or she will take the medicine. Tell the child it is time to take the medicine.
2. Give choices when possible. *Example*: Ask which medicine he or she wants to take first or what he or she wants to drink with the medicine.
3. Infants will frequently suck medication from a nipple.
4. A syringe may be used to administer liquid medicine to an infant. Gently squeeze the infant's cheeks to prevent medicine from being pushed from the mouth, and administer small amounts into the side of the child's mouth. (Medicine placed on top of the tongue is likely to be pushed from the mouth.)
5. Do not add medication to the infant's formula.
6. Never blow into a child's face or pinch his or her nose closed in an attempt to make him or her swallow medication, as this may cause the child to gasp and aspirate medicine into the airway.
7. When giving IM medications, be sure to have assistance in holding the child. Be honest about pain, and finish the procedure as quickly as possible.

PEDIATRIC IV MEDICATION ADMINISTRATION METHODS

NOTE: *Heparin locks* are frequently used to administer medications. With a heparin lock, IV fluids are discontinued after medication infusion, and the IV device is flushed with enough diluted heparin to prevent clotting. The amount of diluted heparin administered depends on the size of the IV device but is usually 1 to 2 mL.

Usual methods of medication administration include.

1. IV *push or bolus*: Medication is administered manually or by a secondary pump.
2. *Buretrol*: Medication is placed in the Buretrol. When this method is used, the medication must be followed by enough flush to remove all medication from the IV tubing. The amount of flush needed is equal to

the amount of fluid in the IV line itself (usually 15 to 25 mL).

> Example: *To infuse medication* in 1 hour: If the medication and the fluid in the Buretrol equal 10 mL and the IV tubing holds 15 mL of fluid, the IV rate would be 25 mL/h or 25 gtt/min. A minimum of 25 mL fluid must be administered to clear all medication from the tubing.

3. *Retrograde method*: This method is used when it is desirable to limit fluid intake. The IV line is clamped, and medication is injected at a Y port above the clamped site. This results in the medication's going "backward" into the line. The displaced fluid goes into a receptacle on the line (these receptacles are commercially available) or into an empty syringe placed at another Y site above the injection site. (To avoid losing medication into the empty syringe, the tubing volume between the medication and empty syringes must be greater than the amount of medication injected.) The line clamp is released to allow infusion. To ensure that the child receives all medication in the IV line, calculate the total volume of fluid to be infused by adding the volume of fluid below the injection site to the volume injected.

To determine the best method of IV medication administration to use:

- Consider the literature-recommended dilution and rate of flow for the medication.
- Consider the rate of and amount of fluid the child can tolerate (see *Pediatric Maintenance Fluid Calculation*, which follows).
- Consider the compatibility and timing of other ordered IV medications.

PEDIATRIC MAINTENANCE FLUID CALCULATION

Because infants and young children suffer the ill effects of dehydration or fluid overload much more quickly than adults, it is important for the nurse to check the accuracy of all fluid orders with the same care used to check the safety of drug dosage orders. The following formula is widely used to calculate **usual maintenance** fluid requirements for children. *Maintenance fluid* is the amount needed to maintain adequate hydration in a healthy child. More fluid is given to compensate for certain pathologic states, and less fluid may be needed if pathology indicates that fluid should be restricted.

Steps

1. Convert the child's weight in pounds to kilograms by multiplying the number of pounds by 0.45.
2. Calculate 100 mL of fluid per kilogram per 24 hours for the 1st 10 kg of the child's body weight.
3. Calculate 50 mL of fluid per kilogram per 24 hours for the 2nd 10 kg of the child's body weight.
4. Calculate 10 to 25 mL of fluid per kilogram per 24 hours for each kilogram of body weight over 20.
5. Add the products of steps 2, 3, and 4 to determine the milliliters of fluid needed per 24 hours.
6. To calculate the IV rate, divide the sum derived in step 5 by 24 (number of hours in a day). Milliliters per hour will be the same as microdrops per minute.

NOTE: Add 12% maintenance fluid (to the sum of step 5) for every degree (Celsius) of body temp over 37.5°C. Eliminate any step not applicable to the weight of the child.

Examples of Maintenance Fluid Calculation for Children

CALCULATION TO DETERMINE THE MAINTENANCE FLUID FOR A 15-LB INFANT

- Convert 15 lb to kilograms by multiplying 15 × 0.45 = 6.75 kg.
- Allow 100 mL/kg for the 6.75 kg (= 675 mL).
- Divide 675 by 24 to determine the rate of IV if indicated.
- RATE = 28 mL/h or 28 gtt/min (microdrop).

CALCULATION TO DETERMINE THE MAINTENANCE FLUID FOR A 40-LB CHILD

- Convert 40 lb to kilograms by multiplying 40 × 0.45 = 18 kg.

- Allow 100 mL/kg for the 1st 10 kg (= 1000 mL).
- Allow 50 mL/kg for the remaining 8 kg (= 400 mL).
- Add the 1000 mL to the 400 mL (= 1400 mL).
- Divide the total of 1400 by 24 to determine the rate.
- RATE = 58 mL/h or 58 gtt/min (microdrop).

CALCULATION TO DETERMINE THE MAINTENANCE FLUID FOR A 70-LB CHILD

- Convert 70 lb to kilograms by multiplying 70 × 0.45 = 31.5 kg.
- Allow 100 mL/kg for the 1st 10 kg (= 1000 mL).
- Allow 50 mL/kg for the 2nd 10 kg (= 500 mL).
- Allow 20 mL/kg for the remaining 11.5 kg (= 230 mL). (Physician preference and age and condition of child will determine whether more than 10 mL/kg is given for each kilogram over 20.)
- Add 1000 mL + 500 mL + 230 mL (= 1730 mL).
- Divide 1730 by 24 to determine the rate.
- RATE = 72 mL/h or 72 gtt/min (microdrop).

PEDIATRIC IV ADMINISTRATION TIPS

- It is essential that the nurse check every IV order to ensure that a safe amount of fluid has been ordered. See preceding *Pediatric Maintenance Fluid Calculation.*
- The microdrop or minidrop equipment is usually used when administering IV fluids to children. When this equipment is used, the microdrops per minute rate is the *same* as the milliliters per hour rate.

> Example: An IV that is to infuse at 20 mL/h will run at 20 gtt/min. If it is desirable to give 20 mL in 30 minutes, then the IV rate would be 40 gtt/min. Similarly, to give 20 mL in 15 minutes, the rate would be 80 gtt/min. (The principle is the same as driving an automobile at 20 mph to travel 20 miles in 1 hour, or at 40 mph to travel 20 miles in 30 minutes.)

- A volume control chamber such as the Buretrol should be hung below the IV bag.
- To prevent accidental fluid overload, never add over 2 hours' worth of fluid to the Buretrol at any time.

- If possible, place the IV on a pump to decrease the possibility of accidental fluid overload. Monitor closely for infiltration when pump is used.
- Isotonic solution for the child younger than age 5 is usually D5.2NS, which differs from adult isotonic solution because of the greater amount of extracellular fluid in a child.
- Isotonic solution for the child 5 years and older is usually D5.45NS.
- Potassium is not added to a child's IV until after the child has voided.

CHILDREN'S FEARS RELATED TO HOSPITALIZATION

Age	*Common Fears*	*Nursing Indications*
5 mo–3 yr	Separation from mother or usual caregiver	Encourage rooming in. Encourage patient to bring familiar objects (e.g., toys, blanket) from home.
1–18 yr	Bodily harm (A 3-yr-old may view hospitalization as punishment. A schoolaged child or an adolescent may fear harm that may cause him or her to "look different" [body mutilation].)	Explain procedure in simple terms. Do not inform the child of painful procedures far in advance. Demonstrate procedures with dolls. Be honest regarding pain that may be experienced during procedures. Do not discourage crying. Allow parents to be with child during painful procedures when possible.
6–18 yr	Separation from parents, separation from peers, loss of control	Encourage visits from family and friends. Encourage use of the telephone to maintain family and peer contact. Allow choices when possible. Explain procedures in simple terms. Do not discourage crying.
	Loss of control	If necessary to restrain child for a procedure, say this will be done to help him or her hold still.

CHILDREN AND DEATH

Age	*Usual Understanding of Death*
Birth–1 yr	No concept.
1–3 yr	Believes death is temporary and reversible. May believe his or her thoughts or unrelated actions caused another's death.
4–8 yr	Begins to understand permanence of death. May view death as separation. May worry about effect of own death on family.
8 and older	Understands permanence of death and begins to face reality of own mortality.

NURSING CONSIDERATIONS

The dying child should be allowed to ask questions regarding his or her condition. Before formulating specific answers, the nurse should determine the child's understanding of his or her condition and his or her understanding of death, as well as his or her coping strategies and the family's wishes.

Siblings as well as parents of the dying child often feel great guilt and may believe that they are responsible for the child's condition. It is important for both siblings and parents to be allowed liberal visitation privileges.

The nurse should be certain that the family and the child have access to support from a member of the clergy of their religious preference and that the performance of religious activities not be hindered.

AGE-APPROPRIATE PLAY AND DIVERSIONAL ACTIVITIES FOR HOSPITALIZED CHILDREN

Age	*Activity*
Birth–1 mo	Cuddle. Rock. Smile at and talk to the infant in a soft voice. Provide music. Place a mobile over the bed.

(continued on the following page)

Age	*Activity*
2–3 mo	Place a small rattle in the infant's hand. Place infant in a swing or car seat. Provide a crib mobile.
4–6 mo	Provide a nonbreakable mirror. Provide stuffed dolls or animals.
6–9 mo	Play peekaboo by momentarily covering your face with a towel. Provide brightly colored toys. Show pictures in a book. Provide noise-making toys.
9–12 mo	Provide blocks and demonstrate stacking. Provide a ball and demonstrate how to roll it on the floor. Place the child on a waterproof surface with a basin containing an inch of water and demonstrate how to stir the water (constant supervision needed). Provide toys and large container into which the toys can be placed and demonstrate placing the toys into the container and pouring them out. Play "Where is your nose?", "Where is your mouth?"
1–3 yr	Provide push and pull toys (especially useful when therapeutic ambulation is indicated). Hold a wand filled with a commercial "bubble" solution and have child blow bubbles (useful when deep breathing is desirable). Provide art supplies (supervise carefully). Provide modeling clay or dough (supervise carefully). Provide a doll and syringes without needles, bandages, tape, and other equipment used in the care of the child (supervise carefully). Provide a tea set or small pitcher and allow the child to pour and drink or eat from the small dishes (especially helpful when increased fluid or food intake is desirable). Read to the child.

Age	*Activity*
3–6 yr	Provide simple puzzles. Provide simple board or card games. Fill a cup half full of water and liquid soap mixture. Provide a straw and allow the child to blow bubbles into the glass (to encourage deep breathing). Tell the beginning of a story and ask the child to complete the story. See *Activities for 1–3 yr*.
School age or adolescent	Provide books. Provide board games. Provide supplies for letter writing. Provide free access to telephone if possible. Allow noninfectious children in these age groups to interact with each other and eat meals together.

ENCOURAGING CHILDREN TO EAT

1. Ask about food preferences, then request that dietary send favorite foods.
2. Foods that can be picked up with the fingers are often most acceptable to younger children.
3. Serve food lukewarm. Children usually object to very hot or very cold foods.
4. Keep in mind that most children like grain products best, vegetables least.
5. Most children dislike spicy foods.
6. Make meals a special occasion. Celebrate holidays, especially days that are meaningful to the child—his dog's birthday!
7. A nurse can always suggest an "Un-Birthday celebration"—as in *Alice in Wonderland*—on any day of the year, except, of course, the child's birthday.
8. Decorate "place mats" made from almost any kind of paper with crayons, pencils, etc.
9. Make an effort to schedule procedures after meals or at least an hour before mealtime.
10. Make paper hats—the triangle sort—out of any type of paper for the celebration of eating. Or

perhaps make paper airplanes. Use your imagination plus the child's imagination!

11. A flower, any kind, including one made of paper, is effective in making mealtime fun.
12. Use a small pitcher and allow the child to pour from it into his or her cup or glass—seems to improve intake tremendously.
13. A clean "play" tea set used for serving real food or liquid is fun for most children.
14. Keep the child company at mealtime, even if he or she is self-feeding.
15. Allow children to eat with other children if possible. The playroom helps to distract them from the "sick" atmosphere in their own rooms.

SAFETY PRECAUTIONS FOR HOSPITALIZED INFANTS AND TODDLERS

INFANT

- Keep side rails up or your hand on the infant at **all** times.
- Do not prop bottles.
- Keep pillows out of the bed.
- Make certain the mattress fits snugly into the crib to avoid entrapment.
- Make sure that the infant's head, arms, and legs cannot be trapped in any part of the crib.
- Keep objects small enough to fit into the infant's mouth out of his or her bed and reach.
- Keep syringes and open safety pins out of the infant's bed.
- Be certain the infant cannot reach cords or electrical outlets from the crib.
- Check the placement of IV lines and monitor the cords frequently.
- Place "bubble" top or "cage" top on bed if the child attempts to climb over crib rail.
- Empty all bottles after the feeding is completed.

TODDLER

- Never refer to medication as "candy."
- Never leave medication or ointments in the child's room.
- If the child climbs on tables or other objects, remove them from the room.
- Be aware of the child's whereabouts when opening and closing doors. (Finger entrapment is a common cause of injury.)
- Be certain the child is *constantly* attended when out of the crib.
- See also the preceding precautions for infants.

CARDIAC MURMURS

DEFINITION

A soft blowing sound (similar to a breath sound) caused by movement of blood within the heart and adjacent large blood vessels.

TYPES

Functional—does not indicate organic disease of the heart and may disappear upon return to health. (Example: hypertension)

Innocent—vibrations in normal valves because of rapid blood flow. (Examples: following exercise or with fever).

NOTE: Approximately 30% of all children have functional or innocent murmurs. These murmurs are always systolic and may disappear with a change in position. They are grade I or II.

Organic—murmur caused by structural changes in heart or vessels.

GRADING OF MURMUR

Grading indicates volume (loudness) or intensity and is usually based on a system with six values, as follows:

Grade	*Intensity*
I/VI	Barely audible
II/VI	Faint, but easily heard
III/VI	Soft to moderately loud without thrill (palpable vibration)
IV/VI	Moderate to loud with thrill
V/VI	Loud: heard with stethoscope barely on chest with easily palpable thrill
VI/VI	Heard with stethoscope lifted from chest (Thrill is present.)

Grading of cardiac murmurs may also be based on a system with four values:

Grade	*Intensity*
I/IV	Faintest
II/IV	Soft
III/IV	Loud
IV/IV	Very loud

Other noteworthy components of murmur classification are:

Location: Aortic, pulmonic, tricuspid, mitral area
Radiation: Of sound
Timing: Early, mid, or late systole or diastole
Character: Crescendo, that is, gradual increase in volume, or decrescendo, that is, gradual decrease in volume
Quality: Blowing, harsh, rumbling
Pitch: High, medium, low
Variance: With respiration or position change

SIGNS OF AIR HUNGER (HYPOXIA) IN CHILDREN

1. Restlessness, which is the earliest sign of air hunger
2. Anorexia
3. Nasal flaring
4. Head bobbing

5. Retractions, that is, the sinking in of soft tissue of the chest on inspiration. *Types*:
   Supraclavicular: Above the clavicles
   Suprasternal: Above the sternum
   Intercostal: Between the ribs
   Subcostal: Under the rib cage
   Substernal: Under the sternum
6. Dyspnea, that is, labored breathing
7. Upright or forward-leaning (tripod) position of the child
8. Respiratory rate increased for age (see *Vital Signs*).
9. Pulse rate increased for age (see *Vital Signs*).
10. Cyanosis
11. SaO_2 less than 95%

NOTE: Because the young child's airway is anatomically smaller than the adult's, the airway can quickly become obstructed by mucus or inflammation. It is, therefore, essential that the nurse frequently monitor children with respiratory problems, as their conditions can deteriorate rapidly.

SIGNS OF SHOCK IN CHILDREN

1. Apprehension and irritability, which are early signs
2. Thirst
3. Tachycardia for age (see *Vital Signs,* p. 372).
4. Tachypnea for age (*see Vital Signs,* p. 373).
5. Pallor, that is, paleness
6. Decreased tissue perfusion in the hands and feet
7. Decreased urine output (should be at least 0.5 mL/kg/h)
8. Narrowed pulse pressure (difference between systolic and diastolic blood pressure decreases)
9. Decreased blood pressure for age (see Table 4–1 and 4–2), which is a late sign. (Blood pressure does not drop early in pediatric shock because of the elasticity of the child's blood vessels, which adjust readily to decreased vascular volume.)

NOTE: Children develop hypovolemic shock more quickly than adults because of their small blood volumes and large amounts of extracellular fluid that normally undergo rapid turnover.

RESPIRATORY AND CARDIAC MONITORING

Infants who are born prematurely, have a history of apnea, respiratory problems, or cardiac problems, or who are seriously ill are often placed on continuous cardiac monitors.

MONITOR SETTINGS

Cardiac: Set alarm limits 15 beats per minute above and below normal, age-appropriate resting limits (see *Vital Signs*).

Respiratory: Set alarm limits 15 breaths per minute above and below normal, age-appropriate limits (see *Vital Signs*).

MONITOR LEAD PLACEMENT

White: Top right
Green: Lower right
Black: Top left
Red: Lower left (Red is sometimes omitted.)

NOTE: If snap-on lead wires are used, they should be attached to the electrodes *prior* to placing the electrodes on the child.

NOTES

NOTES

NOTES

NOTES

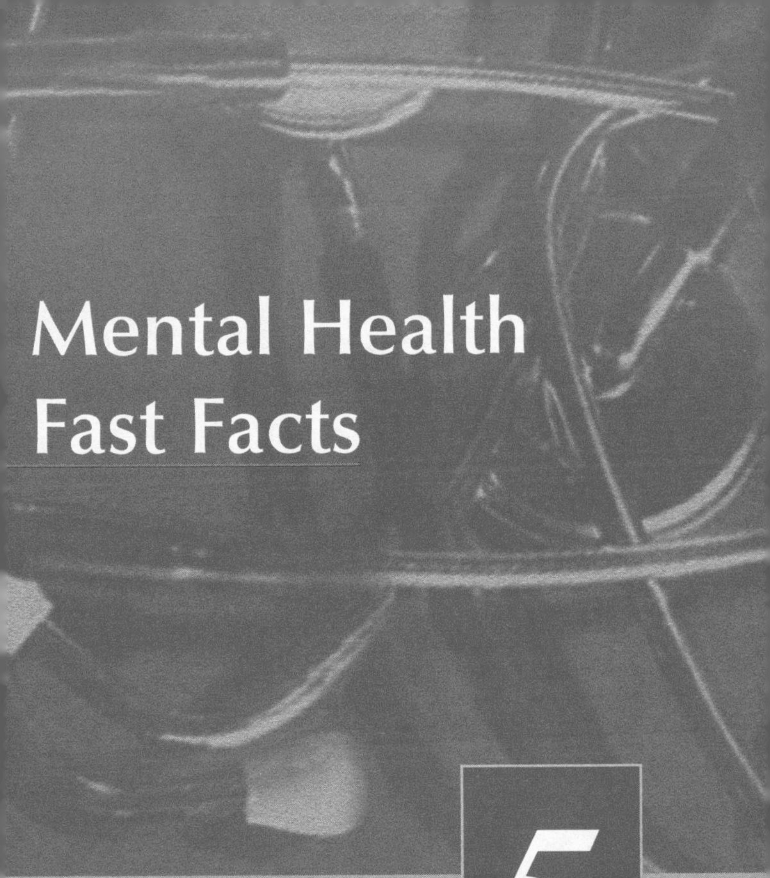

Mental Health Fast Facts

Section

5

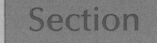

THERAPEUTIC COMMUNICATION TECHNIQUES

Technique	*Use*	*Example*
Clarifying	Gives voice to what has been suggested; increases the accuracy of the listener's understanding of the message	Patient, "It's no use taking this medicine anymore." Nurse, "You're concerned that the medication isn't helping you?"
Encouraging/accepting/acknowledging	Helps the patient verbalize feelings	"Tell me what you are feeling." "How does that seem to you?"
Exploring	Pursues the topic in more detail	"Tell me more about that."
Focusing	Keeps the conversation goal directed; specific and concrete.	"What does that mean to you?" Nonverbal: eye contact and attentive body posture. When using or evaluating nonverbal communication, be familiar with patient's culture and customs.
Hypothetical question	Determines whether a patient has accurate information or determines how a particular situation might be handled; can provide an opportunity to determine cognitive abilities	"What would you do if you felt dizzy?"

(continued on the following page)

Mental Health

Technique	*Use*	*Example*
Mirroring/ Reflecting/ Restating	Establishes rapport	Nurse assumes same physical posture as patient or statement made by patient is said back to him/her.
Offering broad general leads	Encourages the patient to continue	"And then?" "Go on," "I see" (should not be overused and should not be used when the patient is rambling or does not make sense).
Offering self	Increases patient's feeling of self-worth	Making time/self available to patient. "I'll stay with you."
Open-ended question	Avoids placing limits on the patient's response	"How do you feel about your new medication?"
Broad opening statement	Encourages patient to take initiative in communication	Nurse might say, "Where would you like to begin?"
Reflecting	Clarifies meaning or encourages patient to elaborate	Nurse may use a questioning tone to repeat what the patient just said.
Silence	Allows patient to collect thoughts; express emotions; conveys acceptance	Patient may pause while discussing a subject that causes him or her to feel strong emotions. The nurse remains silent.
Voicing doubt and presenting reality	Describes reality from another view; expresses different perspective	"I understand the voices seem real to you, but I do not hear voices."

Technique	*Use*	*Example*
Verbalizing the implied or translating	Interpreting the unspoken meaning of patient's behavior or what is unsaid.	Patient: "I'm lost at sea." Nurse: "You are feeling abandoned?"

NONVERBAL CLUES

Watch for nonverbal clues (symbolic messages, tone of voice, use of touch, reaction to touch, use of space, facial expression, mannerisms). Be aware of cultural influence; for example, in some cultures, it is considered disrespectful to make eye contact with an authority figure.

AVOID

- Closed-ended questions that can have only a specific response. Use such questions only if specific or factual information is needed.
- "Why" questions, as these may appear blaming or may distract from emotions by forcing thoughts into cognitive mode.

DEFENSE (COPING) MECHANISMS

By definition, a *defense mechanism* is an attempt (usually unconscious) to resolve or conceal conflicts or anxieties. They may be adaptive or maladaptive.

Compensation: Attempts to escape real or imagined inferiority by achievement or exaggerated statements regarding self or achievements.

Conversion reaction: Expresses a psychologic conflict through the loss of a physical function.

Denial: Keeps anxiety-producing realities out of conscious awareness

Displacement: Transfers an emotion from the original to a different idea.

Fantasy: Escapes stress by focusing on unreal mental images in which his or her wishes are fulfilled.

Identification: Patterns himself or herself after another person.

Intellectualization: Deals with problem on an intellectual basis to avoid discomfort of emotions.

Introjection: Identifies self with another and assumes the supposed behavior and attitudes of the other.

Projection: Displaces own undesirable actions or feelings to another person.

Rationalization: Attempts to become comfortable by substituting acceptable reason(s) for the actual reason(s) for behavior.

Reaction formation: Acts in a way that is the opposite of actual feelings.

Regression: Stress results in behavior characteristic of an earlier developmental period.

Repression: Unconsciously inhibits an idea or desire.

Restitution: See *Undoing.*

Sublimation: Converts unacceptable desires and impulses into acceptable behavior.

Suppression: Consciously inhibits an idea or desire.

Undoing: Attempts to cancel misdeeds by atonement ("making-up-for") activities (restitution).

CHARACTERISTICS AND MANAGEMENT OF INDIVIDUALS WITH MALADAPTIVE BEHAVIOR

Behavior	*Characteristics*	*Management*
Addictive behavior	Negative self-concept • Sense of loneliness, guilt, shame, and despair • Personality types vary • Extensive use of defense mechanisms • Chemicals, food, sex, gambling, or other behavior may be involved (multiple addictions are common)	Convey acceptance of person but nonacceptance of addiction • Correct misconceptions regarding substance abuse • Confront pathologic defenses • Encourage self-esteem • Plan for discharge and follow-up
Aggressive/Assertive behavior	Forceful physical, verbal, or symbolic actions; may be appropriate (assertiveness) or inappropriate (destructive toward self or others)	Set limits • Be consistent and firm • Confront behavior • Encourage constructive expressions of aggression • Avoid retaliation
Altered eating behavior (anorexia nervosa)	Intense fear of becoming obese that does not diminish as weight loss progresses • Refusal to eat • Preoccupation with food • Compulsive behavior • Attempts to get full control of body	Encourage expression of feelings and support assertiveness • Avoid arguments about weight or food • Monitor intake and observe for at least 1 h following meals • Set time limit for

(continued on the following page)

CHARACTERISTICS AND MANAGEMENT OF INDIVIDUALS WITH MALADAPTIVE BEHAVIOR (continued)

Behavior	*Characteristics*	*Management*
Altered eating behavior (anorexia nervosa) (continued)	• Generally attention seeking, high achiever with low self-concept; from middle or upper income family with controlling parents	meals to be ingested to prevent eating behavior from gaining further attention • Monitor exercise • Parenteral or nasogastric feeding if intake refused • Extended follow-up
Anxious behavior (generalized)	Feeling of worry, uneasiness, or dread (patient is usually unaware of cause)	Reduce stimuli • Encourage expression of feelings • Assist in identification and reduction or removal of stressors if possible • Identify problem-solving methods successfully used in the past and encourage use if appropriate • Avoid offering false reassurance • Reinforce reality if necessary
Codependent behavior	Low self-esteem • Difficulty setting boundaries • Own needs and desires ignored because of	Encourage to write a self-affirmation, such as "I am valuable" and "I deserve to be happy"

Codependent behavior (continued)	extreme involvement (enmeshment) in other's behavior • Attempts to use caring behaviors to control dysfunctional environment • Physical symptoms such as aches, ulcers, or hypertension • Difficulty accepting help	and to read these at least 3 times a day • Encourage journal-keeping to increase awareness of own needs and feelings • Encourage participation in group recovery programs
Delusional behavior	Fixed, false belief(s) that cannot be changed by reasoning • Feelings of rejection, inadequacy, and inferiority • Lack of trust • Hypersensitive • May use defense mechanisms such as projection • Manipulative • Difficulty in admitting own errors	Assess potential for harm to self or others, and use appropriate preventive measures • Note events preceding delusional behavior • Reinforce reality • Set limits for actions and discussions • Educate family and patient regarding stress triggers, management, and medication therapy
Dependent behavior	Reliance on others to meet needs and desires • Denial of behavior • Lack of self-confidence • Avoidance of making demands on others to maintain relationship	See *Manipulative behavior* and *Hypochondriacal behavior*

(continued on the following page)

CHARACTERISTICS AND MANAGEMENT OF INDIVIDUALS WITH MALADAPTIVE BEHAVIOR (continued)

Behavior	***Characteristics***	***Management***
Depressed behavior	Loss of interest in pleasurable outlets such as food, sex, work, friends, or hobbies • Change in eating or sleeping habits • Weight loss or gain • Psychomotor agitation or retardation • Fatigue • Feelings of hopelessness, worthlessness, self-reproach, or excessive or inappropriate guilt • Thoughts of death	Evaluate potential for self-injury • Provide nutrition and fluids, and monitor intake • Assist with ADL • Use positive reinforcement • Reduce support gradually as patient improves • Also see *Withdrawn behavior*
Hallucinatory behavior	Appears to look at, listen to, smell, or taste something that is not present, or appears to respond to nonexistent stimuli	Stay with patient during hallucinations • Offer empathy, but let the patient know that you do not, hear or see what he or she hears or sees • Do not argue about the reality of the patient's perceptions • Engage patient in reality-based conversation or activities

Hyperactive behavior	Constant overactivity • Distractibility • Impulsiveness • Inability to concentrate • Aggressiveness	Provide opportunity for noncompetitive physical activity • Decrease external stimuli • Set and enforce limits regarding intrusive or destructive behavior • Keep instructions and explanations brief • Provide finger foods and frequent snacks • Monitor intake and weight • Assess, and avoid stimuli that appear to cause increase in characteristic behaviors
Hypochondriacal behavior	Excessive interest in illness • Fear and complaints of disease • Discomfort in dealing with daily stressors	Evaluate physical complaints • Listen to but do not dwell on statements regarding illness • Assist patient to identify ways of dealing with conflict
Manic behavior	Psychomotor overactivity • Elation • Delusions of grandeur • Hypersexual • Bizarre clothing or makeup • Loud voice • Shopping	See *Hyperactive behavior*
Manipulative behavior	Exploitation (use or misuse) of others to have personal needs or desires met	Collaborate with staff to identify manipulative behaviors, and set limits • Inform patient of identified behaviors and limits • Refuse to be influenced by favors from the patient

(continued on the following page)

CHARACTERISTICS AND MANAGEMENT OF INDIVIDUALS WITH MALADAPTIVE BEHAVIOR (continued)

Behavior	*Characteristics*	*Management*
Manipulative behavior (continued)		• Help patient identify why manipulation is used • Assist in identification of direct and acceptable means of having needs met • Reinforce attempts to alter own behavior
Obsessive-compulsive behavior	Obsessions are persistent ideas or thoughts. Compulsions are repetitive and intentional stereotyped behavior (rituals) in response to an obsessive impulsive, thought	Initiate conversation or introduce stimuli to distract patient when ritual begins • Negotiate progressively less frequent times for performance of rituals • Do not physically interfere with rituals
Passive aggressive behavior	Procrastination • Sulkiness • Slowness at work • Claims of having forgotten obligations	Identify underlying feelings and needs • Encourage responsible behavior • Encourage to express needs directly

	• Masochism • Constant criticism and demeaning of those in authority • Unaware of own underlying anger	
Phobic behavior	Irrational fear of an object, activity, or situation • Compelling desire to avoid feared stimulus	Desensitization • Reciprocal inhibition
Suicidal behavior	Anger • Withdrawal • Depression • Suicidal threats or attempts • Expression of uselessness • Giving away cherished possessions	Provide safe environment • Always take overt or covert suicide threats or attempts seriously • Observe closely, especially when in bathroom • Encourage expression of feelings • Assign tasks to increase feelings of usefulness • Provide full schedule of activities • Show acceptance, respect, and appreciation • Do not argue with patient, but remind him or her that there are alternatives to suicide
Suspiciousness	Lack of self-trust and of trust of others • Uses projection as defense mechanism	Begin with one-on-one interactions and gradually expand to include groups • Allow expression of feelings without rebuttal • Be precisely honest, and explain procedures and treatments

(continued on the following page)

CHARACTERISTICS AND MANAGEMENT OF INDIVIDUALS WITH MALADAPTIVE BEHAVIOR (continued)

Behavior	*Characteristics*	*Management*
Suspiciousness (continued)		• Avoid any action that patient is likely to misinterpret (such as whispering or mixing medications with food) • Allow patient to set bounds of physical closeness • Provide noncompetitive activities in which he or she is likely to experience success, and give positive reinforcement
Withdrawn behavior	Avoids interaction and relationships with others • Daydreams • Stares into space • Diminished capacity to tolerate feelings that occur in relationships	Avoid withdrawing from patient • Attempt to interact with patient, but do not demand a response • Attempt to identify and limit stimuli that increase withdrawal • Protect from intrusive individuals • Attempt to involve patient in activities in which he or she will experience success and receive positive feedback • Monitor intake and weight

CHARACTERISTICS AND MANAGEMENT OF FREQUENTLY ENCOUNTERED SITUATIONS AND DISORDERS

Situation or Disorder	*Characteristics*	*Management*
Alcohol withdrawal (also known as *Delirium Tremens* or DTs)	Restlessness • Irritability • Confusion • Tremulousness • Insomnia • Possible convulsions • Dilated pupils • Fever • Tachycardia • Profuse sweating	Protect patient and those around him or her (be alert for sudden responses to hallucinations) • Keep room well lighted and quiet to reduce hallucinations • Monitor vital signs, cardiopulmonary and liver function (be alert for fever and shock)
Crisis situation	Anxiety • Short attention span • Decreased awareness of environment • Impulsive • Unproductive • Obsessive preoccupation with situation	Support right to have whatever feelings are expressed • Assist in resolving immediate problem by exploring methods of dealing with stress and reinforcing strengths (do not make decisions *for* patient unless he or she is suicidal or homicidal) • Provide anticipatory guidance to avoid future crises

(continued on the following page)

CHARACTERISTICS AND MANAGEMENT OF FREQUENTLY ENCOUNTERED SITUATIONS AND DISORDERS (continued)

Situation or Disorder	*Characteristics*	*Management*
Family violence (battering)	Delay between injury and seeking attention • Hesitancy to provide information regarding injury • Inconsistent or unlikely report of how injury occurred • Minimization of injury • History or signs of other injury • Repeated reporting of "vague" or nonspecific symptoms between battering episodes • May avoid socialization	Provide privacy for interview • Explain all planned actions to family (if report will be filed, family is told) • Avoid judgmental attitude or statements of blame • If child is victim, he or she should be interviewed alone by a person trained to interview children. (be aware that abuser may retaliate if victim is interviewed alone) • Make appropriate referrals and file reports • Long-term intervention involves having family identify needed changes and goals as well as appropriate follow-up

Post-traumatic stress syndrome	History of traumatic event such as rape, assault, combat, or disaster • Nightmares • Flashbacks • Obsessive ruminations • Withdrawal • Avoidance of stimuli associated with the trauma • Hyperalertness • Insomnia • Memory impairment • Difficulty concentrating • Stress intolerance • Explosiveness • Substance abuse	Careful history taking, as patient frequently does not volunteer information related to traumatic event • Encourage ventilation of feelings • See *Crisis situation*

PSYCHOTHERAPEUTIC TREATMENT MODALITIES

Aversion therapy: An undesired behavior (such as drinking alcohol) is presented to the patient at the same time as an unpleasant or painful stimulus.

Behavior modification: Use of various techniques such as positive reinforcement, aversive therapy, and modeling to change maladaptive behaviors.

Bibliotherapy: Psychotherapeutic technique in which the patient reads self-help books or writes a daily journal.

Brief therapy: A method of short-term therapy (8–10 sessions) designed to resolve a special problem or symptom. Problem solving and providing information are methods used.

Cognitive therapy (rational–emotive behavioral therapy): A therapy method which helps the patient understand erroneous thoughts that cause nonproductive behavior. The counselor educates the patient regarding healthy thoughts to change pessimistic, self-degrading, or other negative thoughts.

Covert rehearsal: Therapy in which the patient imagines himself or herself calmly engaged in an activity that usually causes him or her to experience anxiety.

Crisis intervention: A therapy method used with victims of a sudden stressful event. Interventions focus on situational support, directive information, and improving functioning in the client's life tasks and roles.

Desensitization: Patient is gradually exposed to real or imagined anxiety-producing stimuli until it no longer produces anxiety.

Electroconvulsive therapy: Use of electric shock to produce convulsions. May be especially useful in people with acute depression and psychosis not responsive to medications.

Family therapy: Treatment of the members of a family together.

Group therapy: Simultaneous psychotherapy involving two or more patients and one or more psychotherapists for the purpose of treating each patient's mental illness.

Insight-oriented therapy: The therapist assists the patient to understand the underlying motivation or subconscious drives for behavior.

Life review therapy: Therapy that helps the patient improve his or her self-image through development of an extensive autobiography.

Milieu therapy: Control of the patient's environment to provide interpersonal contacts that will develop trust, assurance, and personal autonomy.

Modeling: Therapy in which patient is rewarded for socially acceptable behavior that is acquired by following another's example.

Play therapy: Therapy in which the patient discharges emotionally repressed or unconscious experiences through play, toys, or dolls. Usually conducted with children.

Psychoeducation: Therapy that explores the patient's and family's reactions to mental illness and educates the family regarding the patient's disorder and its treatment.

Psychopharmacology: Use of drugs to alter behavior and emotional states.

Psychotherapy: Treatment of disorders by verbal rather than pharmacological or surgical methods.

Reality therapy: Therapy in which the therapist largely uses goal setting and plan formation for taking productive action to solve problems.

Reciprocal inhibition: Anxiety-producing stimulus is paired with anxiety-suppressing stimulus until stimuli no longer produces anxiety.

Relaxation therapy: Use of progressive muscular relaxation and deep-breathing exercises to reduce anxiety.

MONITORING FOR REACTIONS TO PSYCHOTROPIC MEDICATIONS

The nurse must monitor for and report reactions to psychotropic drugs. The table below lists selected reactions to specific types of psychotropic drugs.

Reaction—Possible Causes	***Characteristics***
Alpha blockade—TCAs	Sedation, orthostatic hypotension
Anticholinergic phenomena—TCAs	Dry mouth, constipation, blurred vision
Cardiac arrhythmias—TCAs	Irregular heart rhythm
Extrapyramidal effects (EPS)—neuroleptics (antipsychotics), high doses of TCAs	Four syndromes—the first three may occur soon after initiation of neuroleptic therapy and are treatable; the fourth may not appear until after years of neuroleptic use and may be irreversible 1. Dystonia—hypertonicity of muscles of neck and back, difficulty swallowing, spasms of jaw muscles 2. Akathisia—motor restlessness, anxiety 3. Parkinsonian syndrome—unchanging facial expression, drooling, tremors, disturbances in posture and gait, rigidity, akinesia (decreased motor activity) 4. Tardive dyskinesia—involuntary movements of the tongue, face, mouth, and jaw

Reaction—Possible Causes	***Characteristics***
Hypertensive crisis (***potentially life threatening***)—MAOIs with coadministration of sympathomimetics such as pseudoephedrine and phenylpropanolamine or meperidine, dextromethorphan, or tyramine-containing foods	Occipital headache, nausea, palpitations, tachycardia/bradycardia, chest pain
Hypotension—TCAs, neuroleptics	Blood pressure drops when patient changes positions; dizziness and transient loss of consciousness may occur (***Note: use particular caution with the elderly or when there is preexisting impairment of the cerebrovascular circulation.***)
Seizures (increased risk for) occur with use of SSRIs, TCAs, bupropion, neuroleptics	
Neuroleptic malignant syndrome (NMS) (***potentially fatal***)—antipsychotics such as chlorpromazine or haloperidol, withdrawal of drugs that increase CNS dopamine levels; i.e., levodopa or carbidopa	Hyperthermia, catatonic rigidity, altered mental status, profuse sweating; occasionally rhabdomyolysis, renal failure, seizures, death

(continued on the following page)

Reaction—Possible Causes	*Characteristics*
Sedation—TCAs, neuroleptics, especially piperidine phenothiazines	Decreased mental alertness, drowsiness
Serotonin syndrome (SS)—SSRIs with risk increased by co-use of sympathomimetics such as pseudoephedrine	Mental status changes, seizures, myoclonus, blood dyscrasias
SSRI toxicity—SSRIs with risk increased with couse of TCAs	Seizures, nausea, vomiting, excessive agitation, restlessness
Tardive dyskinesia (TD)—phenothiazines such as prochlorperazine or promethazine	Repeated tongue rolling, pill-rolling movements of the hands, thrusting, ticklike movements of the face; movements are not present during sleep

For abbreviations, refer to abbreviations in *Medical-Surgical Fast Facts.*

Note: All patients on psychotropics should be monitored for significantly increased temperature, body and facial rigidity, stiff movements, and involuntary movements including tremor.

NOTES

NOTES

NOTES

NOTES

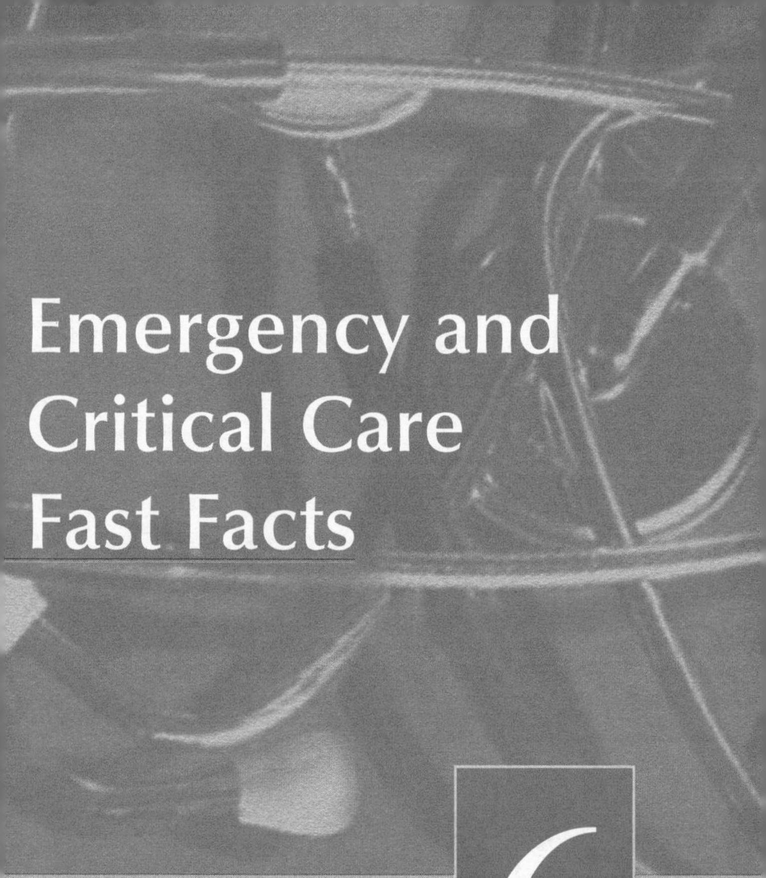

Emergency and Critical Care Fast Facts

Section 6

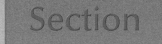

The purpose of triage is to classify severity of illness or injury and determine priority needs for efficient use of health care providers and resources. Most emergency care systems use three categories of classification:

1. *Emergent*: Conditions that are life threatening and require immediate attention. *Examples*: Cardiopulmonary arrest, pulmonary edema, chest pain of cardiac origin, and multisystem trauma. These patients frequently arrive by ambulance. **Treatment must be immediate.**
2. *Urgent*: Conditions that are significant medical problems and require treatment as soon as possible. Vital signs are stable. *Examples*: fever, simple lacerations, uncomplicated extremity fractures, significant pain, and chronic illnesses such as cancer or sickle cell disease.
   Treatment may be delayed for several hours if necessary.
3. *Nonurgent*: Minor illnesses or injuries such as rashes, sore throat, or chronic low back pain. **Treatment can be delayed indefinitely.**

Emergency

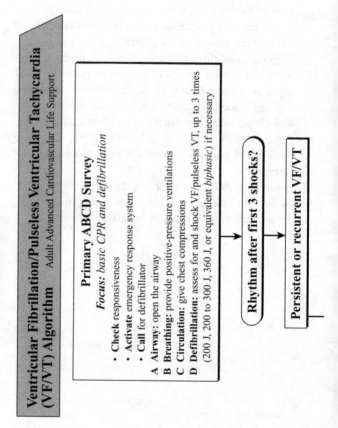

Ventricular Fibrillation/Pulseless Ventricular Tachycardia (VF/VT) Algorithm

Adult Advanced Cardiovascular Life Support

Primary ABCD Survey

***Focus:** basic CPR and defibrillation*

- **Check** responsiveness
- **Activate** emergency response system
- **Call** for defibrillator

A **Airway:** open the airway
B **Breathing:** provide positive-pressure ventilations
C **Circulation:** give chest compressions
D **Defibrillation:** assess for and shock VF/pulseless VT, up to 3 times (200 J, 200 to 300 J, 360 J, or equivalent *biphasic*) if necessary

↓

Rhythm after first 3 shocks?

↓

Persistent or recurrent VF/VT

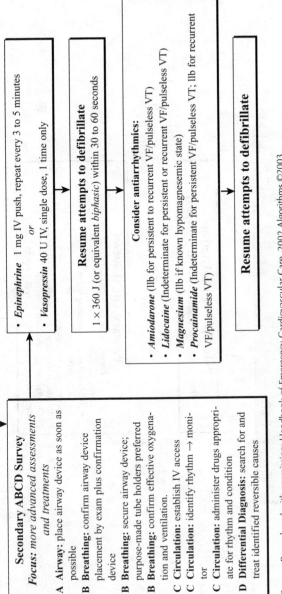

Secondary ABCD Survey
Focus: *more advanced assessments and treatments*

- **A Airway:** place airway device as soon as possible
- **B Breathing:** confirm airway device placement by exam plus confirmation device
- **B Breathing:** secure airway device; purpose-made tube holders preferred
- **B Breathing:** confirm effective oxygenation and ventilation.
- **C Circulation:** establish IV access
- **C Circulation:** identify rhythm → monitor
- **C Circulation:** administer drugs appropriate for rhythm and condition
- **D Differential Diagnosis:** search for and treat identified reversible causes

→

- ***Epinephrine*** 1 mg IV push, repeat every 3 to 5 minutes

or

- ***Vasopressin*** 40 U IV, single dose, 1 time only

↓

Resume attempts to defibrillate
1 × 360 J (or equivalent *biphasic*) within 30 to 60 seconds

↓

Consider antiarrhythmics:

- ***Amiodarone*** (llb for persistent to recurrent VF/pulseless VT)
- ***Lidocaine*** (Indeterminate for persistent or recurrent VF/pulseless VT)
- ***Magnesium*** (llb if known hypomagnesemic state)
- ***Procainamide*** (Indeterminate for persistent VF/pulseless VT; llb for recurrent VF/pulseless VT)

↓

Resume attempts to defibrillate

Source: Reproduced with permission: Handbook of Emergency Cardiovascular Care, 2002 Algorithms ©2003, Copyright American Heart Association

Pulseless Electrical Activity Algorithm

Adult Advanced Cardiovascular Life Support

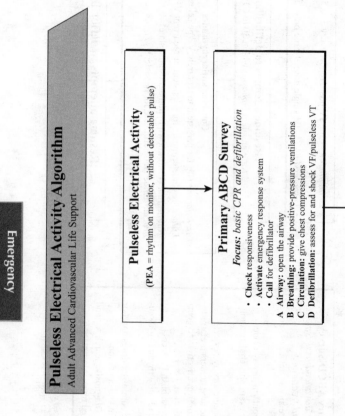

Pulseless Electrical Activity

(**PEA** = rhythm on monitor, without detectable pulse)

↓

Primary ABCD Survey

Focus: *basic CPR and defibrillation*

- **Check** responsiveness
- **Activate** emergency response system
- **Call** for defibrillator

A **Airway:** open the airway
B **Breathing:** provide positive-pressure ventilations
C **Circulation:** give chest compressions
D **Defibrillation:** assess for and shock VF/pulseless VT

↓

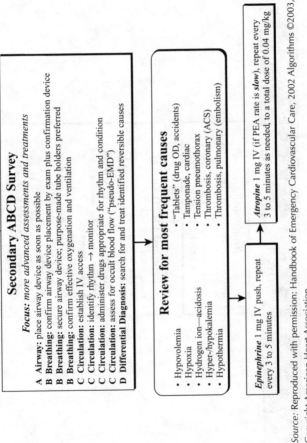

Secondary ABCD Survey

***Focus:** more advanced assessments and treatments*

- A **Airway:** place airway device as soon as possible
- B **Breathing:** confirm airway device placement by exam plus confirmation device
- B **Breathing:** secure airway device; purpose-made tube holders preferred
- B **Breathing:** confirm effective oxygenation and ventilation
- C **Circulation:** establish IV access
- C **Circulation:** identify rhythm → monitor
- C **Circulation:** administer drugs appropriate for rhythm and condition
- C **Circulation:** assess for occult blood flow ("pseudo-EMD")
- D **Differential Diagnosis:** search for and treat identified reversible causes

↓

Review for most frequent causes

- Hypovolemia
- Hypoxia
- Hydrogen ion—acidosis
- Hyper-/hypokalemia
- Hypothermia
- "Tablets" (drug OD, accidents)
- Tamponade, cardiac
- Tension pneumothorax
- Thrombosis, coronary (ACS)
- Thrombosis, pulmonary (embolism)

↓

Epinephrine 1 mg IV push, repeat every 3 to 5 minutes

→ ***Atropine*** 1 mg IV (if PEA rate is ***slow***), repeat every 3 to 5 minutes as needed, to a total dose of 0.04 mg/kg

Bradycardia Algorithm (Patient Not in Cardiac Arrest)

Adult Advanced Cardiovascular Life Support

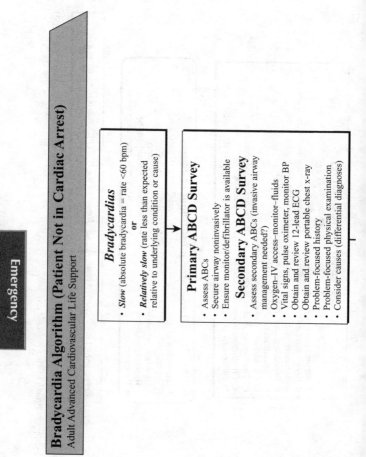

Bradycardias

- ***Slow*** (absolute bradycardia = rate <60 bpm)

or

- ***Relatively slow*** (rate less than expected relative to underlying condition or cause)

↓

Primary ABCD Survey

- Assess ABCs
- Secure airway noninvasively
- Ensure monitor/defibrillator is available

Secondary ABCD Survey

- Assess secondary ABCs (invasive airway management needed?)
- Oxygen–IV access–monitor–fluids
- Vital signs, pulse oximeter, monitor BP
- Obtain and review 12-lead ECG
- Obtain and review portable chest x-ray
- Problem-focused history
- Problem-focused physical examination
- Consider causes (differential diagnoses)

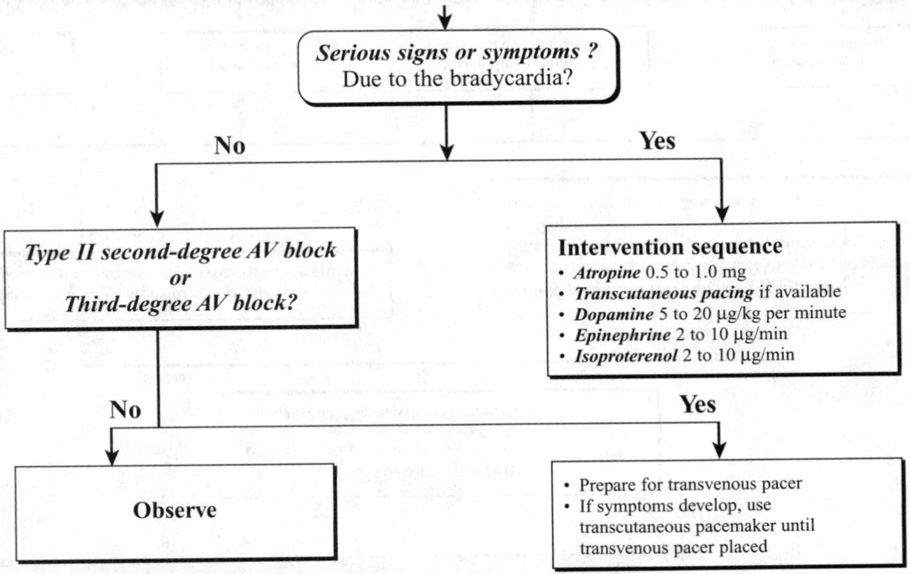

Source: Reproduced with permission: Handbook of Emergency Cardiovascular Care, 2002 Algorithms ©2003, Copyright American Heart Association

The Tachycardias: Overview Algorithm

Adult Advanced Cardiovascular Life Support

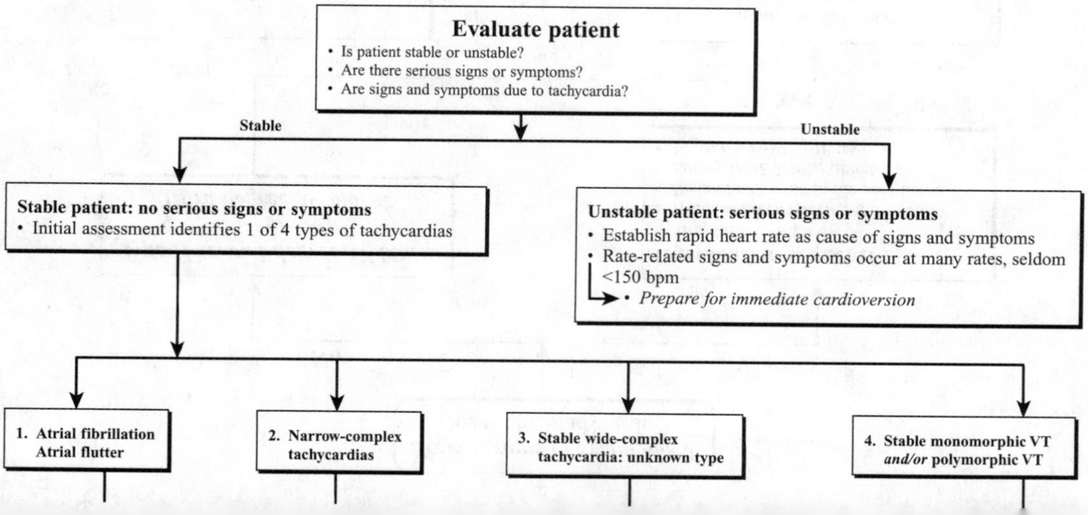
Evaluate patient
• Is patient stable or unstable?
• Are there serious signs or symptoms?
• Are signs and symptoms due to tachycardia?
Stable
Unstable
Stable patient: no serious signs or symptoms
• Initial assessment identifies 1 of 4 types of tachycardias
Unstable patient: serious signs or symptoms
• Establish rapid heart rate as cause of signs and symptoms
• Rate-related signs and symptoms occur at many rates, seldom <150 bpm
• Prepare for immediate cardioversion
1. Atrial fibrillation Atrial flutter
2. Narrow-complex tachycardias
3. Stable wide-complex tachycardia: unknown type
4. Stable monomorphic VT and/or polymorphic VT

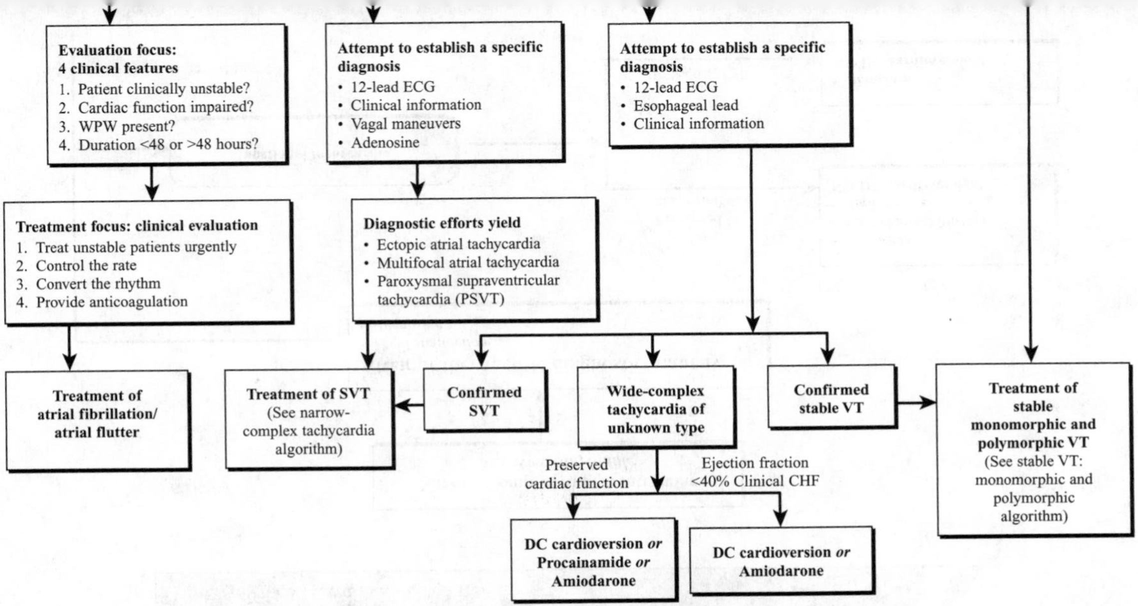
Evaluation focus:
4 clinical features
1. Patient clinically unstable?
2. Cardiac function impaired?
3. WPW present?
4. Duration <48 or >48 hours?
Attempt to establish a specific diagnosis
• 12-lead ECG
• Clinical information
• Vagal maneuvers
• Adenosine
Attempt to establish a specific diagnosis
• 12-lead ECG
• Esophageal lead
• Clinical information
Treatment focus: clinical evaluation
1. Treat unstable patients urgently
2. Control the rate
3. Convert the rhythm
4. Provide anticoagulation
Diagnostic efforts yield
• Ectopic atrial tachycardia
• Multifocal atrial tachycardia
• Paroxysmal supraventricular tachycardia (PSVT)
Treatment of atrial fibrillation/ atrial flutter
Treatment of SVT (See narrow-complex tachycardia algorithm)
Confirmed SVT
Wide-complex tachycardia of unknown type
Confirmed stable VT
Treatment of stable monomorphic and polymorphic VT (See stable VT: monomorphic and polymorphic algorithm)
Preserved cardiac function
Ejection fraction <40% Clinical CHF
DC cardioversion or Procainamide or Amiodarone
DC cardioversion or Amiodarone

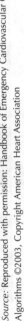

Source: Reproduced with permission: Handbook of Emergency Cardiovascular Care, 2002 Algorithms ©2003, Copyright American Heart Association

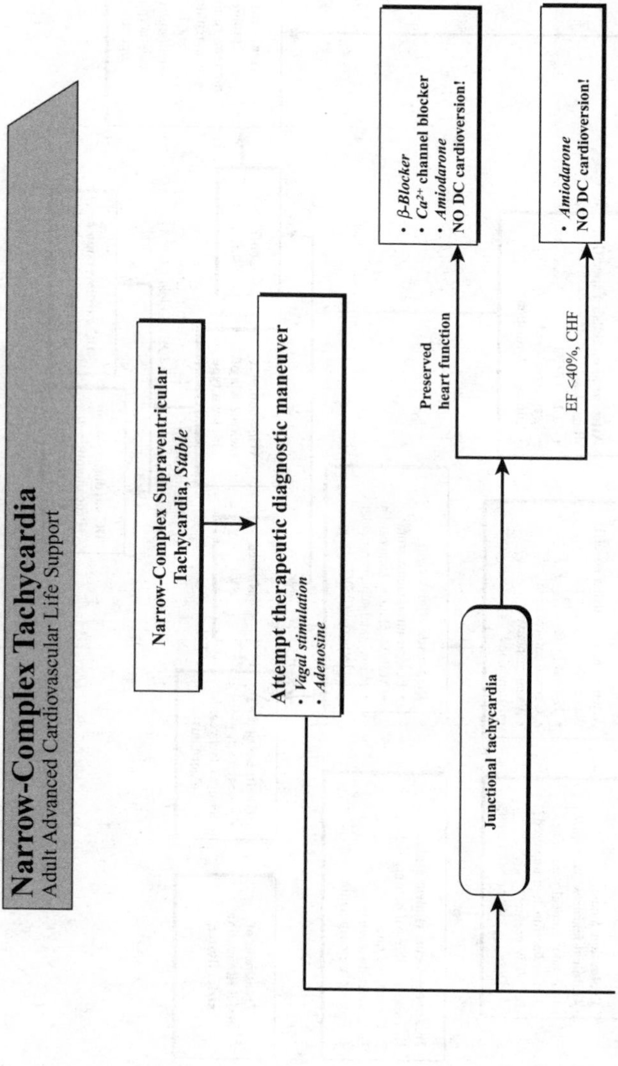

Narrow-Complex Tachycardia
Adult Advanced Cardiovascular Life Support
Narrow-Complex Supraventricular Tachycardia, *Stable*
Attempt therapeutic diagnostic maneuver
• *Vagal stimulation*
• *Adenosine*
Junctional tachycardia
Preserved heart function
• *β-Blocker*
• *Ca²⁺ channel blocker*
• *Amiodarone*
NO DC cardioversion!
EF <40%, CHF
• *Amiodarone*
NO DC cardioversion!

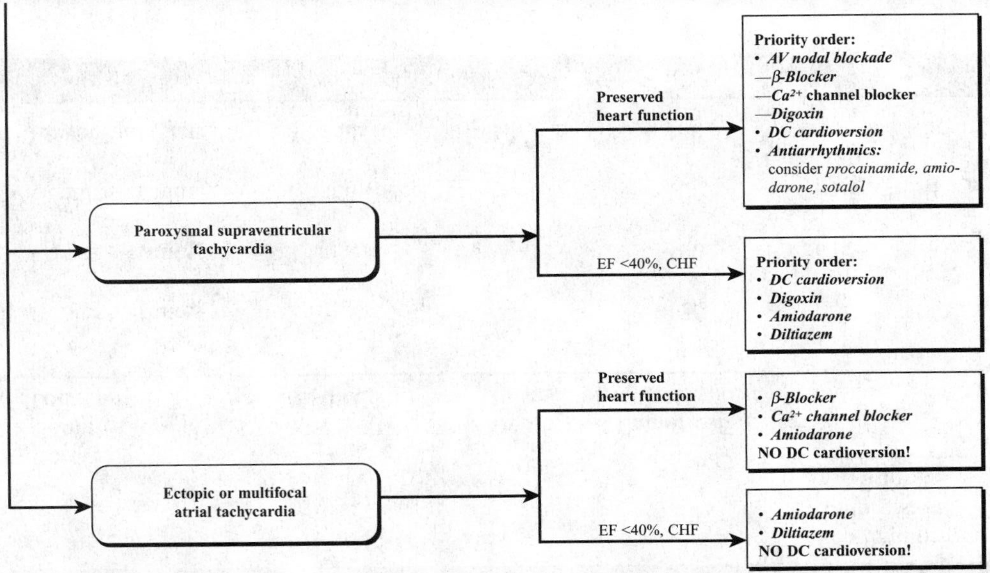

Source: Reproduced with permission: Handbook of Emergency Cardiovascular Care, 2002 Algorithms ©2003, Copyright American Heart Association

Table 6–1. CPR GUIDELINES

Age	Cardiac Compression Location	Method	Depth, Inches	Compression, Rate/Min	Ventilation: Compression Ratio		Number of Ventilation Cycles/Min	
					1 Man	2 Men	1 Man	2 Men
Neonate	Center sternum	2 fingers	$^1/_2$–1	120				
Infant <1 yr	Center sternum	2 fingers	$^1/_2$–1	100	1 : 5	1 : 5	20	20
Child 1–8 yr	Center sternum	1 hand (heel)	1–1 $^1/_2$	100	1 : 5	1 : 5	20	20
Adult	Lower half, sternum	2 hands	1 $^1/_2$–2	100	2 : 15*	2 : 15	4	4

*Adults who are intubated may receive ventilation: compression ratio of 1:5.

MULTIPLE-TRAUMA PATIENT IN THE EMERGENCY DEPARTMENT*

PRIMARY SURVEY

1. *Airway maintenance with cervical spine immobilization*: Use jaw thrust, clear secretions, and insert artificial airway as needed.
2. *Breathing*: Intubate if needed. Administer high-flow oxygen.
3. *Circulation with hemorrhage control*: Use pressure as needed, establish two large-bore IVs, and draw blood for cross-match.
4. *Neurologic status*: Assess and document LOC, assess pupil reaction to light, and assess for head and neck injuries.
5. *Injuries*: Expose patient to completely assess for injuries.
6. *Assess and document* VS (*and* ECG *if indicated*).
7. *Assign trauma score*: See Table 6–4.

As life-threatening problems are identified, each must be dealt with immediately.

SECONDARY SURVEY

The secondary survey consists of a history and a complete head-to-toe assessment. The purpose of the survey is to identify problems that may not have been identified as life threatening. **If, at any time during the secondary survey, the patient's condition worsens, return to the steps in the primary survey.**

1. Take history and complete head-to-toe assessment.
2. Splint fractures.
3. Insert urinary catheter unless there is gross blood at meatus.
4. Assess urinary output and check urine for blood.

**References*: Kitt, S, and Kaiser, I: Emergency Nursing Physiologic and Clinical Perspectives. WB Saunders, Philadelphia, 1990, and American College of Surgeons Committee on Trauma, October 1979.

5. Insert NG tube (OG if facial fractures are involved).
6. Obtain CXR.
7. Administer tetanus prophylaxis (see *Tetanus Prophylaxis*) and antibiotics (question regarding allergies first) if indicated.
8. Continue to monitor components under primary survey as well as adequacy of urine output, and document findings.

Certain mechanisms of trauma result in predictable injuries; therefore, the history of the event may reveal information to enable rapid diagnosis and treatment.

Table 6–2. PREDICTABLE INJURIES IN THE TRAUMA PATIENT

Trauma	Predictable Injuries
Pedestrian hit by car	
Child	Head, chest, abd injuries
Adult	Fractures of femur, tibia, and fibula on side of impact
Pedestrian hit by large vehicle or dragged under vehicle	Pelvic fractures
Front seat occupant (lap and shoulder restraint worn)	Head, face, chest, ribs, aorta, pelvis, and lower abdomen
Front seat occupant (lap restraint only)	Cervical or lumbar spine, laryngeal fracture, head, face, chest, ribs, aorta, pelvis, and lower abdomen
Unrestrained driver	Head, chest, abd, pelvis
Front seat passenger (unrestrained, head-on collision)	Fractures of femurs and/or patellas, posterior dislocation of acetabulum

Table 6–2. PREDICTABLE INJURIES IN THE TRAUMA PATIENT (continued)

Trauma	Predictable Injuries
Back seat passenger (without head restraints, rear-end collision)	Hyperextension of neck with associated high cervical fractures
Fall injuries with landing on feet	Compression fractures of lumbosacral spine and fractures of calcaneus (heel bone)

Source: Adapted from Trauma Nursing Core Course Provider Manual, ed 2. Emergency Nurses Association, Award Printing Corporation, Chicago, 1986, with permission.

INCREASED INTRACRANIAL PRESSURE

Increased intracranial pressure (ICP) is defined as intracranial pressure above 15 mm Hg. It can result from head injury, brain tumor, hydrocephaly, meningitis, encephalitis, or intracerebral hemorrhage. Increased ICP should be treated as a medical emergency.

MANIFESTATIONS OF INCREASED ICP

- Headache
- Change in level of consciousness
- Irritability
- Increased systolic BP
- Decreased HR (early)
- Increased HR (late)
- Decreased RR
- Hemiparesis
- Loss of oculomotor control
- Photophobia (light sensitivity)
- Vomiting (with subsequent decreased headache)
- Diplopia (double vision)

- Papilledema (optic disk swelling)
- Behavior changes
- Seizures
- Bulging fontanel in infant

MANAGEMENT OF INCREASED ICP

1. Elevate head of bed 15 to 30 degrees. Keep head in neutral alignment. Do not flex or rotate neck.
2. Establish IV access.
3. Insert Foley catheter. (Output may be profound if diuretic is given.)
4. Meds that may be used include osmotic diuretics, sedatives, neuromuscular blocking agents, corticosteroids, and anticonvulsants.
5. Restrict fluids.
6. Closely monitor vital signs and perform neuro checks. Monitor fluids and electrolytes (diuretic administration can predispose the patient to hypovolemic shock).
7. Schedule all procedures (including bathing and especially suctioning) to coincide with periods of sedation.
8. Discourage patient activities that result in use of Valsalva's maneuver.
9. Keep environment as quiet as possible.
10. Ventilator may be used to maintain $PaCO_2$ between 25–35.
11. Ventricular tap may be performed if unresponsive to other measures.
12. ICP monitoring via a fiberoptic catheter may be used to continuously assess changes in ICP.

Table 6–3. GLASGOW COMA SCALE FOR INFANTS AND TODDLERS

Eye opening	Spontaneous	4	
	To sounds and speech	3	
	To Pain	2	
	None	1	
	INFANT		**TODDLER**
Verbal response	Smiles, interacts, follows objects	5	Interacts appropriately
	Cries, is consolable	4	Interacts inappropriately
	Cries, is inconsistently consolable	3	Moans, uses inappropriate words
	Cries, inconsolable	2	Restless, irritable
	No response	1	No response
Best Motor response	Obeys command to move body part	6	
	Localizes pain	5	
	Tries to remove painful stimuli	4	
	Flexes arm in response to pain	3	
	Extends arm in response to pain	2	

NOTE: A score of 7 or less generally indicates coma; a score of 3 indicates deep coma or death.

Source: Adapted from Hahn, YS, et al: Head injuries in children under 36 months of age. Childs Nerv Syst 4:34, 1988, with permission.

Table 6–4. ADULT TRAUMA SCORE

Cardiopulmonary*

Respiratory rate	10–24/min	4	
	24–35/min	3	
	36/min or greater	2	
	1–9/min	1	
	None	0	
Respiratory expansion	Normal	1	
	Retractive	0	
Systolic blood pressure	90 mm Hg or greater	4	
	70–89 mm Hg	3	
	50–69 mm Hg	2	
	0–49 mm Hg	1	
Pulse	None	0	

Neurological† (Glasgow Coma Scale)

Eye opening	Spontaneous	4	
	To Voice	3	
	To Pain	2	
	None	1	
Verbal response	Oriented	5	
	Confused	4	
	Inappropriate speech	3	
	Incomprehensible sounds	2	
	None	1	
Motor response	Obeys command	6	
	Localizes pain	5	
	Withdraws (pain)	4	
	Flexion (pain)	3	
	Extension (pain)	2	
	None	1	
Glasgow Coma Score Total ______			

Capillary refill	Normal	2		**Total Glasgow Coma Scale Points**	
	Delayed	1		14–15 = 5 11–13 = 4 8–10 = 3 5–7 = 2 3–4 = 1	Conversion = Approximately one third total value
	None	0			

Cardiopulmonary assessment ________ Neurological assessment ________

Total trauma score = Cardiopulmonary + Neurological

*Adapted from Champion, HR, Sacco, WJ, Carnazzo, AJ, et al: Trauma score. Crit Care Med 9(9):672–676, 1981.

†Adapted from Teasdale, G, and Jennett, B: Lancet II, 1974, p. 81, and Teasdale, G, et al: Acta Neurochirurgia Suppl. 28, 1979, pp 13–16.

Source: Thomas, CL (ed): Taber's Cyclopedic Medical Dictionary, ed 18. FA Davis, Philadelphia, 1997, p 1989, with permission.

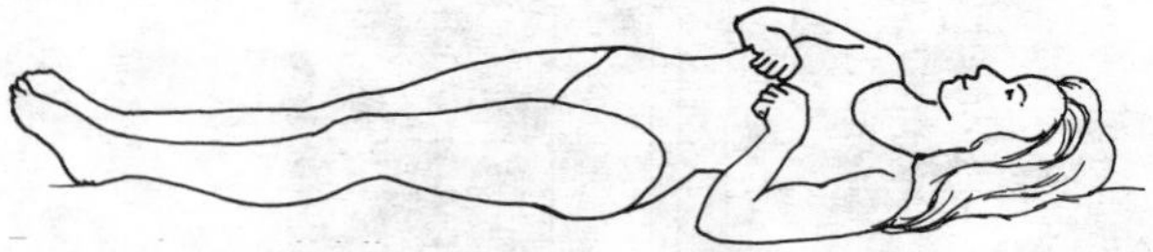

Decorticate rigidity

Decorticate rigidity: Flexion of the arm, wrist, and fingers, with adduction of upper extremities. Extension, internal rotation, and vigorous plantar flexion of lower extremities indicate lesion in cerebral hemisphere, basal ganglia, and/or diencephalon or metabolic depression of brain function.

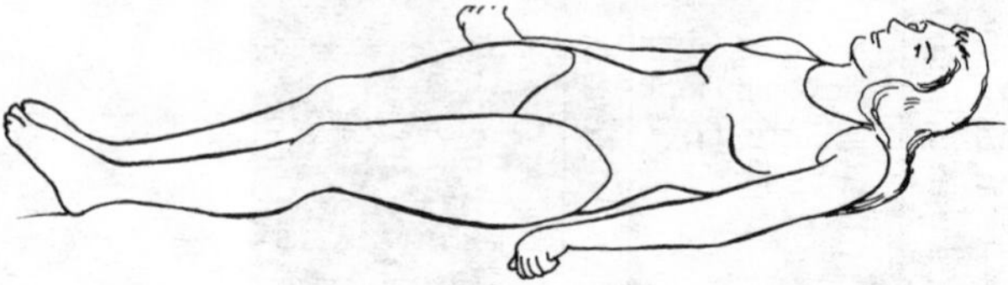

Decerebrate rigidity

Decerebrate rigidity: Arms are stiffly extended, adducted, and hyperpronated. Legs and feet are stiffly extended with feet plantar flexed. Teeth may be clenched (may be seen with opisthotonos). Indicates brain stem pathology and poor prognosis.

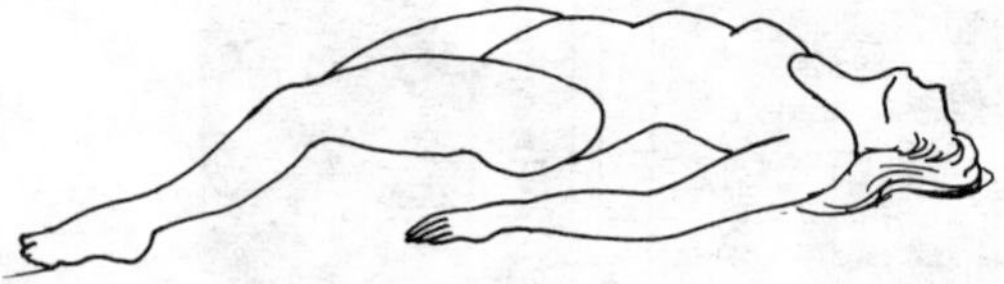

Opisthotonos

Opisthotonos: Rigid hyperextension of the spine. The head and heels are forced backward and the trunk is pushed forward. Seen in meningitis, seizures, tetanus, and strychnine poisoning.

Figure 6–1. Rigid postural responses to neurologic conditions.

EMERGENCY CARE OF PATIENT DURING SEIZURE ACTIVITY

1. If the patient is standing or sitting when seizure begins, ease him or her to the floor to prevent fall.
2. Move furniture and other objects on which the patient may injure himself or herself during uncontrolled movements.
3. Do not put objects (e.g., tongue blades, depressors) into the patient's mouth.
4. After the seizure, turn the patient to the side and ascertain patency of airway.
5. Allow the patient to rest or sleep without disturbance.

DOCUMENTATION

Facts that should be recorded when a seizure occurs include:

1. Documentation and description of aura if reported by the patient
2. Circumstances in which the seizure activity occurred
3. Time of the onset of seizure activity
4. Muscle groups involved (and whether unilateral or bilateral)
5. Total length of seizure activity
6. Vital signs
7. Behavior after seizure
8. Neurologic status in postictal period (weakness or inactivity of a body part, sleep, amnesia, confusion, or headache)
9. Documentation and assessment of any injury and documentation that injury has been reported to the proper person

Table 6–5. SHOCK

Type	Pathology	Causes	Signs and Symptoms	Treatment
Anaphylactic shock	Dilation of blood vessels, fluid shifts, edema, and spasms of respiratory tract.	Allergic reaction	Respiratory distress Hypotension Edema Rash Pale, cool skin Convulsions possible	O_2 Epinephrine Corticosteroids Antihistamine IV fluids Aminophylline
Cardiogenic shock	Failure to maintain blood supply to circulatory system and tissues because of inadequate cardiac output.	Acute left or right ventricular failure Acute mitral regurgitation Acute ventricular septal defect Acute pericardial tamponade Acute pulmonary embolism Acute myocardial infarction	Increased pulse rate Weak pulses Cardiac dysrhythmias Prolonged capillary fill time Cool, clammy skin Cyanosis Altered mental ability	IV fluids O_2 Dopamine Norepinephrine Nitroprusside if BP adequate Dobutamine

Hypovolemic shock	Decrease in intravascular volume relative to vascular capacity. Results from blood volume deficit of at least 25% and larger interstitial fluid deficit.	Hemorrhage Vomiting Diarrhea Any excess loss of body fluids	Hypotension Decreased pulse pressure Tachycardia Rapid respiratory rate Pale, cool skin Anxiety	Control bleeding IV fluids (Replace type F&E lost if known.) O_2 Elevate legs Volume expanders
Neurogenic shock	Increase in vascular capacity and subsequent decrease in blood volume:space ratio resulting from profound vasodilation.	Anesthesia Spinal cord injury	Hypotension Bradycardia Bounding pulse Pale, warm, and dry skin	Supine position O_2 IV fluids Possibly vasopressors
Septic shock	Circulatory failure and impaired cell metabolism associated with septicemia. Divided into "early warm" (increased cardiac output) and "later cold" (decreased cardiac output).	Endotoxins released most commonly by gram-negative organism	Elevated temperature Flushed, warm skin Vasodilation (early) Vasoconstriction (late) Decreased WBC at first Normal urinary output (early) Decreased urinary output (late)	O_2 IV fluids Culture, e.g., blood, urine, sputum, wounds. Antibiotics Possibly vasopressors

FRACTURES

SIGNS AND SYMPTOMS

- Obvious deformity (in alignment, contour, or length)
- Local and/or point tenderness that increases in severity until splinting
- Localized ecchymosis
- Edema
- Crepitus (grating sound) on palpation
- False movement (unnatural movement at fracture site)
- Loss of function related to pain

EMERGENCY MANAGEMENT

- Assess and document:
  - Alignment
  - Warmth
  - Tenderness
  - Sensation
  - Motion
  - Circulatory status distal to injury
  - Intactness of skin
- Cover open fractures with a sterile dressing.
- Remove rings from fingers immediately if upper extremity is involved (progressive swelling may make it impossible to remove rings without cutting).
- Splint injured extremity.
  Never attempt to force bone or tissue back into wound.
- Elevate injured extremity and apply ice (do not apply ice directly to skin).
- Assess for and document frequently the five Ps:
  - Pain
  - Pulselessness
  - Pallor
  - Paralysis
  - Paresthesia (e.g., sensation of numbness, burning, tingling)

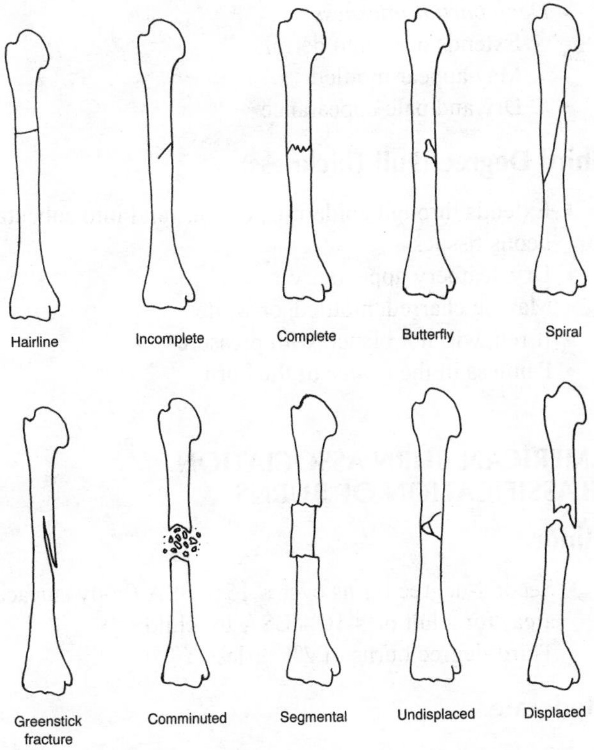

Figure 6–2. Types of fractures.

BURNS

CLASSIFICATION CATEGORIES

First Degree

- Involves epidermis only
- Erythematous and painful skin
- Looks like sunburn

Second Degree (Partial Thickness)

- *Superficial partial thickness*
  Extends beyond epidermis superficially into dermis
  Red and weepy appearance
  Very painful
  Formation of blisters

- *Deep partial thickness*
  Extends deep into dermis
  May appear mottled
  Dry and pale appearance

Third Degree (Full Thickness)

- Extends through epidermis, dermis, and into subcutaneous tissues
- Dry, leathery appearance
- May be charred, mottled, or white
- If red, will not blanch with pressure
- Painless in the *center* of the burn

AMERICAN BURN ASSOCIATION CLASSIFICATION OF BURNS

Minor

- Second-degree burns over <15% BSA (body surface area) for adult or <10% BSA for child
- Third-degree burns of 2% or less

Moderate

- Second-degree burns over 15 to 25% BSA for adult or 10 to 20% BSA for child
- Third-degree burns of 2% to 5% BSA
- Burns not involving eyes, ears, face, hands, feet, or perineum

Major

- Second-degree burns >25% BSA for adult or >20% BSA for child
- Third-degree burns ≥10% BSA
- All burns of hands, face, eyes, ears, feet, or perineum
- All inhalation injuries
- Electric burns
- All burns with associated complications of fractures or other trauma
- All high-risk patients (with such conditions as diabetes, COPD, or heart disease)

EMERGENCY CARE OF BURN INJURIES

- First, evaluate respiratory system for distress or smoke inhalation (any abnormal respiratory findings in rate, effort, noise, or observations of smoky odor of breath or soot in nose or mouth).
- Assess cardiovascular status. (Look for symptoms of shock.)
- Assess percentage and depth of burns, as well as presence of other injuries.
- Flush chemical contact areas with sterile water; 20 to 30 minutes of flushing may be needed to remove chemical. Fifteen to 20 minutes of normal saline irrigation is preferable for chemical burns to eyes. Contact lens must be removed prior to eye irrigation.
- Insert IV line(s) for major and some moderate burns. (Establish more than one large-bore IV site if possible.) Attempt to insert IV(s) in unburned area(s).
- Weigh patient to establish baseline and assist in determination of fluid needs.
- Fluid resuscitation with Ringer's lactate or Hartmann's solution for the first 24 hours as follows:

  4 mL fluid × kilograms of body weight × percent of burned BSA.

  Administer $^1/_2$ of fluid in first 8 hours.
  Administer $^1/_4$ of fluid in second 8 hours.
  Administer $^1/_4$ of fluid in third 8 hours.

NOTE: Time is calculated from time of injury, not time of admission.

- Administer analgesics as indicated.
- Remove easily separated clothing. Soak any adherent clothing to facilitate removal.

NOTE: Keep patient warm. Removal of clothing may result in rapid and dangerous drop in temperature.

- Cover burn area with sterile dressing.
- Hold NPO until function of GI system is evaluated.
- Insert NG tube for gastric decompression if indicated.
- Insert Foley catheter (to monitor urine output) for severe and some moderate burns.

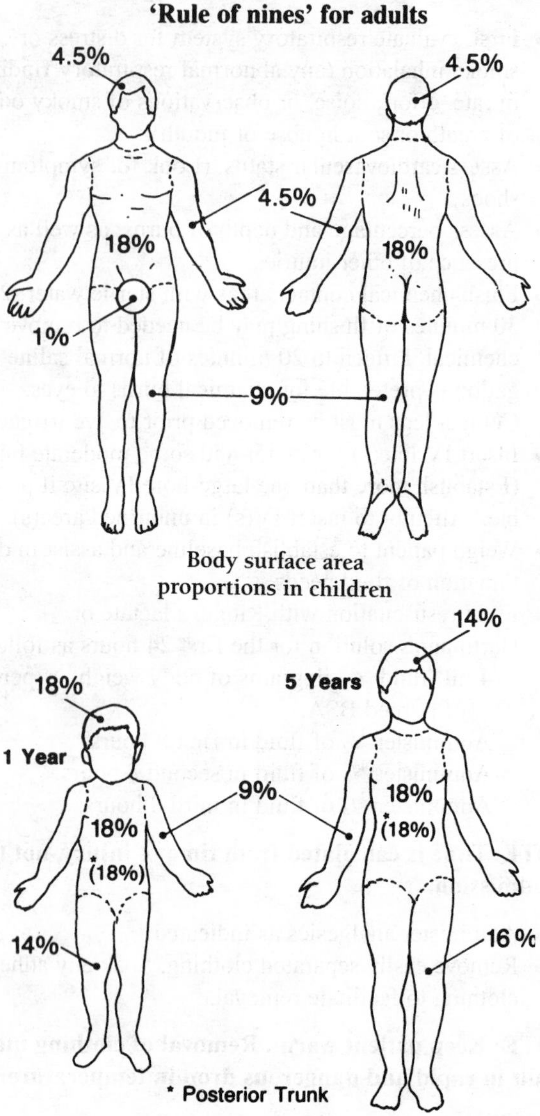

Figure 6–3. Estimation of burned body surface area for adults and children. (From Fulde, GWO [ed]: Emergency Medicine: The Principles of Practice, ed 2. MacLennan & Petty Pty Limited, Sydney, Australia, 1992, p 375, with permission.)

- Assess need for and administer tetanus prophylaxis (see *Tetanus Prophylaxis*).
- Frequently monitor vital signs (be aware that patients who have inhaled smoke are subject to progressive swelling of the airway for several hours following injury), ABGs, and serum electrolytes.
- Monitor urine output and titrate fluids to maintain:
  30 to 50 mL urine/h in the adult
  0.5 to 2 mL urine/kg of body weight/h in the child

TETANUS PROPHYLAXIS

Recommendations for tetanus prophylaxis are based on:

1. The condition of the wound, as related to its susceptibility to tetanus
2. The patient's history of tetanus immunization

Table 6–6. WOUND CLASSIFICATION (TETANUS-PRONE VERSUS NON–TETANUS-PRONE WOUNDS)

Clinical Features	Tetanus-Prone Wounds	Non–Tetanus-Prone Wounds
Age of wound	>6 hours	≤6 hours
Configuration	Stellate wound, avulsion, abrasion	Linear wound
Depth	>1 cm	≤1 cm
Mechanism of injury	Missile, crush, burn, frostbite	Sharp surface (e.g., knife, glass)
Signs of infection	Present	Absent
Devitalized tissue	Present	Absent
Contaminants (e.g., dirt, feces, soil, saliva)	Present	Absent

Source: American College of Surgeons Committee on Trauma Prophylaxis Against Tetanus in Wound Management, April 1984, with permission.

The wound classification table (Table 6–6) and immunization schedule that follow are from the American College of Surgeons Committee on Trauma Prophylaxis Against Tetanus in Wound Management.

IMMUNIZATION SCHEDULE (TETANUS)

Verify a history of tetanus immunization from medical records so that appropriate tetanus prophylaxis can be accomplished.

History of Tetanus Immunization (Doses)	Tetanus-Prone Wounds		Non–Tetanus-Prone Wounds	
	*Td[1]	†TIG	*Td[1]	†TIG[2]
Uncertain	Yes	Yes	Yes	No
0 or 1	Yes	Yes	Yes	No
2	Yes	No[3]	Yes	No
3 or more	No[5]	No	No[4]	No

*Td: Tetanus and diphtheria toxoids adsorbed (for adult use).

†TIG: Tetanus immune globulin (human).

[1]For children younger than 7 years old, diphtheria and tetanus toxoids and pertussis vaccine adsorbed (or diphtheria and tetanus toxoids adsorbed, if pertussis vaccine is contraindicated) is preferable to tetanus toxoid alone. For persons 7 years old and older, Td is preferable to tetanus toxoid alone.

[2]When administering TIG and Td concurrently, use separate syringes and separate sites.

[3]Yes, if wound is more than 24 hours old.

[4]Yes, if more than 10 years since last dose.

[5]Yes, if more than 5 years since last dose. (More frequent boosters are not needed and can accentuate side effects.)

Table 6–7. ACID-BASE DISORDERS (ARTERIAL BLOOD GASES)

ABG Values	Disorder	Causes	Interventions
pH: 7.35–7.45 $PaCO_2$: 35–45 HCO_3: 22–26	None	Normal ABGs	None
pH: <7.35 $PaCO_2$: >45 HCO_3: 22–26 or >26 if kidneys compensating	Respiratory acidosis	CNS depression Asphyxia Hypoventilation	Treat underlying cause IV fluids Bronchodilators Mechanical ventilation O_2
pH:<7.35 $PaCO_2$: 35–45 or <35 if lungs compensating HCO_3: <22	Metabolic acidosis	Tissue hypoxia Diarrhea Renal failure Salicylates Excess alcohol Shock DKA	Correct underlying cause IV sodium bicarb Seizure precautions Monitor and correct electrolyte imbalances

(continued on the following page)

Table 6–7. ACID-BASE DISORDERS (ARTERIAL BLOOD GASES) (continued)

ABG Values	Disorder	Causes	Interventions
pH:>7.45 $PaCO_2$:<35 HCO_3:22–26 or <22 if kidneys compensating	Respiratory alkalosis	Hyperventilation Gram-negative bacteremia CHF Early salicylate intoxication	Treat underlying cause Breathe into paper bag to >$PaCO_2$ Sedatives and calm environment
pH:>7.45 $PaCO_2$:35–45 or >45 if lungs compensating HCO_3:>29	Metabolic alkalosis	Vomiting GI suction Potassium loss Hypercalcemia Excessive alkali Ingestion	Correct cause IV normal saline IV potassium, as indicated Seizure precautions Monitor and correct electrolyte imbalances

NOTE: Acceptable values for PaO_2 range from 60 to 100 mm Hg.
Newborn values:
- pH: 7.29 to 7.45
- $paCO_2$: 27 to 45
- pO_2: 60 to 90
- HCO_3: Similar to adult

POISONING MANAGEMENT

1. Focus initially on the ABCs of life support:
   A = Establish and maintain airway.
   B = Assess RR, and provide oxygen and respiratory support PRN.
   C = Assess HR and BP, establish IV access, and keep warm (shock may occur).
2. Attempt to identify poison.
3. Contact poison control center for directions. **Phone numbers for poison control centers in the U.S. and Canada are listed in the appendices of Taber's Cyclopedic Medical Dictionary.** The phone number for your state should be determined and listed here for quick reference:

   ____

4. *Vomiting* is to be induced *only if the patient is conscious* and *nonconvulsive* and *only if the ingested substance is noncorrosive* (corrosives will further damage esophagus if vomited and may also be aspirated into the lungs). Vomiting may be induced by tickling the back of the throat or administering ipecac syrup in the following dosages:
   Ipecac syrup (PO)
   Child under 1 *year*: 5–10 mL followed by 100 to 200 mL water
   Child 1 *year or older*: 15 mL followed by 100 to 200 mL water
   Adult: 15 mL followed by 100 to 200 mL water
   Dose may be repeated after 20 minutes if patient does not vomit.
5. *Gastric lavage* with NG tube can be used to remove poison but *must not be attempted if corrosive has been ingested* (corrosives severely damage tissue and NG tube may cause perforation). Corrosives include strong acids and alkalies such as drain cleaners, detergents, and many household cleaners as well as strong antiseptics such as bichloride of mercury, phenol, Lysol, cresol compounds, tincture of iodine, and arsenic compounds.
6. Corrosives should be diluted with water and the poison control center contacted immediately. Activated charcoal may be given via NG tube. Destruction

and/or swelling of esophageal and airway tissue is likely with corrosive ingestion. Monitor respiratory status closely.

7. If several hours have passed since poison ingestion, large quantities of IV fluids are given to promote diuresis. Peritoneal dialysis or hemodialysis may be required.
8. Continue ABCs of life support and monitor fluids, electrolytes, and urine output.

CHEMICAL EYE CONTAMINATION

Flush eye with sterile water for 15 to 20 minutes, allowing water to drain away from uncontaminated eye.

INHALED POISONS

Move victim away from toxic fumes and refer to steps 1, 2, and 3 of poisoning management.

Table 6–8. WARNING "SIGNS" OF ILLNESS AND INJURY

Sign	Observation	Associated Diagnoses
Aaron's	Pain or distress occurs near heart or stomach when McBurney's point (about halfway between umbilicus and head of femur) is palpated	Appendicitis
Ballance's	Flank area dullness to percussion that disappears with position change	Peritoneal irritation
Battle's	Bruising behind one or both ears	Head trauma or skull fracture
Beck's triad	Systemic hypotension, muffled heart tones, elevated venous pressure, neck vein distention	Cardiac tamponade

Sign	Observation	Associated Diagnoses
Brudzinski's	With patient in dorsal recumbent position, forward flexion of head results in flexion of hip and knee	Meningeal irritation (meningitis)
Chvostek's	Facial muscle spasm in cheek and around mouth, elicited by light percussion of facial nerve adjacent to ear	Tetany (acute hypocalcemia or hypomagnesemia)
Cullen's	Bluish discoloration around umbilicus	Hemorrhagic pancreatitis or ectopic pregnancy
Cushing's triad	Increased systolic BP, decreased heart rate, widened pulse pressure	Increased intracranial pressure
Grey Turner's	Subcutaneous bruising around flanks and umbilicus	Retroperitoneal hematoma
Hamman's crunch	Crunching sound auscultated over precordium during heartbeat	Alveolar rupture, esophageal tear, tracheal tear, bronchial tear, hemothorax, pneumothorax, or respiratory failure
Homans's	Pain in calf elicited by passive dorsiflexion of foot	Deep vein thrombosis of lower leg
Kehr's	Pain in subscapular area; usually on left side	Splenic rupture, ectopic pregnancy, or GI diseases
Kernig's	With patient supine, flex leg at hip and knee, then attempt to straighten knee joint; pain & resistance noted	Meningeal irritation (meningitis)

(continued on the following page)

Emergency

Table 6–8.	WARNING "SIGNS" OF ILLNESS AND INJURY (continued)	
Sign	**Observation**	**Associated Diagnoses**
McBurney's	Sharp pain when examiner palpates deeply about halfway between umbilicus and head of femur, then suddenly withdraws hand	Appendicitis
Murphy's	Pain when examiner presses fingers under rib cage and patient inhales deeply	Gallbladder inflammation
Psoas	Pain in abdomen when right leg is extended while patient lies on left side, or when legs are flexed while supine	Appendicitis
Raccoon eyes	Bruising and swelling around one or both eyes	Head trauma, basilar skull fracture, or facial fracture
Rovsing's	Pain in RLQ when pressure applied to LLQ	Appendicitis
Trousseau's	Flexion of wrist, adduction of thumb, and extension of one or more fingers after tourniquet applied to arm	Tetany (hypocalcemia or hypomagnesemia), osteomalacia

Source: Adapted from Revere, C, and Hasty, R: Clinical notebook diagnostic and characteristic signs of illness and injury. J Emerg Nurs 19:137, 1993, with permission.

Table 6–9. EVALUATION OF NONSPECIFIC PRESENTING SYMPTOMS

Many patients present to the emergency room with vague symptoms that may be associated with any one or more of a number of specific diagnoses. It is important to closely observe these patients and ask questions that facilitate timely diagnosis and treatment of the underlying disorder.

Presenting Symptom	Possible Causes	Information Needed
Fever	Infection, hot environment, dehydration, thyroid storm, breakdown of necrotic tissue (such as postop or after an MI). Injury to the hypothalamus. Many meds have the ability to cause fever.	*Ask:* Pain? How long febrile? Anyone in family sick? Recent surgery or injury? Recent chest pain? Meds taken in last several days? *Observe for:* Guarding of any body area, dehydration, redness, lesions, or injury
Wheezing or SOB	Asthma, CHF, tumor, aspiration of foreign body, TB, COPD, acute allergic reaction. In infant, bronchiolitis. In child, croup.	*Ask:* History or family history of breathing problems? Allergies? How long wheezing? Meds taken in past few days? Exposure to harsh chemicals? Any episode of coughing in past few days (which may indicate aspiration especially in young child)? Worried?

(continued on the following page)

Emergency

Table 6–9.	EVALUATION OF NONSPECIFIC PRESENTING SYMPTOMS (continued)	
Presenting Symptom	**Possible Causes**	**Information Needed**
Wheezing or SOB (continued)		*Observe:* All VS, color of lips and nail beds, O_2 saturation, preferred position, chest shape and movement with respirations, lung sounds during auscultation, facial expression.
Chest pain	Acute MI, angina, pericarditis, costochondritis, pulmonary embolism, pneumothorax, pleurisy, indigestion.	*Ask:* Describe pain. Point to location of pain. Are there other symptoms? Does the pain radiate? If so, where? Rate pain 1–10. Any previous trauma? Anything make pain better or worse? Worried? *Observe:* All VS, color of lips and nail beds, O_2 sat, facial expression.
Abdominal pain	Indigestion, ulcer, gastroenteritis, cholecystitis, UTI, PID, ectopic pregnancy, cyst or tumor. With children, also suspect volvulus, intussusception, strep throat, or pneumonia.	*Ask:* Describe pain. Point to pain. Rate pain 1–10. Other symptoms? Last BM? Appearance of stool? Previous abdominal surgery or trauma? Worried? Anything make pain better or worse? Last menstrual period? *Observe:* All VS, guarding, bowel sounds, appearance of abdomen, palpable masses, facial expression.

Table 6–10. CAUSES OF ABNORMAL VITAL SIGNS

	Increased (Causes)	Decreased (Causes)
TEMPERATURE Norm: 97.7–99.5 (oral)	See *Fever* in Table 6–9.	Exposure, shock, brain lesions, cancer
HEART RATE Adult norm: 60–100 1 mo avg: 130 12 mo avg: 115 2–4 yr avg: 105	Exercise, anxiety, fever, caffeine intake, anemia, hypoxia, pain, thyroid abnormalities, shock	Acute MI, meds, thyroid abnormalities, ICP
RESPIRATIONS Adult: 14–20 1 mo avg: 35 2–4 yr avg: 24	Fever, pain, anxiety, hypoxia, anemia, metabolic acidosis, diabetic ketoacidosis, brain lesions, late ICP	CNS depression, meds, anesthesia, CO_2 narcosis, metabolic alkalosis, early ICP

(continued on the following page)

Table 6–10. CAUSES OF ABNORMAL VITAL SIGNS (continued)

	Increased (causes)	Decreased (causes)
BLOOD PRESSURE Adult: 120/80 1 mo avg: 84/52 2–4 yr avg: 90/56	Kidney disorders, essential hypertension, arteriosclerosis, congestive heart failure, anxiety, ICP, fluid overload, vasoconstricting meds	Acute MI, left-sided heart failure, dehydration, shock, heat exhaustion, burns, Addisonian crisis

NOTE: Some factors that normally cause variations in vital signs include time of day, position of patient, activity level, and emotional and physical status. A child's pulse and respiratory rate are markedly affected by these variables.

Table 6–11. COMPARISON OF DIABETIC KETOACIDOSIS AND HYPOGLYCEMIA

	Diabetic Ketoacidosis	Hypoglycemia
Onset	Gradual	Often sudden
History	Often acute infection in a diabetic or insufficient insulin intake Previous history of diabetes may be absent	Recent insulin injection, inadequate meal, or excessive exercise after insulin
Musculoskeletal	Muscle wasting or weight loss	Weakness Tremor Muscle twitching
Gastrointestinal	Abdominal pains or cramps, sometimes acute Nausea and vomiting	Nausea and vomiting
Central nervous system	Headache Double or blurred vision Irritability	Convulsions Coma

(continued on the following page)

Table 6–11. COMPARISON OF DIABETIC KETOACIDOSIS AND HYPOGLYCEMIA (continued)

	Diabetic Ketoacidosis	Hypoglycemia
Cardiovascular	Rapid, feeble pulse Decrease in blood pressure Flushed, dry skin	Pallor Diaphoresis Decrease in pulse rate followed by increase Decrease in blood pressure followed by increase Palpitations
Respiratory	Air hunger Acetone odor of breath Dyspnea	Air hunger Increased respiratory rate
Laboratory values	Elevated blood glucose (>200 mg/dL) Glucose and acetone in urine	Subnormal blood glucose (20–50 mg/dL) Absence of glucose and acetone in urine unless bladder is full

Source: Venes, D, and Thomas, CL (eds): Taber's Cyclopedic Medical Dictionary, ed 19. FA Davis, Philadelphia, 2001, p. 578, with permission.

THE OB PATIENT IN THE EMERGENCY DEPARTMENT

Type Emergency	*Manifestations*
Abruptio placentae	Bleeding, pain, contractions, rigid and tender abdomen, excessive fetal movement, possible shock
Eclampsia	Hypertension, headache, dizziness, spots before eyes, convulsions, coma
Ectopic pregnancy	Acute pain, referred shoulder pain, possible flank pain, N/V, faintness, tender abdomen, possible bleeding, possible shock
Imminent birth	See *Signs of imminent birth.*
Placenta praevia	Painless bleeding, usually in last trimester
Prolapsed cord	Rupture of membranes, "something in vagina"

INITIAL ASSESSMENT OF OB PATIENT

ASK
Due date?
Contractions?
Frequency?
Duration?
Ruptured BOW?
Bleeding?
Number of previous pregnancies (gravida)?
Number of births (para)?
Problems with past deliveries?
Problems with pregnancy?
Has the baby moved today?

OBSERVE
Size of abdomen
Fundal height
Presentation (cephalic or breech)
Fetal heart tones (not assessed if birth is imminent)

Emergency

SIGNS OF IMMINENT BIRTH*

- Mother is experiencing tension, anxiety, diaphoresis, and intense contractions.
- With a contraction, the mother catches her breath and grunts with involuntary pushing (with inability to respond to questions).
- A blood "show" is caused by a rapid dilatation of the cervix.
- The anus is bulging, evidencing descent.
- Bulging or fullness occurs at the perineum.
- "Crowning" of the head at the introitus of a multiparous mother means that the birth is very imminent. In nulliparous birth, it means that the birth may be up to 30 minutes later. (Birth is near when the head stays visible between contractions.)

EMERGENCY BIRTH DO'S AND DON'TS

DO:

Keep calm.

Allow the baby to emerge slowly.

Clear the airway.

Dry the baby off.

Hold the baby at or slightly above the level of introitus.

Put the baby next to the mother's skin and allow nursing.

Wait for the placenta to separate.

Inspect the placenta for completeness.

DO NOT:

Do not put your fingers into the birth canal.

Do not force rotation of the baby's head after the head emerges.

Do not try to pull out the baby's arm.

Do not overstimulate the baby by slapping.

Do not put traction on the cord or pull on the cord.

---

*Signs of imminent birth and emergency birth "do's and don'ts" with permission from: Roberts, J: Emergency birth. J Emerg Nurs 11(3):125, 1985.

Do not hold the baby up by the ankles.
Do not allow the baby to become cold.
Do not hold the baby below the mother's perineum.
Do not "strip" or "milk" the umbilical cord.
Do not push on the uterus to try to deliver the placenta.
Do not cut the cord unless you have sterile equipment.
Do not allow the mother's bladder to become distended.

DOMESTIC VIOLENCE

Clues of abuse in patient history:

- frequent injuries reported as "accidental"
- history of repeated miscarriages
- vague or changing description of pain or injury
- lack of patient cooperation during collection of subjective and/or objective data

Common sites of injuries caused by physical abuse:

- head and neck (most common)
- breasts
- chest
- abdomen

Signs of *possible* abuse:

- multiple injuries
- bilateral distribution of injuries
- injuries at different stages of healing
- fingernail marks
- bruises shaped like a handprint or instrument
- rope burns
- cigarette burns
- bites
- spiral fractures
- burns

Appropriate nursing actions:

Question and examine the patient in privacy.
Assure confidentiality.
Examine entire body.
Ask specific questions related to suspected abuse.

Be aware that the perpetrator may retaliate if exposed by the patient.
Encourage patient to seek shelter if abuse is suspected.
Give patient contact information for community resources.
Call law enforcement immediately if violence is threatened (do not warn the perpetrator of this action).

CLUES TO POSSIBLE CHILD ABUSE AND/OR NEGLECT

None of the clues listed here is diagnostic of child abuse. When evaluating the behavior of parents, it is important to remember that the actions and speech of many parents can be negatively affected by the stress of having a child in the emergency department. Although all 50 states require that health professionals report any suspicion of child abuse, state statutes define child abuse. A copy of state laws and forms for reporting abuse should be available in the emergency department. If the child appears to be in imminent danger, the child should not be discharged to the parents; instead, appropriate steps should be taken to detain the child until further assessment can be made. (In most hospitals, Social Services should be contacted.)

1. Reported cause of injury does not seem likely.

> *Example:* A 1-year-old with multiple skull fractures is reported to have fallen down a flight of stairs. The child has no other injuries on his or her body.

2. Details of injury change when reported by different informants or to different personnel.
3. History is inconsistent with developmental abilities.

> *Example:* A 3-month-old falling into a hot bathtub.

4. A child less than 3 years of age has a bone fracture. (A child less than 3 years of age is not

usually involved in activities that might result in a fracture.)

5. Parent emphasizes that child or sibling is to blame for injury.
6. Parent seems angry that child is injured.
7. Parent is hostile toward health care workers.
8. Exaggeration or absence of emotional response from parent to child's injury.
9. Child has injuries or untreated illness unrelated to present injury.
10. Child exhibits signs of the "failure to thrive" syndrome.
11. Child has areas of baldness (from hair being pulled).
12. Child has bruises in various stages of healing (more suspicious if near genitalia).
13. Burns are evident, especially on the feet or buttocks.
14. Child has lesions that resemble bites, fingernail marks, or cigarette tip burns.
15. The genital area is irritated.
16. The vaginal or rectal orifice is enlarged.
17. Radiographs reveal old fractures.
18. Parent does not attempt to comfort child, and/or child does not turn to parent for comfort.
19. Toddler or preschooler does not protest if parents leave the room.
20. Child does not prefer parent over health care worker.
21. Child withdraws as if fearful when approached.

QRST COMPLEX OF ELECTROCARDIOGRAM

Figure 6–4 indicates the actual location of designated intervals. (Note that some interval names seem to be misnomers because the intervals do not actually begin and end at obvious points.)

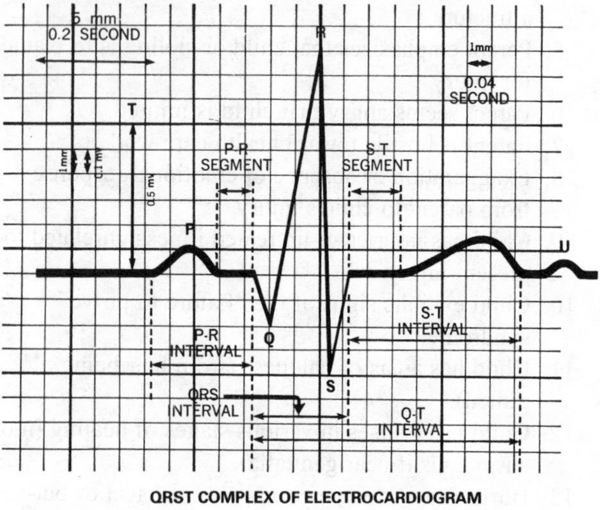

Figure 6–4. QRST complex of ECG. (From Venes, D, and Thomas, CL [eds]: Taber's Cyclopedic Medical Dictionary, ed 19. FA Davis, Philadelphia, 2001, p. 673, with permission.)

ECG HEART RATE PER MINUTE CALCULATION

METHOD 1, FOR REGULAR RATES ONLY

Count the number of whole and parts of (such as 4.5) large boxes that separate any two consecutive R waves, and divide that number into 300.

METHOD 2, KNOWN AS THE DUBIN METHOD, FOR REGULAR RATES ONLY

First, find an R wave that peaks on a heavy black line. Next, name the consecutive heavy black lines in the following manner:

300, 150, 100, 75, 60, 50, 43

The heart rate is equal to the number named where the next R wave occurs.

METHOD 3, FOR REGULAR OR IRREGULAR RATES

Note standard markings on top of the ECG strip:

- Marks on every 5th heavy line indicate 1-second intervals.
- Marks on every 15th line indicate 3-second intervals.
- Marks on every 30th line indicate 6-second intervals.

Use one R wave as starting point (do not count this wave), and count all consecutive R waves in a 6-second interval. Multiply the number of R waves in a 6-second interval by 10 to determine rate.

HEART RATE CALCULATION TOOL

NOTE: A handy duplicate of Figure 6–5 can be found inside the front cover of this book.

To use the tool, place arrow at an appropriate point on one cycle of the ECG, and measure to the corresponding point in the next cycle. Follow the line downward to read the rate.

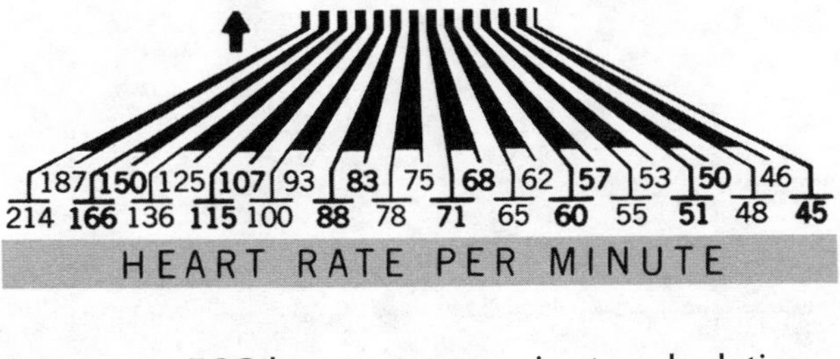

Figure 6–5. ECG heart rate per minute calculation tool.

NOTE: A handy duplicate of Figure 6–6 can be found inside the front cover of this book.

To use the tool, place "0.00" at the appropriate point in the cycle and follow the line (downward) that falls at the end of the interval being measured. (Measures are in hundredths of a second.) Refer to dysrhythmia tables for more information.

Norms: P–R interval = 0.12 − 0.20
QRS = 0.06 − 0.10
Q−T = 0.32 − 0.4

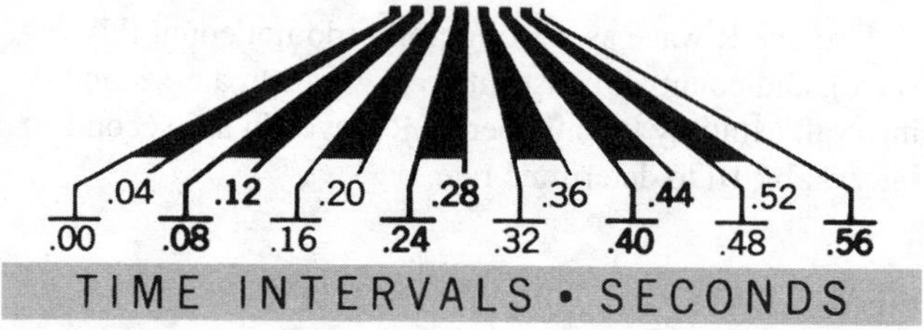

Figure 6–6. ECG interval assessment tool.

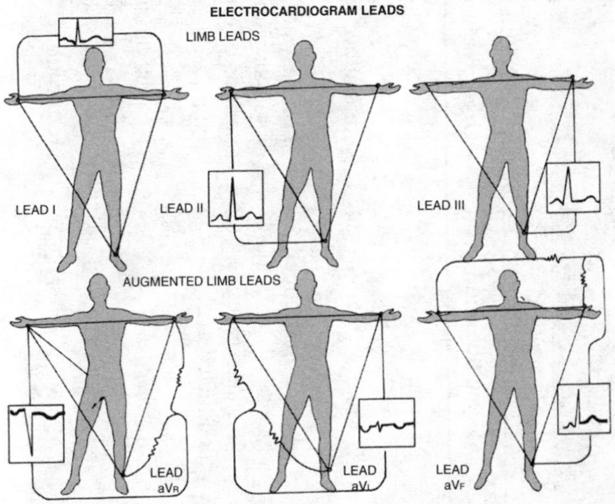

Figure 6–7. ECG leads. (From Venes, D, and Thomas, CL [eds]: Taber's Cyclopedic Medical Dictionary, ed 19. FA Davis, Philadelphia, 2001, p. 673, with permission.)

Table 6–12. IDENTIFICATION OF CARDIAC DYSRHYTHMIAS

A. Sinus Dysrhythmias

	P Waves	QRS Complexes	AV Relationship	Other Features
1. Sinus bradycardia	Normal	Normal	Normal	Rate below 60/min
2. Sinus tachycardia	Normal	Normal	Normal	Rate above 100/min
3. Sinus arrest/SA exit block	Missing in dropped cycles Normal in conducted cycles	Missing in dropped cycles Normal for conducted cycles	Missing in dropped cycles Normal for conducted cycles	Long asystolic R-R intervals during periods of arrest
4. Sinus dysrhythmia	Normal shape	Normal shape	Normal	Benign variation of NSR Varies with phases of respiration

B. Supraventricular Tachycardias

	P Waves	QRS Complexes	AV Relationship		Key Features
Atrial flutter	Absent, replaced by regular F waves Atrial rate of 250–350/min	Normal Usually regular	Usually a fixed AV conduction greater than 1: 1, e.g., 2 : 1, 3 : 1, 4 : 1	Sawtooth pattern	Stepwise decrease in rate with return to previous rate with offset of pressure
Atrial fibrillation	Absent; replaced by irregular f waves. Atrial rate of 350–600/min (not countable)	Normal Irregularly irregular; rate is under 100/min (treated) or above 100/min (untreated)	Random AV conduction	Fibrillatory/ chaotic baseline Irregularly irregular R-R intervals	No response or transient slowing of ventricular response
Multifocal atrial tachycardia	Sinus P waves plus P′ waves of at least three shapes	Irregular rhythm	1 : 1	Changing shapes of ectopic P waves	None

(continued on the following page)

Table 6–12. IDENTIFICATION OF CARDIAC DYSRHYTHMIAS (continued)

B. Supraventricular Tachycardias (continued)

	P Waves	QRS Complexes	AV Relationship		Key Features
Paroxysmal supraventricular tachycardia (PSVT)	Absent P′ waves are missing If present, found preceding, following, or in the QRS complex	Normal Regular R-R interval	1 : 1 if P′ wave visible S2 : 1, 3 : 1 conduction, suspect digitalis toxicity	Abrupt onset and termination Occur in bursts	No response or conversion to NSR
Sinus tachycardia	Normal	Normal	1 : 1	Gradual return to slower rates	None, or transient slowing
AV junctional tachycardia	See PSVT; unable to differentiate from PSVT				

C. AV Heart Block–Induced Dysrhythmias

	P Waves	QRS Complexes	AV Relationship	Key Features
1. First degree	Normal All P waves are conducted	Normal No QRS complexes are dropped	P-R interval over 0.20 sec Only AV block with 1 : 1 AV conduction	Long P-R interval Site of block: within AV node
2. Second degree A. Wenckebach type	Normal Some P waves are not conducted	Normal Some QRS complexes are dropped	Progressive increase in P-R intervals followed by dropped QRS complex Ratio typically 3 : 2, 4 : 3, etc. P-R interval of first beat in each cycle often greater than 0.20 sec	Grouped beating Increasing P-R intervals The longest R-R interval is equal to less than twice the shortest one Site of blocks: intranodal
B. Mobitz type 2	Normal Some P waves are not conducted	Wide Some QRS complexes are dropped	Fixed P-R interval prior to dropped beats Ratio may be 3 : 2, 4 : 3 or higher degrees (4 : 2, 5 : 3, etc.) P-R interval usually normal	Fixed P-R intervals Site of block: infranodal

(continued on the following page)

Table 6–12. IDENTIFICATION OF CARDIAC DYSRHYTHMIAS (continued)

C. AV Heart Block–Induced Dysrhythmias (continued)

	P Waves	QRS Complexes	AV Relationship	Key Features
3. Third degree	Normal shape, regular intervals No P waves are conducted More P waves than QRS complexes	Escape rhythm depends on level of block Usually wide and distorted if low in ventricle Narrow if high in ventricle Regular R-R intervals Rate slower than atrial (usually below 50/min)	Complete dissociation Activities are independent of one another	Site of block: infranodal AV dissociation

NOTE: Not all second-degree blocks with 2 : 1 AV conduction are type 2 blocks.

D. Ventricular Rhythms

	P Waves	QRS Complexes	AV Relationship	Other Features
1. Escape idioventricular rhythm	Absent	Depends on level of escape focus High in ventricle are narrow and 40–50/min Low in ventricle are wide and 20–40/mm	Absent	Life-sustaining in event of sinus arrest and third-degree heart block
2. Accelerated idioventricular rhythm	Absent	Wide, distorted Rate 50–100/min	Absent or AV dissociation Occasional ventricular capture complexes	Originally thought to be benign; now considered pathologic
3. Ventricular tachycardia	Absent or sporadically present	Wide and bizarre Rate: Above 100/min (commonly about 150/min)	Absent	Resembles a string of PVCs

(continued on the following page)

Table 6–12. IDENTIFICATION OF CARDIAC DYSRHYTHMIAS (continued)

D. Ventricular Rhythms (continued)

	P Waves	QRS Complexes	AV Relationship	Other Features
4. Torsades de pointes (variation of ventricular tachycardia)	Absent	Wide and slurred QRS axis constantly changing in the same lead	Absent	Prolonged Q-T interval in NSR prior to or following episode of ventricular tachycardia
5. Ventricular fibrillation	Absent	No defined pattern	Absent	Chaotic tracing with complexes of varying heights and shapes
6. Asystole	Absent	Absent	Absent	Flat line

E. Ectopic Complexes

	P Waves	QRS Complexes	AV Relationship	Key Features
1. Premature complexes				
A. PAC/atrial	Premature ectopic P′ wave	Normal if conducted May be blocked or aberrantly conducted	1 : 1 AV conduction P-R interval differs from sinus complexes	Noncompensatory pause Normal T waves
B. PJC/junctional	Retrograde P′ wave just before or after QRS complex Often P′ wave missing	Normal	May be 1 : 1 or missing P-R interval often shortened	Noncompensatory pause Normal T waves
C. PVC/ ventricular	Absent	Wide, bizarre	Absent	Compensatory pause Abnormal T waves (slope opposite aberrant QRS)
2. Escape complexes				
A. Atrial	P′ wave	Normal	Variable	Occur in cases of sinus depression

(continued on the following page)

Table 6–12. IDENTIFICATION OF CARDIAC DYSRHYTHMIAS (continued)

E. Ectopic Complexes (continued)

	P Waves	QRS Complexes	AV Relationship	Key Features
2. Escape complexes (continued)				
B. Junctional	Retrograde P′ wave or missing	Normal Sustained rhythm at rate of 40–60/min	Variable	Occur when sinus node is depressed
C. Ventricular	Missing	Wide, bizarre Sustained rhythm at rate of 20–40/min	Missing	Occur when sinus and AV junction fail as pacemaker

NOTES: Premature beats occur early in the R-R interval, whereas escape beats occur late. Premature beats compete with sinus node for pacemaker role (interrupt R-R cycles of dominant rhythm); escape beats "reluctantly" assume pacemaker role when SA node fails (end R-R cycles longer than dominant rhythm).

Source: Brown, K, and Jacobson, S: Mastering Dysrhythmias: A Problem-Solving Guide. FA Davis, Philadelphia, 1988, pp 53, 54, 95, 130, 131, with permission.

INDICATIONS FOR USE

- Failure of SA node to generate spontaneous impulse
- Failure of cardiac conduction system to transmit impulses from the SA node to ventricles
- Failure of SA node to maintain control of cardiac pacing

NOTE: Artificial pacing can be temporary or permanent.

THREE MAJOR MEANS OF ARTIFICIAL PACING

Type	*Method*	*Comments*
External (transcutaneous)	Two surface electrode patches administer about 50–125 mA.	Temporary, noninvasive. Can be instituted immediately. Patient may feel tingling sensation at electrode site.
Epicardial	Lead wires inserted through chest directly to epicardial surface.	Invasive. Almost always present immediately after coronary artery bypass surgery.
Endocardial (transvenous)	Lead wires threaded through subclavian, or femoral artery, through right atrium, into right ventricular wall.	Invasive.

Source: Data from Dolan, JT: Critical Care Nursing. FA Davis, Philadelphia, 1991, p 858.

DEFINITION

To terminate ventricular fibrillation by electric countershock.

INDICATIONS FOR USE

- Ventricular fibrillation
- Pulseless ventricular tachycardia

NOTE: CPR efforts should be enacted during preparation for defibrillation.

METHOD

1. Place two gel pads on the patient's bare chest or apply gel to entire surface of paddles. (To prevent burns and improper conduction, remove gel from your hands and the sides of the paddles, and remove any gel that may have fallen on the patient's chest.)
2. Temporarily discontinue oxygen (if applicable).
3. Apply one electrode below right clavicle just to the side of the upper sternum. Apply second electrode just below and lateral to left nipple.
4. Set defibrillator at 200 joules (J) (AHA recommendation).
5. Grasp paddles by insulated handles only.
6. Give "Stand Clear" command, and ascertain that no one is touching patient or bed.
7. Push discharge buttons in both paddles simultaneously, using pressure to ensure firm contact with the patient's skin.
8. Remove paddles and assess patient and ECG pattern.
9. Successive attempts at defibrillation may deliver 200 to 300 J, then 360 J. Energy levels for biphasic models are 50 J, 100 J, 150 J.

AHA recommends that, if three rapidly administered shocks fail to defibrillate, CPR should be continued, IV access accomplished, epinephrine given, and then shocks repeated.

Cardioversion differs from defibrillation in that it is synchronized to avoid the T wave of the cardiac cycle.

CALCULATED HEMODYNAMIC PARAMETERS AND NORMAL PRESSURE MEASUREMENTS

Type of Measurement	*Adult Norms*
Arteriovenous oxygen difference (a $-vDO_2$)	3.5–5.5 vol%
Aortic pressure	
Systolic	100–140 mm Hg
Diastolic	60–80 mm Hg
Mean	70–90 mm Hg
Cardiac output (CO)	4–8 L/min
Cardiac index (CI)	2.5–4 L/min m^2
Central venous pressure (CVP)	2–6 mm Hg
Coronary artery perfusion pressure (CAPP)	60–80 mm Hg
Left atrial mean pressure	4–12 mm Hg
Left ventricular systolic pressure	100–140 mm Hg
Left ventricular diastolic pressure	0–5 mm Hg
Left ventricular stroke work index (LVSWI)	30–50 g/beat/m^2
Mean arterial pressure (MAP)	70–90 mm Hg

(continued on the following page)

CALCULATED HEMODYNAMIC PARAMETERS AND NORMAL PRESSURE MEASUREMENTS (continued)

Type of Measurement	*Adult Norms*
Oxygen content of blood	
Arterial	17.5–20.5 vol%
Venous	12.5–16.5 vol%
Oxygen consumption (VO_2)	200–250 mL/min
Oxygen delivery (DO_2)	900–1100 mL/min
Pulmonary artery systolic pressure	20–30 mm Hg
Pulmonary artery diastolic pressure	10–20 mm Hg
Pulmonary artery mean pressure	10–15 mm Hg
Pulmonary capillary mean wedge pressure (PCW)	4–12 mm Hg
Right atrial mean pressure	2–6 mm Hg
Right ventricular pressure	
Systolic	20–30 mm Hg
Diastolic	0–5 mm Hg
End Diastolic	2–6 mm Hg
Pulmonary ventricular stroke work index (PVSWI)	5–10 g/beat/m^2
Stroke index (SI)	40–50 mL/beat/m^2
Stroke volume (SV)	70–130 mL/beat
Superior vena cava mean pressure (SVC)	2–6 mm Hg

Type of Measurement	*Adult Norms*
Systemic vascular resistance (SVR)	900–1600 dyn/s/cm^{-5}
Systemic venous oxygen saturation (SVO_2)	60–80%

From Dolan, JT: Critical Care Nursing. F.A. Davis, Philadelphia, 1991, P. 841, with permission.

NOTE: To convert millimeters of mercury to centimeters of H_2O, multiply the millimeters of mercury by 1.34.

REFERENCES

Dolan, J: Critical Care Nursing Clinical Management through the Nursing Process. FA Davis, Philadelphia, 1991, p 841.

Long, B, and Phipps, W: Medical-Surgical Nursing: A Nursing Process Approach. CV Mosby, St. Louis, 1993, p. 1567.

NOTES

NOTES

NOTES

NOTES

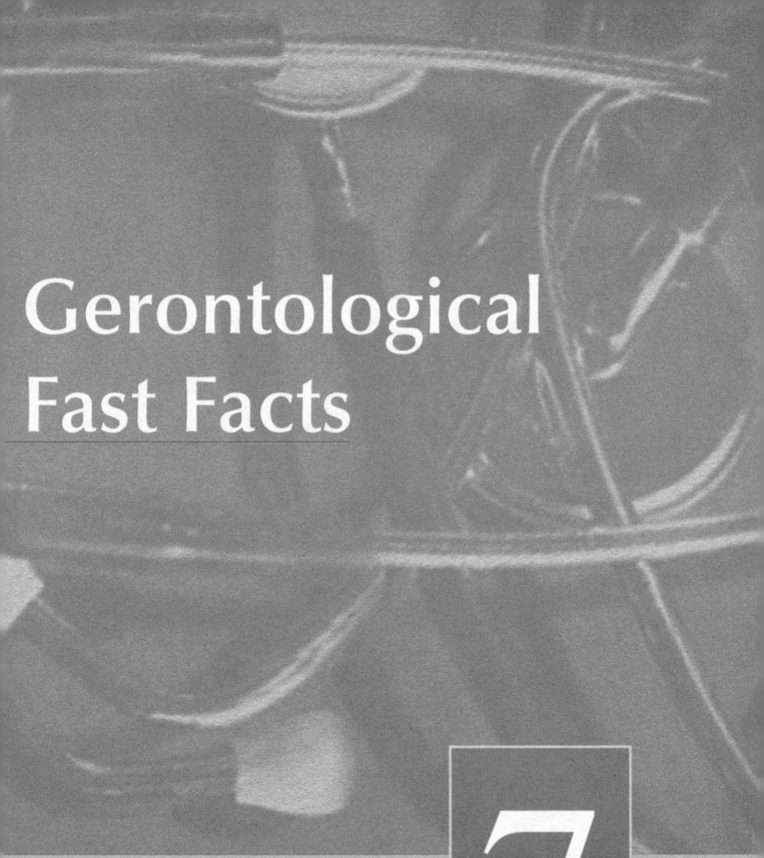

Gerontological Fast Facts

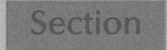

Section 7

AGE-RELATED CHANGES AND THEIR NURSING IMPLICATIONS

Age-Related Change	*Appearance or Functional Change*	*Nursing Implication*
INTEGUMENTARY SYSTEM		
Loss of dermal and epidermal thickness	Paper-thin skin	Prone to skin breakdown and injury
Flattening of papillae	Shearing and friction force more readily peels off the epidermis	
	Diminished cell-mediated immunity in the skin	
Atrophy of the sweat glands	Decreased sweating	Frequent pruritus
Decreased vascularity	Slower recruitment of sweat glands by thermal stimulation	Alteration in thermoregularity response
		Fluid requirements may change seasonally

(continued on the following page)

AGE-RELATED CHANGES AND THEIR NURSING IMPLICATIONS (continued)

Age-Related Change	*Appearance or Functional Change*	*Nursing Implication*
INTEGUMENTARY SYSTEM (continued)		
	Decreased body odor	Loss of skin water
	Decreased heat loss	Increased risk of heat stroke
	Dryness	
Collagen cross-linking	Increased wrinkling	Potential effect on one's morale and feeling of self-worth
Elastin regression	Laxity of skin	
Loss of subcutaneous fat	Intraosseous atrophy, especially of back of hands and face	Loss of fat tissue on soles of feet—trauma of walking increases foot problems
Decreased elasticity		
Loss of subcutaneous tissue	Purpuric patches after minor surgery	Reduced insulation against cold temperatures; *prone to hypothermia*
		Check why injury is occurring; be alert—potential abuse or falls

Decreased number of melanocytes	Loss of pigment Pigment plaque appears	Teach importance of using sun block creams; refer to dermatologist as needed
Decline in fibroblast proliferation	Decreased epidermal growth rate Slower re-epithelialization Decreased vitamin D production and synthesis	Decreased tissue repair response
Decreased hair follicle density	Loss of body hair	
Decreased growth phase of individual fibers	Thin, short villous hairs predominate Slower hair growth	
Loss of melanocytes from the hair bulb	Graying of the hair	Potential effect on self-esteem
Alternating hyperplasia and hypoplasia of nail matrix	Longitudinal ridges Thinner nails of the fingers Thickened, curled toenails	Nails prone to splitting Advise patient to wear gloves, keep nails short, avoid nail polish remover (causes dryness); refer to podiatrist May cause discomfort

(continued on the following page)

AGE-RELATED CHANGES AND THEIR NURSING IMPLICATIONS (continued)

Age-Related Change	*Appearance or Functional Change*	*Nursing Implication*
RESPIRATORY SYSTEM		
Decreased lung tissue elasticity	Decreased vital capacity Increased residual volume Decreased maximum breath capacity	Reduced overall efficiency of ventilatory exchange
Thoracic wall calcification	Increased anteroposterior diameter of chest	Obscuration of heart and lung sounds Displacement of apical impulse
Cilia atrophy	Change in mucociliary transport	Increased susceptibility to infection
Decreased respiratory muscle strength	Reduced ability to handle secretions and reduced effectiveness against noxious foreign particles Partial inflation of lungs at rest	Prone to atelectasis

CARDIOVASCULAR SYSTEM		
Heart valves fibrose and thicken	Reduced stroke volume, cardiac output may be altered Slight left ventricular hypertrophy	Decreased responsiveness to stress Increased incidence of murmurs, *particularly aortic stenosis and mitral regurgitation*
Mucoid degeneration of mitral valve	S_4 commonly heard Valve less dense; mitral leaflet stretches with intrathoracic pressure	
Fibroelastic thickening of the sinoatrial (SA) node; decreased number of pacemaker cells Increased subpericardial fat Collagen accumulation around heart muscle	Slower heart rate Irregular heart rate	Increased prevalence of arrhythmias
Elongation of tortuosity and calcification of arteries	Increased rigidity of arterial wall	Aneurysms may form

(continued on the following page)

AGE-RELATED CHANGES AND THEIR NURSING IMPLICATIONS (continued)

Age-Related Change	*Appearance or Functional Change*	*Nursing Implication*
CARDIOVASCULAR SYSTEM (continued)		
Elastin and collagen cause progressive thickening and loss of arterial wall resiliency	Increased peripheral vascular resistance	Decreased blood flow to body organs Altered distribution of blood flow
Loss of elasticity of the aorta dilation		Increased systolic blood pressure, contributing to coronary artery disease
Increased lipid content in artery wall	Lipid deposits form	Increased incidence of atherosclerotic events, such as *angina pectoris*, stroke, gangrene
Decreased baroreceptor sensitivity (stretch receptors)	Decreased sensitivity to change in blood pressure Decreased baroreceptor mediation to straining	Prone to loss of balance—potential for falls Valsalva's maneuver may cause sudden drop in blood pressure

GASTROINTESTINAL SYSTEM		
Liver becomes smaller	Decreased storage capacity	
Less efficient cholesterol stabilization of absorption	Increased evidence of gall stones	
Dental enamel thins	Staining of tooth surface occurs	Tooth and gum decay; tooth loss
Gums recede	Teeth deprived of nutrients	
Fibrosis and atrophy of salivary glands	Prone to dry mucous membranes	Shift to mouth breathing is common Membrane more susceptible to injury and infection
	Decreased salivary ptyalin	May interfere with breakdown of starches
Atrophy and decrease in number of taste buds	Decreased taste sensation	Altered ability to taste sweet, sour, and bitter Change in nutritional intake Excessive seasoning of foods
Delay in esophageal emptying	Decline in esophageal peristalsis Esophagus slightly dilated	Occasional discomfort as food stays in esophagus longer
Decreased hydrochloric acid secretion	Reduction in amount of iron and vitamin B_{12} that can be absorbed	Possible delay in vitamin and drug absorption, *especially calcium and iron*

(continued on the following page)

AGE-RELATED CHANGES AND THEIR NURSING IMPLICATIONS (continued)

Age-Related Change	*Appearance or Functional Change*	*Nursing Implication*
GASTROINTESTINAL SYSTEM (continued)		
Decrease in gastric acid secretion		Altered drug effect Fewer cases of gastric ulcers
Decreased muscle tone	Altered motility	Prone to constipation, functional bowel syndrome, esophageal spasm, diverticular disease
Atrophy of mucosal lining	Decreased colonic peristalsis Decreased hunger sensations and emptying time	
Decreased proportion of dietary calcium absorbed	Altered bone formation, muscle contractility, hormone activity, enzyme activation, clotting time, immune response	Symptoms more marked in women than in men
Decreased basal metabolic rate (rate at which fuel is converted into energy)		May need fewer calories Possible effect on lifespan

GENITOURINARY AND REPRODUCTIVE SYSTEMS		
Reduced renal mass Loss of glomeruli	Decreased sodium-conserving ability Decreased glomerular filtration rate Decreased creatinine clearance Increased blood urea nitrogen concentration	Administration and dosage of drugs may need to be modified
Histologic changes in small vessel walls Sclerosis of supportive circulatory system	Decreased renal blood flow	
Decline in number of functioning nephrons	Decreased ability to dilute urine concentrate	Altered response to reduced fluid load or increased fluid volume
Reduced bladder muscular tone	Decreased bladder capacity or increased residual urine	Sensation of urge to urinate may not occur until bladder is full Urination at night may increase
Atrophy and fibrosis of cervical and uterine walls	Menopause; decline in fertility	

(continued on the following page)

AGE-RELATED CHANGES AND THEIR NURSING IMPLICATIONS (continued)

Age-Related Change	*Appearance or Functional Change*	*Nursing Implication*
GENITOURINARY AND REPRODUCTIVE SYSTEMS (continued)		
Reduced number and viability of oocytes in the aging ovary	Narrowing of cervical canal	
Decreased vaginal wall elasticity	Vaginal lining thin, pale, friable Narrowing of vaginal canal	Potential for discomfort in sexual intercourse
Decreased levels of circulating hormones	Reduced lubrication during arousal state	Increased frequency of sexual dysfunction
Degeneration of seminiferous tubules	Decreased seminal fluid volume Decreased force of ejaculation Reduced elevation of testes	

Proliferation of stromal and glandular tissue	Prostatic hypertrophy	Potentially compromised genitourinary function; *urinary frequency, and increased risk of malignancy*
Involution of mammary gland tissue	Connective tissue replaced by adipose tissue	Easier to assess breast lesions
NEUROMUSCULAR SYSTEM		
Decreased muscle mass	Decreased muscle strength Tendons shrink and sclerose	Decreased tendon jerks Increased muscle cramping
Decreased myosin adenosine triphosphatase (ADT) activity	Prolonged contraction time, latency period, relaxation period	Decreased motor function and overall strength
Deterioration of joint cartilage	Bone makes contact with bone	Potential for pain, crepitation, and limitation of movement
Loss of water from the cartilage	Narrowing of joint spaces	Loss of height
Decreased bone mass Decreased osteoblastic activity	Decreased bone formation and increased bone resorption, leading to osteoporosis	More rapid and earlier changes in women Greater risk of fractures

(continued on the following page)

AGE-RELATED CHANGES AND THEIR NURSING IMPLICATIONS (continued)

Age-Related Change	*Appearance or Functional Change*	*Nursing Implication*
NEUROMUSCULAR SYSTEM (continued)		
Osteoclasts resorb bone	Hormonal changes	Gait and posture accommodate to changes
Increased proportion of body fat	Centripetal distribution of fat and invasion of fat in large muscle groups	Anthropometric measurements required
Regional changes in fat distribution		Increased relative adiposity
Thickened leptomeninges in spinal cord	Loss of anterior horn cells in the lumbosacral area	Leg weakness may be correlated
Accumulation of lipofuscin	Altered RNA function and resultant cell death	
Loss of neurons and nerve fibers	Decreased processing speed and vibration sense	Increased time to perform and learn

	Altered pain response	Possible postural hypotension
	Decreased deep tendon, Achilles' tendon	Safety hazard
Decreased conduction of nerve fibers	Decreased psychomotor performance	Alteration in pain response
Few neuritic plaques		Possible cognitive and memory changes
Neurofibrillary tangles in hippocampal neurons		Heavy tangle formation and neuritic plaques in cortex of those with Alzheimer's disease
Changes in sleep-wake cycle	Decreased stage 4, stage 3, and rapid eye movement phases	Increased or decreased time spent sleeping
	Deterioration of circadian organization	Increased nighttime awakenings Changed hormonal activity
Slower stimulus identification and registration	Delayed reaction time	Prone to falls
Decreased brain weight and volume		May be present in absence of mental impairments

(continued on the following page)

AGE-RELATED CHANGES AND THEIR NURSING IMPLICATIONS (continued)

Age-Related Change	Appearance or Functional Change	Nursing Implication
SENSORY SYSTEM		
Morphologic changes in choroid, epithelium, retina	Decreased visual acuity Visual field narrows	Corrective lenses required Increased possibility of disorientation and social isolation
Decreased rod and cone function		Slower light and dark adaptation
Pigment accumulation		
Decreased speed of eye movements	Difficulty in gazing upward and maintaining convergence	
Sclerosis of pupil sphincter	Difficulty in adapting to lighting changes	Glare may pose an environmental hazard
	Increased threshold for light perception	Dark rooms may be hazardous

Increased intraocular pressure		Increased incidence of glaucoma
Distorted depth perception		Incorrect assessment of height of curbs and steps; potential for falls
Ciliary muscle atrophy Nuclear sclerosis (*lens*) Reduced accommodation Increased lens size Accumulation of lens fibers	Altered refractive powers Presbyopia Hyperopia Myopia	Corrective lenses often required Near work and reading may become difficult
Lens yellows	Color vision may be impaired	Less able to differentiate lower color tones: blues, greens, violets
Diminished tear secretion	Dullness and dryness of the eyes	Irritation and discomfort may result Intactness of corneal surface jeopardized
Loss of auditory neurons	Decreased tone discrimination and voice localization High-frequency sounds lost first	Suspiciousness may be increased because of paranoid dimensions secondary to hearing loss Social isolation
Angiosclerosis calcification of inner ear membrane	Progressive hearing loss, especially at high frequency Presbycusis	Difficulty hearing, particularly under certain conditions such as *background noise, rapid speech, poor acoustics*

(continued on the following page)

AGE-RELATED CHANGES AND THEIR NURSING IMPLICATIONS (continued)

Age-Related Change	*Appearance or Functional Change*	*Nursing Implication*
SENSORY SYSTEM (continued)		
Decreased number of olfactory nerve fibers	Decreased sensitivity to odors	May not detect harmful odors Potential safety hazard
Alteration in taste sensation		Possible changes in food preferences and eating patterns
Reduced tactile sensation	Decreased ability to sense pressure, pain, temperature	Misperceptions of environment and safety risk
ENDOCRINE SYSTEM		
Decline in secretion of testosterone, growth hormone, insulin, adrenal androgens, aldosterone, thyroid hormone	Decreased hormone clearance rates	Increased mortality associated with certain stresses (burns, surgery)

Defects in thermoregulation	Shivering less intense	Susceptibility to temperature extremes (*hypothermia/hyperthermia*)
Reduction of febrile responses	Poor perceptions of changes in ambient temperature	Unrecognized infectious process operative
	Reduced sweating; increased threshold for the onset of sweating	
	Fever not always present with infectious process	
Alteration in tissue sensitivity to hormones	Decreased insulin response, glucose tolerance, and sensitivity of renal tubules to antidiuretic hormone (ADH)	
Enhanced sympathetic responsivity		
Increased nodularity and fibrosis of thyroid		Increased frequency of thyroid disease
Decreased basal metabolic rate	Alteration in carbohydrate tolerance	Increased incidence of obesity

(continued on the following page)

AGE-RELATED CHANGES AND THEIR NURSING IMPLICATIONS (continued)

Age-Related Change	*Appearance or Functional Change*	*Nursing Implication*
HEMATOLOGIC SYSTEM		
Decreased percentage of marrow space occupied by hematopoietic tissue	Ineffective erythropoiesis	Risky for patient who loses blood
IMMUNE SYSTEM		
Thymic involution and decreased serum thymic hormone activity	Decreased number of T cells Production of anti-self reactive T cells	Less vigorous and/or delayed hypersensitivity reactions
Decreased T-cell function	Impairment in cell-mediated immune responses	Increased risk of mortality

Appearance of autoantibodies	Decreased cyclic adenosine monophosphate (AMP) and glucose monophosphate (GMP) Decreased ability to reject foreign tissue Increased laboratory autoimmune parameters	Increased incidence of infection Reactivation of latent infectious diseases Increased prevalence of autoimmune disorders
Redistribution of lymphocytes	Impaired immune reactivity	Increased prevalence of infection
Changes in serum immunoglobulin	Increased immunoglobulin A (lgA) levels Decreased immunoglobulin G (lgG) levels	

Source: From Kennedy-Malone, L, Fletcher, KR, and Plank, LM: Management Guidelines for Gerontological Nurse Practitioners. FA Davis, Philadelphia, 2000, pp 536–543, with permission.

ALTERED MENTAL STATES OF THE OLDER ADULT

It is important to recognize and report signs and symptoms of altered mental states to protect the elderly patient from accidental or intentional self-harm. Three of the most common altered mental states of the older adult are dementia, delirium, and depression.

Dementia: A broad term that refers to cognitive deficits, such as memory, reasoning, judgment, and perception impairment. The patient is disoriented. Short-term memory is impaired first.

- **Causes** include Alzheimer's disease, vascular and/or circulatory problems, brain tumors, head trauma, AIDS, Parkinson's disease, and substance abuse.
- **Onset** is gradual, usually worsening over months to years.
- **Improvement** generally does not occur and the condition worsens. Eventually the patient is unable to perform self-care.

Delirium: A state of mental confusion and excitement marked by disorientation to time and place, usually with illusions (an inaccurate perception or misinterpretation of a real sensory stimulus) and hallucinations (a false perception not accounted for by any exterior stimulus; it may be visual, tactile, auditory, gustatory, or olfactory). Speech is often incoherent and there may be continual aimless physical activity.

- **Causes** may be fever, shock, exhaustion, anxiety, drug overdose, or alcohol withdrawal.
- **Onset** is sudden and is thus a distinguishing feature from some other altered mental conditions; in the elderly, the onset may fluctuate with periods of mental clarity over 2 to 3 days.
- **Improvement** is possible if the cause is corrected, but the condition may be fatal, especially when alcohol withdrawal or serious coexisting illness is present.

Depression: A mental disorder marked by altered mood. There is diminished interest or pleasure in most or all activities. The patient may have poor appetite, psychomotor agitation or retardation, feelings of hopelessness, loss of energy, feelings of worthlessness or guilt, a diminished ability to concentrate, impaired memory, and recurrent thoughts of and wishes for death.

Causes may include reaction to a major life event such as loss of a loved one, a home, or one's independence. Some medications have a side effect of depression. Many times there is no obvious cause for depression, but current theories have a strong emphasis on neurobiologic causes and indicate that depression tends to run in families.

Onset is generally rapid but may take days to weeks to be obvious.

Improvement is possible with time, situation change, and/or medical treatment.

Table 7–1. DIFFERENCES AMONG DELIRIUM, DEMENTIA, AND DEPRESSION

	Delirium	Dementia	Depression
Onset	Rapid	Slow	Rapid
Duration	Short	Long	Short or long
Night symptoms	May worsen	Frequently worsen	Usually do not worsen
Cognitive functions	Variable	Stable	Variable
Physical causes	Common	None	Possible
Recent changes	Common	None or minimal	Common
Suicidal ideation	Rare	Rare	Common
Low self-esteem	Rare	Rare	Common

(continued on the following page)

Table 7–1. DIFFERENCES AMONG DELIRIUM, DEMENTIA, AND DEPRESSION (continued)

	Delirium	Dementia	Depression
History of psychiatric symptoms	Not usually	Rare	Common
Mood	Labile	Labile	Depressed
Behavior	Labile	Labile	Slowed thought and motor processes

Source: Anderson, MA: Caring for Older Adults Holistically, ed. 3. FA Davis, Philadelphia, 2003, p. 224, with permission.

MEDICATIONS AND THE OLDER ADULT

FACTS

The older patient typically takes more than six medicines per day.

Older patients with several comorbid conditions may take more than six medicines per day.

Drug toxicity is a common problem.

POTENTIAL PREDISPOSING FACTORS FOR DRUG TOXICITY IN THE ELDERLY

Drug interactions are possible because of multiple drugs being used to treat several conditions.

Reduced hepatic function results in altered drug metabolism.

Reduced hepatic and renal function may lead to drug accumulation with subsequent toxicity (reduced dosages are often appropriate).

Over-the-counter and herbal preparations may interact with prescribed medications.

RELATED NURSING CARE

Determine whether the drug dosage ordered is safe for the age and condition of the patient.

Assess medications for potential interactions.

Assess for proper medication use with respect to indication, time of administration, and with respect to food and water ingestion.

Avoid polypharmacy by asking the patient to report and show you the containers for every medication he or she is taking (both prescription and over-the-counter).

Know and monitor for signs of drug intolerance, toxicity and side effects. Common signs are:

- Confusion
- Constipation
- Depression
- Exprapyramidal symptoms
- Falls
- GI bleeds
- Incontinence
- Memory loss
- Nausea and vomiting
- Restlessness
- Sedation

SPECIFIC PRESCRIPTION MEDICATIONS COMMONLY USED BY OLDER ADULTS AND POTENTIAL HAZARDS

Medication	*Potential Hazard(s)*
ACE inhibitors	Hypotension, palpitations, elevated serum potassium
Antihistamines	Dizziness, sedation
Aspirin and other NSAIDs	GI bleed, GI upset
Benzodiazepines	Dizziness, significant sedation
Beta-blockers	Hypotension, dizziness, depression

(continued on the following page)

Medication	*Potential Hazard(s)*
Digoxin	Nausea, vomiting, dysrhythmias
Diuretics	Dizziness, decreased serum potassium
Morphine	Palpitations, hypotension
Haloperidol	Extrapyramidal symptoms
Ranitidine, cimetidine, famotidine	Mental confusion, drug interactions
Tricyclic antidepressants	Anticholinergic effects, sedation
Warfarin	Bleeding (watch for co-use of herbals)

SPECIFIC OVER-THE-COUNTER AND HERBAL MEDICINES COMMONLY USED BY OLDER ADULTS AND POTENTIAL HAZARDS

Medication	*Potential Hazard(s)*
Aloe (PO)	Diarrhea, electrolyte imbalances
Antacids	GI upset, electrolyte imbalances, interference with action of other meds
Antihistamines	Sedation, dizziness
Decongestants	Hypertension, nausea
Ephedra	Hypertension, palpitations
Gingko biloba	Palpitations, bleeding
Kava-kava	Excessive sedation

Medication	*Potential Hazard(s)*
Laxatives	Diarrhea, electrolyte imbalances
Licorice root	Hypertension, electrolyte imbalances
Ranitidine, cimetidine, famotidine	Mental confusion, drug interactions

NOTES

NOTES

NOTES

NOTES

Long-Term Care Fast Facts

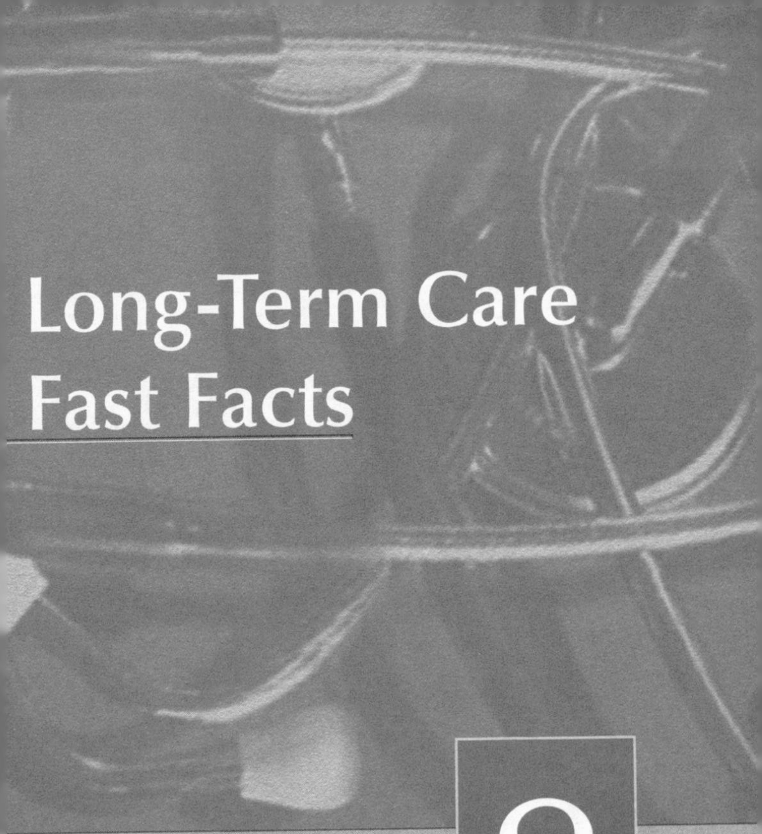

8

Section

Table 8–1.	PROBLEMS COMMONLY ENCOUNTERED IN LONG-TERM CARE AND PREVENTIVE STRATEGIES
Potential Problem	**Prevention**
Constipation due to decreased mobility and certain meds (example: calcium channel blockers, some antidepressants)	Assess: usual bowel habits and monitor for changes Provide and monitor intake of: adequate fluid and fiber Encourage: activity as tolerated
Boredom	Assess: interests and abilities Encourage: diversional activities, liberal visitation
Depression	Monitor for: tearfulness, loss of energy, expressions of guilt or self-criticism, irritability, inability to concentrate, decreased interest in daily activity, changes in appetite or body weight, insomnia or excessive sleep, deficits in social functioning Encourage: self-care, group activities, liberal visitation Listen to: concerns Express: optimism but guard against excessive cheerfulness
Decubitus ulcers	See *pressure (decubitus) ulcers*.
Falls	Assess: vision, gait, balance, orientation Ensure: adequate lighting that eliminates shadows, light switches within patient's reach, shoes that provide proper traction, avoidance of walking in socks or stocking feet, nonslippery floors, handrails in all rooms, electrical cords placed behind furniture or secured to floor, extended toilet seats, correction of vision problems

(continued on the following page)

Table 8–1. PROBLEMS COMMONLY ENCOUNTERED IN LONG-TERM CARE AND PREVENTIVE STRATEGIES (continued)

Potential Problem	Prevention
Falls (continued)	Eliminate: throw rugs and floor clutter
Incontinence	Assess: ability to control bladder and bowel movements Provide: scheduled times for toileting
Infections	Observe: universal precautions Assess: vital signs and lung sounds on a scheduled basis, appearance of urine when a catheter is in use Ensure: patient handwashing before meals, liberal fluid intake, pneumococcal and flu vaccines
Isolation	Monitor for: avoidance of interactions with others Encourage: group activities and dining, liberal visitation and passes when possible
Learned dependence	Encourage: decision making when possible, maximized self-care
Loss of privacy	Assess: usual habits (e.g., hours of sleep, TV viewing) and adaptability of potential roommates when a private room is not possible Knock: before entering room Provide: storage space that can be locked, privacy when requested
Medication side effects and/or interactions	Assess: for potential interactions each time a new drug is ordered Monitor for: changes in appetite, weight, behavior, elimination (bowel and bladder), change in vital signs

Table 8–1. PROBLEMS COMMONLY ENCOUNTERED IN LONG-TERM CARE AND PREVENTIVE STRATEGIES (continued)

Potential Problem	Prevention
	Suspect: drug side effects or interaction when there is any new complaint or change in condition or vital signs
Nutritional deficit	Assess: dentition and related suitability of diet Discuss: preferred diet with patient and significant others Provide: small frequent feedings, preferred food when possible, group dining if tolerated, assistance with feeding if needed Monitor: weight at least weekly; significant findings are: ≥5% involuntary weight loss in 30 days ≥10% involuntary weight loss in 180 days or less BMI ≤21 (See BMI table in Section 10.) Determine reason for any weight loss
Urinary retention	Monitor for: drugs with identified urinary tract side effects, I&O if patient has impaired communication or cognition Ensure: adequate fluids, toileting schedule, and access to facilities

PRESSURE (DECUBITUS) ULCERS

PREVENTION

In the well-nourished patient, pressure ulcers can usually be prevented by implementing the following measures:

- Maintain adequate nutritional and hydration status.
- Do not allow skin to remain in contact with plastic, nylon, or waterproof surfaces.
- Avoid the use of adhesives such as tape on pressure-prone areas or on red or broken skin.
- Keep the skin clean and well moisturized; although it is important to remove urine or fecal material from the skin immediately, older people do not need daily baths.
- Avoid the use of drying soaps, alcohol, and iodine on the skin.
- Rinse the skin well when soap is used.
- Pat rather than rub skin dry after bathing to avoid friction.
- Remove fallen food particles from the bed after each meal.
- Keep the bed free of personal articles such as combs, brushes, or hairpins.
- Change position frequently; every 1 to 2 hours is ideal.
- Lift and do not pull or drag extremities when repositioning to avoid friction on skin.
- Use a draw or lift sheet for moving heavy parts of the body.
- Perform daily range of motion exercises to promote circulation.
- Use pressure-reducing support surfaces such as pillows and air, water, or gel-filled mattresses to avoid pressure on bony prominences.
- Avoid use of rubber donut-shaped support devices, which may impair circulation.
- Avoid the use of irritating straps on heel or elbow protectors.
- Do not massage bony prominences as this could damage delicate skin and/or capillaries.

TREATMENT

For existing pressure ulcers, continue use of the measures cited above and implement the following:

- Assess and record the following characteristics of ulcer initially and at scheduled intervals:
  - width, length, depth
  - drainage or exudate
  - odor
  - condition of surrounding tissue
- Clean ulcer with saline and remove necrotic tissue by irrigating with a prescribed solution.
- Keep a moist dressing over the ulcer to prevent complete drying that may result in bleeding and disrupt newly forming capillaries.
- Monitor for and report signs of infection such as fever, purulent drainage, or redness and swelling of tissue surrounding the ulcer.

NOTES

NOTES

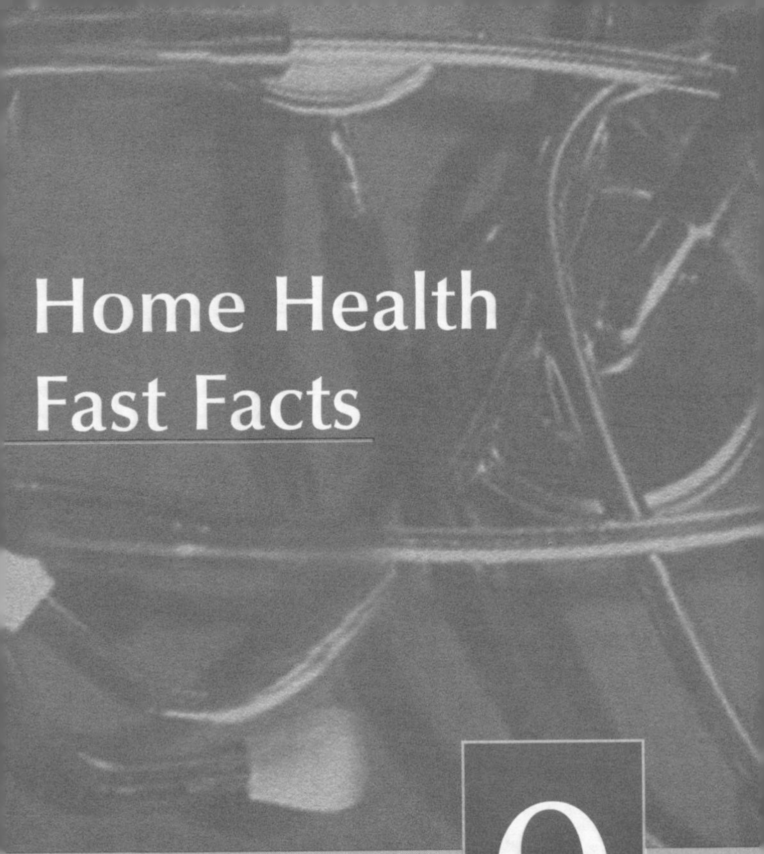

Home Health Fast Facts

Section 9

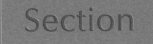

HOME HEALTH TERMINOLOGY AND COMMON ABBREVIATIONS

APHA: American Public Health Association
CDC: Centers for Disease Control and Prevention
COPS: Conditions of Participation (Medicare)
DRG: Diagnosis Related Group
HCFA: Home Care Financing Administration
HHA: Home health agency or home health aide
HHC: Home health care
HIM: Health insurance manual
HME: Home medical equipment
JCAHO: Joint Commission on Accreditation of Healthcare Organizations
MOW: Meals on Wheels
MSS: Medical social services
NIH: National Institutes of Health
OSHA: Occupational Safety and Health Administration
OT: Occupational therapy
POC: Plan of care
PT: Physical therapy
RHHI: Regional home health intermediary
S-LP: Speech-language pathology
SNV: Skilled nursing visit
Title XVIII: The Medicare section of the Social Security Act
Title XIX: The Medicaid section of the Social Security Act
Title XX: The Social Services section of the Social Security Act
VNA: Visiting Nurses Association
WIC: Women, Infants, and Children Program

MEDICARE CERTIFICATION (ACCEPTANCE) FOR HOME CARE

The following criteria must be met for a patient to be eligible for home care under Medicare:

- Patient lives within the service area
- Patient is homebound—physically or mentally unable to go to a facility for care

- Patient has needs that require skilled nursing care
- Improvement can be expected with part-time, intermittent care
- Patient and family accept home health care
- Family and/or another caregiver is available and willing to learn and participate in patient care as required
- Orders/protocols for care have been completed by primary health care provider or referring physician
- Electrical supply is sufficient for equipment
- Water supply is safe for health care procedures
- Residence is physically safe

NOTE
Medicare patients meet eligibility requirements for home care if skilled nursing care is warranted 4 or fewer days per week.
If care is needed 5 or more days per week, eligibility is established only if the care is not needed indefinitely.
Those patients who are incapable of self-injection of daily insulin administration, and for whom there is no care provider available, may receive daily visits while trying to locate a caregiver.

FREQUENCY AND DURATION OF HOME CARE

FREQUENCY

According to the *Health Insurance Manual* (HIM-11), frequency is defined as the number of visits, per discipline, to be rendered and may be expressed in days, weeks, or months.

DURATION

Duration is used to refer to the "length of stay" in home care, such as 60 to 62 days. Recertification by the physician/NP and funding source may need to occur to allow for care beyond the prescribed frequency and duration. The RN must determine if the care can feasibly be carried out in the home, if the patient and family will cooperate, and if the care may reasonably result in patient improvement. If the patient's needs exceed the ability of the agency to provide care, other referrals or arrangements must be made. Admitting a patient for care and then prematurely discharging them may be considered abandonment.

HOME HEALTH VISITS

INITIAL VISIT

- Assessment of patient, family, and environment.
- Determination of need for social service evaluation and other supportive community resources such as Meals on Wheels.
- Signing of informed consent
- Providing the patient or responsible family member with the following:
  - A copy of the signed informed consent
  - Phone numbers for the home health care agency
  - Instructions on how to report complaints
  - Emergency preparedness instructions (See *Home Health Safety*.)
  - An explanation of the plan of care, expected frequency and duration of care, anticipated outcomes, and discharge plans
- Documentation of all actions

SUBSEQUENT VISITS

- Reassessment and evaluation of patient progress
- Provision of care
- Teaching
- Documentation of each action

TERMINATION VISIT

- Assessment and evaluation of patient progress
- Provision of care
- Teaching
- Informing the patient and family regarding discharge plan

- Informing the patient regarding follow-up visits with any other member of the health care team
- Arranging follow-up with referring professional and other agencies to which the patient has been referred
- Assessing the patient's and family's understanding and acceptance of discharge plan
- Documenting each action

THE HOME HEALTH RECORD

PURPOSE

The home health record plays a critical role in the communication and documentation processes needed to ensure legality and quality of home health care. The home health record also plays an essential role in the reimbursement process for home health care. Third-party payers, including Medicare and Medicaid, require that each of certain components be included in the home health record and will not pay for cases that do not include these.

REQUIRED COMPONENTS

1. Diagnoses and/or problems requiring skilled nursing care must be listed with identification of the principal or acute problem. Diagnoses are usually submitted by the referring health care provider. (Skilled care can be provided only by an RN or supervised by an RN. Skilled care includes advanced care procedures, complex assessments, care evaluations, and teaching. Supervision visits are those in which an RN provides skilled care and observes and evaluates the care being provided by a home health aide. Supervision visits are required every 2 weeks as a condition of participation under Medicare.)
2. Orders and/or protocols for care, submitted by the referring health care provider to include:
   Frequency—the number of visits per discipline to be rendered, expressed in days, weeks, or months

Duration—the length of stay (for the patient) in home care, such as 60 to 62 days

3. Any limitations for length of care or number of visits.
4. Patient or guardian informed consent for care (updates are required when there are changes in the plan of care).
5. Admission assessment by an RN (See the description of this assessment that follows.)
6. Referral reports from therapists or community agencies.
7. Agency contact information (one copy to remain in the agency and one in the patient's home).
8. Plan of care (labeled "Plan of Treatment" and referred to as "POC" (See *Plan of Care.*)
9. Documentation of home health care rendered (See *Documentation.*)

ADMISSION ASSESSMENT

PATIENT ASSESSMENT

- Holistic assessment: history and physical with emphasis on system/problem area warranting care, as well as cultural, social, and spiritual assessment
- Patient's learning needs and ability
- Homebound status evaluation including ability to perform activities of daily living
- Family/care provider support systems
- Safety and acceptability of home care environment
- Dated nursing diagnoses
- Quantified (measurable) patient goals
- Specific nursing interventions and alternatives
- Plan for number of visits or time frame for care
- Discharge plans

FAMILY ASSESSMENT

- Willingness and ability to participate in care
- Understanding of emergency actions
- Family stress

ENVIRONMENTAL ASSESSMENT

- Electrical wiring
- Rodents/insects
- Safe water supply and accessibility
- Integrity of flooring and steps
- Temperature of room (heating/cooling for high-risk cases)
- Presence of potentially dangerous pets
- Neighborhood crime elements or environmental hazards
- Plan for disposing of biohazardous waste, if needed

NOTE: Special detailed assessments should be done for premature infant care, elderly, disabled, or mentally ill.

PLAN OF CARE (LABELED "PLAN OF TREATMENT")

The treatment plan is referred to as the "POC" in laws and reimbursement guidelines or the Visit Record (HCFA Form 485/6). A copy of the POC is left in the patient's home. The POC includes the following:

- Specific responses (preferably measurable) to nursing interventions.

> Example: "Patient can stand for 30 seconds without assistance."

- Description of homebound status every week, with reference to physical, mental, or emotional limitations, written in specific terms; *homebound is synonymous with "confined primarily to the home as a result of a medical condition."*
- Annotation of continuing need and use of medical equipment.
- Description of calls to physician, nurse practitioner, or agency for orders or referral.
- Description of any "interdisciplinary" discussions/conferences.
- Care-related quotations of patient/family member whenever possible.
- Documentation of any complaints and follow-up actions.

- Record of progress toward anticipated discharge date and goals.
- Time and date for next visit.
- Description of plans for care during next visit.

DOCUMENTATION

At each visit, documentation of the home health care rendered should:

- Describe care rendered
- Describe teaching to patient and/or family
- Describe family member's ability to provide care
- Describe specific responses to nursing interventions

> Example: "Patient walks 15 feet without assistance."

- Describe why progress has not been made, if necessary
- Describe homebound status at least once a week, with reference to physical, mental or emotional limitation, written in specific terms (*Homebound means "confined primarily to the home as a result of a medical condition."*)
- Document continuing need for and use of medical equipment
- Record progress toward anticipated discharge date and goals
- Describe calls to any other health care team members
- Describe plans for care during next planned visit
- Record time and date for next visit

AVOID

- Vague remarks, such as "improved," "unstable," or "reviewed"
- Use of the word "monitor" when continued assessment or evaluation of a condition is needed
- Reference to any incident reports submitted to agency
- Abbreviations, except those approved by the agency
- Making assumptions or blaming
- Negative remarks about the cultural or religious beliefs of the family

ANECDOTAL NOTES

- Keep a brief *personal* and confidential record of patients, dates seen, care provided, and any special events.

HOME HEALTH SAFETY

PERSONAL SAFETY

Home health personnel should never visit a home they believe to be unsafe because of environmental hazards or personal safety risks; it may be necessary to arrange for family, police, or other special escort. Any missed visit should be clearly documented in the record and reported to the agency supervisor.

BIOHAZARDOUS WASTE

The home health agency is responsible for supplying the nurse and aide with gloves, aprons, face shields, and disposable bags used during patient care. The nurse must be informed of the agency procedure for transport and disposal of biohazardous waste.

EMERGENCY PREPAREDNESS INSTRUCTIONS FOR PATIENT/FAMILY (OFTEN REQUIRED BY STATE LAWS)

Hurricane evacuation plan
Fire escape routes
Flood/earthquake readiness
Knowledge of 911 availability
Family contact phone numbers
Home health agency and referring doctor's or nurse practitioner's phone numbers

LEGAL ASPECTS OF HOME HEALTH PATIENT CARE

1. Continually assess patient's needs; if the patient's needs exceed the ability of the agency to provide care, other referrals or arrangements must be made.
2. Notify physician/nurse practitioner of any change in patient's condition.

3. Be familiar with current JACHO Standards for Home Care.
4. Care should reflect current professional standards of practice.
5. Secure consent for any change in procedures; document any approval or refusal by the patient.
6. Inform patient of risks if care is refused and have patient initial record, then notify physician/nurse practitioner.
7. If patient is injured while under your care, do not leave him or her unattended.
8. Discharge: accepting or admitting a patient for care and then prematurely discharging him or her may be considered abandonment.

INCIDENT REPORTING

- Report any unexpected care event, accident, or action according to agency policies.
- Do not put a copy or any reference to an incident report in the patient's record.
- Report witnessed *or* unobserved:
  Falls
  Damage to property
  Equipment failures
  Crimes
  Auto accidents
  Burns
  Treatment injuries
  Possible abuse and/or neglect

ADVANCED DIRECTIVES

Provide patients an opportunity to complete an advance directive according to agency and state policies/laws.

CONFIDENTIALITY AND PRIVACY

- Do not leave any patient record in the patient's home.
- Avoid calling the physician/nurse practitioner from a phone in a public area.
- Do not leave confidential messages on the patient's answering machine.

NOTES

NOTES

NOTES

Nutrition Fast Facts

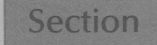

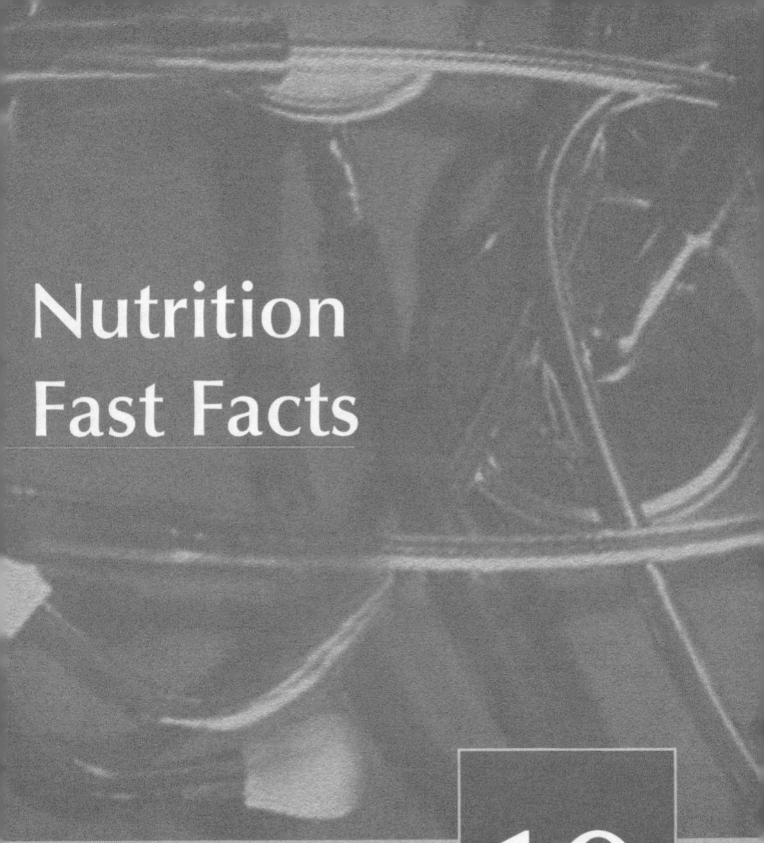

Section

10

DIETARY GUIDELINES FOR HEALTHY ADULTS

Based on The Food Guide Pyramid concept, the U.S. Department of Agriculture makes the following dietary recommendations for adults:

Type Food (Group)	*Number of Daily Servings*
Bread, cereal, rice, pasta	6–11
Vegetable	3–5
Fruit	2–4
Milk, yogurt, cheese	2–3
Meat, poultry, fish, dried beans, eggs, nuts	2–3
Fats, oils, sweets	Use sparingly

The following approximate number of calories are recommended for adults. (Caloric requirements vary according to age and activity level.)

Type Adult	*Number of Calories Needed*
Sedentary women and some older adults	1600
Active women and some sedentary men	2200
Active men and some very active women	2800

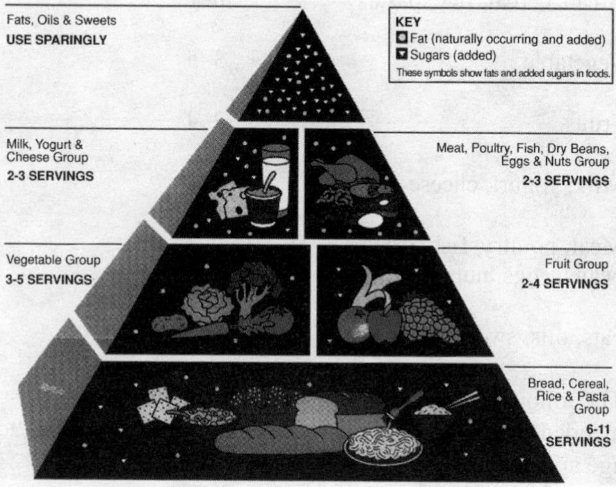

Figure 10–1. Food guide pyramid. (From the U.S. Department of Agriculture, Human Nutrition Information Services; and the U.S. Department of Health and Human Services.)

Table 10–1. RECOMMENDED DIETARY ALLOWANCES (RDAs), * REVISED 2000

Age (yr) and Sex Group	Calcium (mg/d)	Phosphorus (mg/d)	Magnesium (mg/d)	Vitamin (mcg/d)†‡	Fluoride (mg/d)	Thiamine (mg/d)	Riboflavin (mg/d)
INFANTS							
0.0–0.5	210	100	30	5	0.01	0.2	0.3
0.5–1.0	270	275	75	5	0.5	0.3	0.4
CHILDREN							
1–3	500	460	80	5	0.7	0.5	0.5
4–8	800	500	130	5	1	0.6	0.6
MEN							
9–18	1300	1250	240	5	2	0.9	0.9
14–18	1300	1250	410	5	3	1.2	1.3
19–30	1000	700	400	5	4	1.2	1.3
31–50	1000	700	420	5	4	1.2	1.3
51–70	1200	700	420	10	4	1.2	1.3
71+	1200	700	420	15	4	1.2	1.3

(continued on the following page)

Table 10–1. RECOMMENDED DIETARY ALLOWANCES (RDAs), * REVISED 2000 (continued)

Age (yr) and Sex Group	Calcium (mg/d)	Phosphorus (mg/d)	Magnesium (mg/d)	Vitamin (mcg/d)†‡	Fluoride (mg/d)	Thiamine (mg/d)	Riboflavin (mg/d)
WOMEN							
9–13	1300	1250	240	5	2	0.9	0.9
14–18	1300	1250	360	5	3	1	1
19–30	1000	700	310	5	3	1.1	1.1
31–50	1000	700	320	5	3	1.1	1.1
51–70	1200	700	320	10	3	1.1	1.1
71+	1200	700	320	15	3	1.1	1.1
PREGNANT WOMEN							
≤18	1300	1250	400	5	3	1.4	1.4
19–30	1000	700	350	5	3	1.4	1.4
31–50	1000	700	360	5	3	1.4	1.4
LACTATING WOMEN							
≤18	1300	1250	360	5	3	1.5	1.6
19–30	1000	700	310	5	3	1.5	1.6
31–50	1000	700	320	5	3	1.5	1.6

Age (yr) and Sex Group	Niacin (mg/d)§	Vitamin B_6 (mg/d)	Folate (mcg/d)¶	Vitamin B_{12} (mcg/d)	Pantothenic Acid (mg/d)	Biotin (mcg/d)	Choline** (mcg/d)
INFANTS							
0.0–0.5	2	0.1	65	0.4	1.7	5	125
0.5–1.0	4	0.3	80	0.5	1.8	6	150
CHILDREN							
1–3	6	0.5	150	0.9	2	8	200
4–8	8	0.6	200	1.2	3	12	250
MEN							
9–13	12	1.0	300	1.8	4	20	375
14–18	16	1.3	400	2.4	5	25	550
19–30	16	1.3	400	2.4	5	30	550
31–50	16	1.3	400	2.4	5	30	550
51–70	16	1.7	400	2.4	5	30	550
71+	16	1.7	400	2.4	5	30	550

(continued on the following page)

Table 10–1. RECOMMENDED DIETARY ALLOWANCES (RDAs), * REVISED 2000 (continued)

Age (yr) and Sex Group	Niacin (mg/d)§	Vitamin B_6 (mg/d)	Folate (mcg/d)¶	Vitamin B_{12} (mcg/d)	Pantothenic Acid (mg/d)	Biotin (mcg/d)	Choline** (mcg/d)
WOMEN							
9–13	12	1	300	1.8	4	20	375
14–18	14	1.2	400	2.4	5	25	400
19–30	14	1.3	400	2.4	5	30	425
31–50	14	1.3	400	2.4	5	30	425
51–70	14	1.5	400	2.4	5	30	425
71+	14	1.5	400	2.4	5	30	425
PREGNANT WOMEN							
18–50	18	1.9	600	2.6	6	30	450
LACTATING WOMEN							
18–50	17	2	500	2.8	7	35	550

*The allowances, expressed as average daily intakes over time, are intended to provide for individual variations among most normal persons as they live in the United States under usual environmental stresses. Diets should be based on a variety of common foods in order to provide other nutrients for which human requirements have been less well defined.

†As cholecalciferol, 1 mcg cholecalciferol = 40 IU vitamin D.

‡In the absence of adequate exposure to sunlight.

§As niacin equivalents. 1 mg of niacin = 60 mg of tryptophan; 0 to 6 months = preformed niacin.

¶As dietary folate equivalents (DFE). 1 DFE = 1 mcg food folate = 0.6 mcg of folic acid (from fortified food or supplement) consumed with food = 0.5 mcg of synthetic (supplemental) folic acid taken on an empty stomach.

**Although adequate intakes have been set for choline, there are few data to assess whether a dietary supply of choline is needed at all stages of the life cycle, and it may be that the choline requirement can be met by endogenous synthesis at some of these stages.

Source: Deglin, JH, and Vallerand, AH: Davis's Drug Guide for Nurses, ed 8. FA Davis, Philadelphia, 2003, pp 1153–1154, with permission.

Table 10–2. VITAMINS AND MINERALS

Supplement	RDA men	RDA women	Needed for	Food Sources
FAT-SOLUBLE VITAMINS				
A	1000 RE	800 RE	Proper vision, growth	Liver, milk, eggs, beta-carotene found in dark-orange and dark-green fruits and vegetables (carrots, pumpkins, broccoli, spinach)
D	5 μg	5 μg	Proper bone formation, cell function	Fortified milk, liver, fish
E	10 mg	8 mg	Immune system functioning, destruction of free radicals (by-products of metabolism that can cause vascular damage)	Vegetable oils, green leafy vegetables, whole grains

K	80 μg	65 μg	Blood clotting, bone formation	Green leafy vegetables, dairy products
WATER-SOLUBLE VITAMINS				
C	60 μg	60 μg	Collagen synthesis, destruction of free radicals, assistance in iron absorption, infection fighting, healing	Fruits and vegetables (especially citrus fruits)
Thiamine (B_1)	1.5 mg	1.4 mg	Converting carbohydrates and fats to energy	Fortified and whole grains, lean cuts of pork, legumes (beans and peas), seeds, nuts
Riboflavin (B_2)	1.7 mg	1.3 mg	Converting bodily fuels to energy	Dairy products, meat, poultry, fish, whole-wheat and fortified-grain products, green leafy vegetables
Niacin (B_3)	19 mg	15 mg	Converting carbohydrates, fats, and amino acids to energy	Meat, milk, eggs, poultry, fish, enriched breads and cereals

(continued on the following page)

Table 10–2. VITAMINS AND MINERALS (continued)

Supplement	RDA men	RDA women	Needed for	Food Sources
WATER-SOLUBLE VITAMINS (continued)				
B_6	2 mg	1.6 mg	Assistance in at least 50 enzyme reactions—the most important regulate nervous system activity	Chicken, fish, liver, pork, eggs, whole-wheat products, peanuts, walnuts
Folate	200 μg	180 μg	Manufacturing of DNA and new body cells	Liver, leafy vegetables, legumes, fruits
B_{12}	2 μg	2 μg	Manufacturing of new body cells and mature new red blood cells, maintenance of nerve growth, protection of nerve cells	Meat, poultry, fish, dairy products

MINERALS				
Calcium	800 mg	800 mg	Building bone, transmitting nerve impulses, and aiding muscle contractions	Dairy foods, canned sardines and salmon with the bones, fortified orange juice; smaller amounts in some fruits and vegetables (broccoli, tangerines, pumpkins)
Phosphorus	800 mg	800 mg	Building bone, helping the body utilize energy and reproduce cells	In nearly all foods
Magnesium	350 mg	280 mg	Holding calcium in tooth enamel, assistance in relaxing muscles after contractions	Nuts, legumes, cereal grains, green vegetables, seafood
Iron	10 mg	15 mg	Transporting oxygen in red blood cells and muscle cells, DNA synthesis, formation of major enzymes	Meat, poultry, fish, dried beans and peas, fortified grain products

(continued on the following page)

Table 10–2. VITAMINS AND MINERALS (continued)

Supplement	RDA men	RDA women	Needed for	Food Sources
MINERALS (continued)				
Zinc	15 mg	12 mg	Promotion of healing and growth, maintaining immune function, DNA synthesis, and a normal sense of taste	Meats, oysters, milk, egg yolks
Iodine	150 µg	150 µg	Helping the thyroid regulate metabolism	Seafood, iodized table salt
Selenium	70 µg	55 µg	Destruction of free radicals, formation of enzymes	Fish, meat, breads, cereals

Source: Who Needs Vitamins? Special Report 4:10, 1992. Whittle Communications LP, Knoxville, with permission.

BODY MASS INDEX (BMI) TABLE

BMI	***Interpretation***
<18.5	underweight
18.5–24.9	normal
25–29.9	overweight
30–34.9	obesity (class 1)
35–39.5	obesity (class 2)
≥ 40	extreme obesity

For more information, go to:
http://www.nhlbi.nih.gov/guidelines/obesity/ob_gdlns.htm.

BODY MASS INDEX TABLE

	Normal							*Overweight*					*Obese*																							*Extreme Obesity*
BMI	19	20	21	22	23	24	25	26	27	28	29	30	31	32	33	34	35	36	37	38	39	40	41	42	43	44	45	46	47	48	49	50	51	52	53	54
Height (inches)	**Body Weight (pounds)**																																			
58	91	96	100	105	110	115	119	124	129	134	138	143	148	153	158	162	167	172	177	181	186	191	196	201	205	210	215	220	224	229	234	239	244	248	253	258
59	94	99	104	109	114	119	124	128	133	138	143	148	153	158	163	168	173	178	183	188	193	198	203	208	212	217	222	227	232	237	242	247	252	257	262	267
60	97	102	107	112	118	123	128	133	138	143	148	153	158	163	168	174	179	184	189	194	199	204	209	215	220	225	230	235	240	245	250	255	261	266	271	276
61	100	106	111	116	122	127	132	137	143	148	153	158	164	169	174	180	185	190	195	201	206	211	217	222	227	232	238	243	248	254	259	264	269	275	280	285
62	104	109	115	120	126	131	136	142	147	153	158	164	169	175	180	186	191	196	202	207	213	218	224	229	235	240	246	251	256	262	267	273	278	284	289	295
63	107	113	118	124	130	135	141	146	152	158	163	169	175	180	186	191	197	203	208	214	220	225	231	237	242	248	254	259	265	270	278	282	287	293	299	304
64	110	116	122	128	134	140	145	151	157	163	169	174	180	186	192	197	204	209	215	221	227	232	238	244	250	256	262	267	273	279	285	291	296	302	308	314
65	114	120	126	132	138	144	150	156	162	168	174	180	186	192	198	204	210	216	222	228	234	240	246	252	258	264	270	276	282	288	294	300	306	312	318	324

66	118	124	130	136	142	148	155	161	167	173	179	186	192	198	204	210	216	223	229	235	241	247	253	260	266	272	278	284	291	297	303	309	315	322	328	334
67	121	127	134	140	146	153	159	166	172	178	185	191	198	204	211	217	223	230	236	242	249	255	261	268	274	280	287	293	299	306	312	319	325	331	338	344
68	125	131	138	144	151	158	164	171	177	184	190	197	203	210	216	223	230	236	243	249	256	262	269	276	282	289	295	302	308	315	322	328	335	341	348	354
69	128	135	142	149	155	162	169	176	182	189	196	203	209	216	223	230	236	243	250	257	263	270	277	284	291	297	304	311	318	324	331	338	345	351	358	365
70	132	139	146	153	160	167	174	181	188	195	202	209	216	222	229	236	243	250	257	264	271	278	285	292	299	306	313	320	327	334	341	348	355	362	369	376
71	136	143	150	157	165	172	179	186	193	200	208	215	222	229	236	243	250	257	265	272	279	286	293	301	308	315	322	329	338	343	351	358	365	372	379	386
72	140	147	154	162	169	177	184	191	199	206	213	221	228	235	242	250	258	265	272	279	287	294	302	309	316	324	331	338	346	353	361	368	375	383	390	397
73	144	151	159	166	174	182	189	197	204	212	219	227	235	242	250	257	265	272	280	288	295	302	310	318	325	333	340	348	355	363	371	378	386	393	401	408
74	148	155	163	171	179	186	194	202	210	218	225	233	241	249	256	264	272	280	287	295	303	311	319	326	334	342	350	358	365	373	381	389	396	404	412	420
75	152	160	168	176	184	192	200	208	216	224	232	240	248	256	264	272	279	287	295	303	311	319	327	335	343	351	359	367	375	383	391	399	407	415	423	431
76	156	164	172	180	189	197	205	213	221	230	238	246	254	263	271	279	287	295	304	312	320	328	336	344	353	361	369	377	385	394	402	410	418	426	435	443

Source: Adapted from *Clinical Guidelines on the Identification, Evaluation, and Treatment of Overweight and Obesity in Adults: The Evidence Report.* National Institutes of Health.

NEGATIVE INTERACTIONS BETWEEN VITAMINS/MINERALS AND DRUGS

Vitamin/Mineral	*Drug*	*Interaction*
Vitamin A	Isotretinoin	Danger of toxicity
Vitamin B_1	Loop diuretics	Diuretics cause B_1 deficiency
Vitamin B_2	Chlorpromazine	Causes mild B_2 deficiency
Vitamin B_2	Fluphenazine	Causes mild B_2 deficiency
Vitamin B_2	Thioridazine	Causes mild B_2 deficiency
Vitamin B_6	Isoniazid	May cause B_6 deficiency
Vitamin B_6	Levodopa	Decreased efficacy in the presence of B_6
Vitamin B_{12}	Chloramphenicol	Decreased response to B_{12}
Folic Acid	Phenytoin	Increased seizure risk
Folic Acid	Phenobarbital	Increased seizure risk
Folic Acid	Primidone	Increased seizure risk
Folic Acid	Methotrexate	Causes folate deficiency
Folic Acid	Pentamidine	Causes folate deficiency
Folic Acid	Pyrimethamine	Causes folate deficiency

Vitamin/Mineral	*Drug*	*Interaction*
Folic Acid	Trimethoprim	Causes folate deficiency
Vitamin C	Warfarin	Decreased anticoagulant effect
Vitamin D	Phenytoin	Causes vitamin D deficiency
Vitamin D	Phenobarbital	Causes vitamin D deficiency
Vitamin E	Warfarin	Increased anticoagulant effect
Vitamin K	Warfarin	Decreased anticoagulant effect
Calcium	Tetracyclines	Decreased absorption in the presence of calcium
Calcium	Verapamil	Decreased efficacy in the presence of calcium
Beta-carotene	Colestipol	Causes beta-carotene deficiency
Beta-carotene	Cholestyramine	Causes beta-carotene deficiency
Iron	Cholestyramine	Binds iron in GI tract
Iron	Colestipol	Binds iron in GI tract
Iron	Chloramphenicol	Decreased response to iron

(continued on the following page)

Vitamin/Mineral	*Drug*	*Interaction*
Magnesium	Cisplatin	Causes magnesium deficiency
Magnesium	Digoxin	Causes magnesium deficiency
Sodium	Lithium	Antagonized by high sodium, potentiated by low sodium

Source: Published in RN, June 1993.

DIETARY GUIDELINES FOR FOOD SOURCES

Potassium-Rich Foods

avocados
bananas
broccoli
cantaloupe
dried fruits
fish
grapefruit
honey dew
kiwi
lima beans
meats
navy beans
nuts
oranges
peaches
potatoes
prunes
rhubarb
spinach
sunflower seeds
tomatoes

Sodium-Rich Foods

baking mixes
(pancakes, muffins)
barbecue sauce
buttermilk
butter/margarine
canned chili
canned seafood
canned soups
canned spaghetti sauce
cured meats
dry onion soup mix
"fast" foods
frozen dinners
macaroni and cheese
microwave dinners
Parmesan cheese
pickles
potato salad
pretzels, potato chips
salad dressings (prepared)
salt
sauerkraut
tomato ketchup

Calcium-Rich Foods

- bok choy
- broccoli
- canned salmon/sardines
- clams
- cream soups
- milk and dairy products
- molasses (blackstrap)
- oysters
- refried beans
- spinach
- tofu
- turnip greens

Vitamin K–Rich Foods

- asparagus
- beans
- broccoli
- Brussels sprouts
- cabbage
- cauliflower
- cheeses
- collards
- fish
- kale
- milk
- mustard greens
- pork
- rice
- spinach
- turnips
- yogurt

Low-Sodium Foods

- baked or broiled poultry
- canned pumpkin
- cooked turnips
- egg yolk
- fresh vegetables
- fruit
- grits (not instant)
- honey
- jams and jellies
- lean meats
- low-calorie mayonnaise
- macaroons
- potatoes
- puffed wheat and rice
- red kidney and lima beans
- sherbet
- unsalted nuts
- whiskey

Foods That Acidify Urine

- cheeses
- corn
- cranberries
- eggs
- fish
- grains (breads and cereals)
- lentils
- meats
- nuts (Brazil, filberts, walnuts)
- pasta
- plums
- poultry
- prunes
- rice

(continued on the following page)

Foods That Alkalinize Urine

all fruits except cranberries, prunes, plums
all vegetables (except corn)
milk
nuts (almonds, chesnuts)

Foods Containing Tyramine

aged cheeses (blue, Boursault, brick, Brie, Camembert, cheddar, Emmenthaler, Gruyère, mozzarella, Parmesan, Romano, Roquefort, Stilton, Swiss)
American processed cheese
avocados (especially over-ripe)
bananas
bean curd
beer and ale
caffeine-containing beverages (coffee, tea, colas)
caviar
chocolate
distilled spirits
fermented sausage (bologna, salami, pepperoni, summer sausage)
liver
meats prepared with tenderizer
miso soup
over-ripe fruit
peanuts
raisins
rasberries
red wine (especially Chianti)
sauerkraut
sherry
shrimp paste
smoked or pickled fish
soy sauce
vermouth
yeasts
yogurt

Iron-Rich Foods

cereals
clams
dried beans and peas
dried fruit
leafy green vegetables
lean red meats
molasses, blackstrap
organ meats

Vitamin D–Rich Foods

canned salmon, sardines, tuna
cereals
fish
fish liver oils
fortified milk
nonfat dry milk

Source: Deglin, JH, and Vallerand, AH: Davis's Drug Guide for Nurses, ed 8. FA Davis, Philadelphia, 2003, pp 1151–1152, with permission).

FOOD AND DRUG INTERACTIONS

The absorption or action of the drugs listed here is *slowed or reduced in the presence of food.*

NOTE: If the drug causes gastric irritation in individual patients, it may be necessary to give the medication with food even though drug absorption may be slowed or efficacy may be reduced.

Acetaminophen (Tylenol)
Ampicillin
Alendronate (Fosamax)
Aspirin
Azithromycin
Captopril
Chloramphenicol
Digoxin (binds to fiber)
Enoxacin (Penetrex)
Erythromycin (base and stearate forms)
Isosorbide
Lansoprazole (Prevacid)
Levodopa (especially if meal is high in protein)
Nisoldipine (Sular) (especially if meal is high in fat)
Nitroglycerin (oral)
Norfloxacin (Noroxin)
Ofloxacin (Floxin)
Penicillin G
Omeprazole (Prilosec)
Tetracycline

The absorption of bioavailability of the following drugs is *improved in the presence of food*:

Cefuroxime (Ceftin)
Griseofulvin
Hydralazine (Apresoline)
Indinavir (Crixivan)
Ketoconazole (Nizoral)
Lovastatin (Mevacor)
Metoprolol (Lopresor, Toprol-XL)
Propranolol (Inderal)
Spironolactone (Aldactone)
Ticlopidine (Ticlid)
Zalcitabine (ddC)

(continued on the following page)

The following foods *interact negatively with monoamine oxidase inhibitors*. They may induce hypertensive crisis by causing tyramine release.

Aged cheese
Avocados (especially overripe)
Bananas
Chocolate
Cured meats (bologna, salami, pepperoni, summer sausage, smoked sausage)
Distilled spirits
Herring
Overripe fruit
Raisins
Bean pods
Canned figs
Caffeinated beverages
Chicken livers
Raspberries
Red wine (especially Chianti)
Sherry
Soy sauce
Yeast preparations
Yogurt
Vermouth

GRAPEFRUIT–DRUG INTERACTION POTENTIAL

Drugs that utilize the CYP3A4 metabolism pathway may have higher serum drug concentrations and associated adverse effects when taken by a patient who consumes grapefruit or grapefruit juice. This is thought to be due to local inhibition of CYP3A4 in the intestinal wall. Potential for interaction occurs with the drugs listed below. More specific drug interaction information may be accessed at: http://www.powernetdesign.com/grapefruit/.

amiodarone
amlodipine
atorvastatin
buspirone
carbamazepine
carvedilol
cerivastatin
lovastatin
methadone
midazolam
nifedipine
nimodipine
pravastatin
tacrolimus

Anemia, sickle cell	Increase fluids to at least $1\frac{1}{2}$ times usual requirement for weight and age. Folic acid (folate) may be given.	Sickled cells tend to clump together, causing vaso-occlusion. Increased fluid intake results in hemodilution, which impedes the clumping process. Folic acid essential for normal RBC formation.
Arthritis	Maintain ideal body weight by limiting fat and caloric intake.	Excess weight causes stress on joints.
Burns	High kilocaloric and protein intake. Give vitamin and mineral supplements. Enteral or parenteral feedings if PO feedings inadequate.	Calories and protein needed for healing. Decreased level of consciousness, poor appetite, or paralytic ileus may interfere with PO intake.
Calculi, renal	Generous fluid intake. Dietary calcium adequate to maintain serum calcium and prevent excessive bone loss of calcium.	Calculi most often composed of calcium, which is more soluble in acidic urine. Dilute urine less likely to support stone formation.

(continued on the following page)

THERAPEUTIC DIETS (continued)

Health Disorder	Dietary Modification	Rationale or Comments
Cancer	Varies according to site and type of cancer. Generally, increase calories and protein with low to moderate fat. When chemotherapy destroys taste buds, slightly salty or sour tastes are usually accepted best.	Progressive disease causes hypermetabolism, weight loss, negative nitrogen balance, and the use of fat and muscle tissue for energy.
Cardiovascular disease	*Prudent diet*: Control calories in accordance with ideal body weight. Diet to consist of: carbohydrate (mainly complex) = 50% of daily calories, protein = 20% of daily calories, and fat (mostly vegetable) = 30% of daily calories.	These are recommendations of the American Heart Association for prevention and treatment of CV disease. Fat has 9 cal/g, whereas protein and carbohydrates have 4 cal/g.

Diverticulitis	High fiber during remissions. Bland diet during exacerbations. Elemental formulas or parenteral feedings may be used.	High fiber helps to promote peristalsis and may prevent material from remaining in diverticula but is not tolerated during exacerbations. Elemental formulas (predigested) or parenteral feedings allow gut to rest.
Dumping syndrome	Alternate liquids and dry foods. Avoid simple carbohydrates such as fruit juices or sodas. Dilute concentrated tube-feeding formulas.	Alternation of liquid and dry foods puts less food in solution, thereby decreasing osmolarity of gut contents. Simple carbohydrates trigger rapid release of insulin, resulting in hypoglycemia after the GI supply of glucose diminishes. Concentrated tube-feeding formulas attract water to the gut.
Edema	Control sodium. Provide adequate protein.	Edema may be caused by excess sodium or decreased albumin levels, or both.
Esophagitis	Give small, frequent meals. Promote weight loss if overweight. Avoid caffeine, pepper, and any food not well tolerated.	Large meals, obesity, or lying down causes increased abdominal pressure resulting in esophageal reflux.

(continued on the following page)

THERAPEUTIC DIETS (continued)

Health Disorder	***Dietary Modification***	***Rationale or Comments***
Espohagitis (continued)	Chew food thoroughly. Avoid lying down after meals.	Foods avoided are those that cause irritation. Hiatal hernia often results in esophagitis.
Fracture	Adequate protein, calcium, phosphorus, and vitamins A, C, and D. Dairy products are excellent sources for the above nutrients except for vitamin C. Citrus fruits provide vitamin C.	Adequate protein and vitamin C needed for collagen formation. Adequate calcium and phosphorus needed for bone strength. Vitamins A and D necessary for bone cell development, protein synthesis, and mineralization.
Gallbladder disease	See *Cholecystitis*.	
Gastroesophageal reflux disorder (GERD)	Avoid chocolate, fatty foods, peppermint and spearmint oils, caffeine, and alcohol.	Listed foods lower (loosen) esophageal sphincter pressure, which results in reflux.

	Encourage protein-rich foods.	Protein increases (tightens) sphincter pressure.
Gout	Encourage fluids. Limit fats. Decrease high-purine foods such as meats (especially organ meats), fish, fowl, lentils, whole grains, asparagus, mushrooms, spinach, cauliflower, and alcohol.	Extra fluid promotes uric acid excretion and helps prevent renal stone formation. Fats prevent excretion of uric acid. Purine breaks down to form uric acid.
Hepatic encephalopathy	Limit protein intake. Essential amino acids may be used (given IV).	On the limited-protein diet, essential amino acids receive top priority because they cannot be manufactured by the body. Ammonia improperly removed from serum by liver causes abnormal CNS symptoms. See *Cirrhosis*.
Hepatitis	High calorie and protein. Moderate fat. Avoid alcohol.	Anorexia is major problem. Moderation of fat promotes liver regeneration and healing. Alcohol is detoxified by the liver.

(continued on the following page)

THERAPEUTIC DIETS (continued)

Health Disorder	***Dietary Modification***	***Rationale or Comments***
Hiatal hernia	Same indications as *Esophagitis*.	
Hypertension	Control calories to avoid excess weight. Limit sodium. Increase foods high in potassium (fruits and vegetables) and calcium (low-fat dairy products). DASH diet	Obesity increases risk of hypertension. Although the role of sodium in hypertension is debated, research shows that limiting dietary sodium and increasing potassium and calcium can lower blood pressure.
Irritable bowel syndrome	Regular diet when asymptomatic. Bland diet during exacerbation.	Bland diet decreases GI irritation.
Lactose intolerance	Reduce lactose (milk sugar) intake.	Condition may be partial or complete and may be inherited or due to stress or GI irritation.

Nausea/vomiting	Clear liquids. Offer ORS every 20–30 min.	Clear liquids prevent dehydration. ORS replaces electrolytes lost in emesis.
Nephrosis or nephrotic syndrome	Increase protein in diet unless accompanied by renal failure or elevated BUN. No salt added at table.	Protein is lost in urine in this disorder. Salt restriction does not remove edema but may limit its increase.
Obesity	Decrease calories. Modify food habits.	One pound of adipose (fat) tissue is roughly equivalent to 3500 Kcal. An increase or decrease of 500 Kcal a day leads to 1 lb weight gain or loss per week.
Osteoporosis	Ensure adequate dietary calcium by consuming dairy products or by taking supplemental calcium. Encourage exercise as tolerated.	Adequate dietary calcium and adequate exercise thought to be preventive.
Ostomy	Progress from clear liquid to low-residue, high-calorie diet. Maintain until desirable weight attained.	Ostomies result in increased nutrient losses (including electrolyte) from GI tract.

(continued on the following page)

THERAPEUTIC DIETS (continued)

Health Disorder	*Dietary Modification*	*Rationale or Comments*
Ostomy (continued)	Gradually add fiber (individual tolerance varies), avoiding gas-forming foods (based on individual tolerance). Ileal resections make B_{12} injections necessary.	Diet is individualized to avoid foods that cause patient to have excess stooling or gas. Intrinsic factor not available following ileal resection; therefore, B_{12} cannot be absorbed through GI tract.
Pancreatitis	High protein, high carbohydrate with fat added to tolerance. Eliminate gastric stimulants such as coffee, tea, alcohol, and pepper. Withhold oral feedings during exacerbations.	Tolerance of fat is judged by fat in stools, abdominal distention, or abdominal discomfort. Gastric stimulants cause irritating pancreatic enzymes to be secreted.
Peptic ulcer	Bland diet with small, frequent feedings if ulcer is active.	Meat extracts stimulate stomach acid secretion.

	Avoid meat extract, pepper, caffeine, and alcohol.	Obvious irritating foods avoided.
Phenylketonuria	Control phenylalanine (an essential amino acid) in diet. Breast-feeding is contraindicated.	An inborn error results in a lack of enzyme needed to catabolize phenylalanine.
Renal calculi (kidney stones)	See *Calculi, renal*.	
Renal dialysis	Generous calories. Supplement of water-soluble vitamins. Limit fluids, protein, potassium, sodium, and phosphates.	See *Renal failure, acute* and *Renal failure, chronic*.
Renal failure, acute	Restrict protein until BUN and serum creatinine are normal. Restrict fluids during oliguric phase. Replace electrolyte deficits. (Avoid giving potassium during oliguric phase.)	Urea (BUN) and creatinine are the end products of protein metabolism. If kidneys are unable to remove urea, blood levels rise and affect CNS. Serum potassium levels may fluctuate rapidly.

(continued on the following page)

THERAPEUTIC DIETS (continued)

Health Disorder	*Dietary Modification*	*Rationale or Comments*
Renal failure, chronic	Restrict protein proportionate to kidney function. Prevent weight loss by including sufficient calories. Amino acids may be given. Restrict potassium and phosphate intake.	Urea and creatinine accumulate in blood from protein breakdown. Addition of essential amino acids may be indicated if protein tolerance is less than 20 g/24 h. (Monitor BUN and creatinine.) Diseased kidneys do not effectively remove potassium, phosphates, urea, or creatinine from the blood.
Surgery	Adequate protein, calories, iron, and vitamin C.	Listed nutrients are needed for connective tissue (collagen) formation.
Ulcerative colitis	Low-lactose and low-residue diet. (Avoid dairy products and residue, no alcohol, no fried foods, no raw or cooked whole vegetables.) Regular diet during remission.	Stressed mucosa results in impaired ability to produce lactase, which leads to lactose intolerance. Residue (any material that ends up as fecal mass) is irritating.

DASH DIET

Following the Dietary Approaches to Stop Hypertension (DASH) eating plan and reducing the amount of sodium consumed can lower the blood pressure.

The DASH eating plan shown below is based on 2,000 calories a day. The number of daily servings in a food group may vary from those listed, depending on caloric needs. For more information, go to: *http://www.nhlbi.nih.gov/health/public/heart/hbp/dash/new_dash.pdf.*

Food Group	*Daily Servings (except as noted)*	*Serving Sizes*	*Examples and Notes*	*Significance of Each Food Group to the DASH Eating Plan*
Grains and grain products	7–8	1 slice bread 1 oz dry cereal* $^{1}/_{2}$ cup cooked rice, pasta, or cereal	Whole wheat bread, English muffin, pita bread, bagel, cereals, grits, oatmeal, crackers, unsalted pretzels, popcorn	Major sources of energy and fiber

(continued on the following page)

DASH DIET (continued)

Food Group	*Daily Servings (except as noted)*	*Serving Sizes*	*Examples and Notes*	*Significance of Each Food Group to the DASH Eating Plan*
Vegetables	4–5	1 cup raw leafy vegetable $^1/_2$ cup cooked vegetable 6 oz vegetable juice	Tomatoes, potatoes, carrots, green peas, squash, broccoli, turnip greens, collards, kale, spinach, artichokes, green beans, lima beans, sweet potatoes	Rich sources of potassium, magnesium, and fiber
Fruits	4–5	6 oz fruit juice 1 medium fruit $^1/_4$ cup dried fruit $^1/_2$ cup fresh, frozen, or canned fruit	Apricots, bananas, dates, grapes, oranges, orange juice, grapefruit, grapefruit juice, mangoes, melons, peaches, pineapples, prunes, raisins, strawberries, tangerines	Important sources of potassium, magnesium, and fiber

Lowfat or fat free dairy foods	2–3	8 oz milk 1 cup yogurt $1\frac{1}{2}$ oz cheese	Fat-free (skim) or lowfat (1%) milk, fat-free or lowfat buttermilk, fat-free or lowfat regular or frozen yogurt, lowfat and fat-free cheese	Major sources of calcium and protein
Meats, poultry, and fish	2 or less	3 oz cooked meats, poultry, or fish	Select only lean; trim away visible fats; broil, roast, or boil, instead of frying; remove skin from poultry	Rich sources of protein and magnesium
Nuts, seeds, and dry beans	4–5 per week	$\frac{1}{3}$ cup or $1\frac{1}{2}$ oz nuts 2 Tbsp or $\frac{1}{2}$ oz seeds $\frac{1}{2}$ cup cooked dry beans, peas	Almonds, filberts, mixed nuts, peanuts, walnuts, sunflower seeds, kidney beans, lentils,	Rich sources of energy, magnesium, potassium, protein, and fiber
Fats and oils†	2–3	1 tsp soft margarine 1 Tbsp lowfat mayonnaise 2 Tbsp light salad dressing 1 tsp vegetable oil	Soft margarine, lowfat mayonnaise, light salad dressing, vegetable oil (such as olive, corn, canola, or safflower)	DASH has 27% of calories as fat, including fat in or added to foods

(continued on the following page)

DASH DIET (continued)

Food Group	*Daily Servings (except as noted)*	*Serving Sizes*	*Examples and Notes*	*Significance of Each Food Group to the DASH Eating Plan*
Sweets	5 per week	1 Tbsp sugar 1 Tbsp jelly or jam $^1/_2$ oz jelly beans 8 oz lemonade	Maple syrup, sugar, jelly, jam, fruit-flavored gelatin, jelly beans, hard candy, fruit punch, sorbet, ices	Sweets should be low in fat

*Equals $^1/_2$–$1^1/_4$ cups, depending on cereal type. Check the product's Nutrition Facts Label.

†Fat content changes serving counts for fats and oils: For example, 1 tbsp of regular salad dressing equals 1 serving; 1 tbsp of a lowfat dressing equals $^1/_2$ serving; 1 tbsp of a fat-free dressing equals 0 servings.

Source: National Institutes of Health.

NOTES

NOTES

NOTES

NOTES

Pages followed by f indicate a figure. Pages followed by t indicate a table.

O

P